My wonderful neighbor
and valued colleague—
Many thanks for
your advice
through the years,
Seth

TREATING NEURODEVELOPMENTAL DISABILITIES

TREATING NEURODEVELOPMENTAL DISABILITIES

Clinical Research and Practice

Edited by

JANET E. FARMER
JACOBUS DONDERS
SETH WARSCHAUSKY

THE GUILFORD PRESS
New York   London

© 2006 The Guilford Press
A Division of Guilford Publications, Inc.
72 Spring Street, New York, NY 10012
www.guilford.com

All rights reserved

No part of this book may be reproduced, translated, stored in
a retrieval system, or transmitted, in any form or by any means,
electronic, mechanical, photocopying, microfilming, recording,
or otherwise, without written permission from the Publisher.

Printed in the United States of America

This book is printed on acid-free paper.

Last digit is print number: 9   8   7   6   5   4   3   2   1

Library of Congress Cataloging-in-Publication Data

Treating neurodevelopmental disabilities : clinical research and practice / edited by
Janet E. Farmer, Jacobus Donders, and Seth Warschausky.
   p. cm.
Includes bibliographical references and index.
ISBN 1-59385-246-0 (trade cloth)
1. Developmental disabilities—Treatment. 2. Developmentally disabled children—
Rehabilitation. 3. Developmental neurobiology. 4. Children—Diseases—Treatment.
I. Farmer, Janet E. II. Donders, Jacobus. III. Warschausky, Seth
RJ506.D47T74 2006
618.92′8—dc22
                                                  2005017537

With love and gratitude to our spouses—
John Farmer, Arlene Nelson-Donders, and Sandra Finkel

About the Editors

Janet E. Farmer, PhD, is a Professor of Health Psychology and Child Health at the University of Missouri–Columbia. Currently, she directs the Thompson Center for Autism and Neurodevelopmental Disorders, an interdisciplinary initiative that integrates research, service, teaching, and public policy to improve outcomes for children with autism and other brain-based disorders. She also established the Division of Pediatric Psychology and Neuropsychology in the Department of Health Psychology, and she served for 10 years as Clinical Director of a federal interdisciplinary training grant on neurodevelopmental disabilities. Her research investigates community-based interventions designed to enhance health and well-being in children with chronic conditions and their families. Dr. Farmer is a Fellow of the American Psychological Association and a Diplomate in Rehabilitation Psychology.

Jacobus Donders, PhD, is currently the Chief Psychologist at Mary Free Bed Hospital and Rehabilitation Center in Grand Rapids, Michigan. Dr. Donders is board-certified by the American Board of Professional Psychology in both clinical neuropsychology and rehabilitation psychology. He is the coeditor of *Child Neuropsychology*, serves on the editorial boards of several other journals, and has written more than 80 published articles for peer-reviewed journals. His main research interests include construct and criterion validity of neuropsychological test instruments and prediction of outcome after traumatic brain injury. Dr. Donders is a Fellow of the National Academy of Neuropsychology and of Divisions 40 (Clinical Neuropsychology) and 22 (Rehabilitation Psychology) of the American Psychological Association.

Seth Warschausky, PhD, is an Associate Professor of Physical Medicine and Rehabilitation and Director of the Division of Rehabilitation Psychology and Neuropsychology at the University of Michigan. He was formerly President of Division 22, Section 1 (Pediatric Rehabilitation Psychology) of the American Psychological Association. He has served as an advisory board member to the American Psychological Association's Center for Psychology in Schools and Education. Dr. Warschausky's research has included psychometric studies in child neuropsychology, studies of social integration of children with disabilities, and quality-of-life outcomes research.

Contributors

Caroline J. Anderson, PhD, Shriners Hospitals for Children, Chicago, Illinois

Glen P. Aylward, PhD, Department of Pediatrics, Division of Developmental and Behavioral Pediatrics, Southern Illinois University School of Medicine, Springfield, Illinois

Ida Sue Baron, PhD, Independent Private Practice, Potomac, Maryland, and Reston, Virginia

Ronald T. Brown, PhD, Department of Public Health, College of Health Professions, Temple University, Philadelphia, Pennsylvania

Robert W. Butler, PhD, Department of Pediatrics, Division of Pediatric Hematology/Oncology, Oregon Health and Science University, Portland, Oregon

Joshua Cantor, PhD, Department of Rehabilitation Medicine, Mt. Sinai School of Medicine, New York, New York

Elaine Clark, PhD, Department of Educational Psychology, University of Utah, Salt Lake City, Utah

Kathleen K. Deidrick, PhD, Department of Health Psychology, University of Missouri–Columbia, Columbia, Missouri

Jacobus Donders, PhD, Psychology Service, Mary Free Bed Hospital and Rehabilitation Center, Grand Rapids, Michigan

Elena Harlan Drewel, MA, Department of Psychological Sciences, University of Missouri–Columbia, Columbia, Missouri

Ruben J. Echemendía, PhD, Psychological and Neurobehavioral Associates, Inc., State College, Pennsylvania

Janet E. Farmer, PhD, Departments of Health Psychology and Child Health and Director, Thompson Center for Autism and Neurodevelopmental Disorders, University of Missouri–Columbia, Columbia, Missouri

Nora Griffin-Shirley, PhD, Department of Educational Psychology and Leadership, College of Education, Texas Tech University, Lubbock, Texas

Peter C. Hauser, PhD, Department of Psychology, Rochester Institute of Technology, Rochester, New York

Mary R. Hibbard, PhD, Department of Rehabilitation Medicine, Mt. Sinai School of Medicine, New York, New York

Scott J. Hunter, PhD, Pediatric Neuropsychology, Department of Psychiatry, University of Chicago, Chicago, Illinois

Peter K. Isquith, PhD, Department of Psychiatry, Dartmouth Medical School, Lebanon, New Hampshire

William R. Jenson, PhD, Department of Educational Psychology, University of Utah, Salt Lake City, Utah

Tamar Martin, PhD, Department of Rehabilitation Medicine, Mt. Sinai School of Medicine, New York, New York

Alberto I. Moran, PhD, Department of Rehabilitation Medicine, Mt. Sinai School of Medicine, New York, New York

Sylvie Naar-King, PhD, Carmen and Ann Adams Department of Pediatrics, Wayne State University, Detroit, Michigan

Lisa Noll, PhD, Learning Support Center, Texas Children's Hospital, Houston, Texas

Daniel Olympia, PhD, Department of Educational Psychology, University of Utah, Salt Lake City, Utah

Pamela J. Thomas, PhD, Department of Psychology, Paine College, Augusta, Georgia

Lora Tuesday-Heathfield, PhD, Department of Educational Psychology, University of Utah, Salt Lake City, Utah

Lawrence C. Vogel, MD, Department of Pediatrics, Rush Medical Center and Shriners Hospitals for Children, Chicago, Illinois

Shari L. Wade, PhD, Division of Physical Medicine and Rehabilitation, Cincinnati Children's Hospital Medical Center and the University of Cincinnati College of Medicine, Cincinnati, Ohio

Seth Warschausky, PhD, Department of Physical Medicine and Rehabilitation, University of Michigan, Ann Arbor, Michigan

Michael Westerveld, PhD, Department of Neurosurgery and Pediatrics, and Child Study Center, Yale University School of Medicine, New Haven, Connecticut

Karen E. Wills, PhD, Department of Psychology, Children's Hospitals and Clinics, Minneapolis, Minnesota

Preface

Healthy child development is often taken for granted. Parents expect their children to follow a normal developmental trajectory, with at most minor deviations in progress that self-correct over time. However, for children with neurodevelopmental disorders, life course is much less certain. Early delays may resolve in response to intervention, or persist to result in lifelong disability. Parents of these children express a high need for information, and they often have two primary questions: What effect will this condition have on my child's health and development, and what can be done to promote the best possible outcome?

This book is the result of our desire to provide more definitive answers to such questions. We begin by presenting the various categories of neurodevelopmental disabilities, estimates of prevalence, and an overview of psychosocial outcomes. In Part II, experts focus on specific conditions that may result in childhood disability, including acquired neurological injury, congenital and genetic disorders, chronic illness, and sensory impairments. They document the steady growth in descriptive research about physical, cognitive, emotional, and social outcomes in each of these domains over the past two decades. It is our intent to provide a cogent summary of what is known about the effects of neurodevelopmental disorders, highlight gaps in the current knowledge base, and spur additional study.

In our own clinical practice, we experienced a growing frustration over the lack of evidence available to guide interventions for children with disabilities. Therefore, Part III highlights emerging innovations in hospital- and community-based care and empirical support for best practices. As noted in the Epilogue, these new models of care have begun to take into account child, family, and social–ecological factors as they interact to influence child outcomes. These chapters identify specific strategies that can be applied in clinic, hospital, home, and school settings to maximize child and family outcomes, and they also clarify future directions for intervention research.

We greatly appreciate the scholarly contributions of each of the authors to this book, as well as the tremendous support and encouragement of Rochelle Serwator and her colleagues at The Guilford Press. We are indebted to the children and the families who have helped shape our understanding of neurodevelopmental disabilities and who have urged us forward in search of answers. To our own families, we express gratitude for the enthusiastic support and abiding patience that made this book possible.

JANET E. FARMER, PHD
JACOBUS DONDERS, PHD
SETH WARSCHAUSKY, PHD

Contents

Part I. Overview

1 **Introduction to Childhood Disability**   3
    Janet E. Farmer and Kathleen K. Deidrick

Part II. Psychological and Social Aspects of Childhood Disability

2 **Traumatic Brain Injury**   23
    Jacobus Donders

3 **Spinal Cord Injury**   42
    Caroline J. Anderson and Lawrence C. Vogel

4 **Early Medical Risks and Disability**   61
    Glen P. Aylward

5 **Physical Impairments and Disability**   81
    Seth Warschausky

6 **Chronic Illness and Neurodevelopmental Disability**   98
    Ronald T. Brown

7 **Hard-of-Hearing, Deafness, and Being Deaf**   119
    Peter C. Hauser, Karen E. Wills, and Peter K. Isquith

8 **Visual Impairments**   132
    Scott J. Hunter, Nora Griffin-Shirley, and Lisa Noll

Part III. Innovative Treatment Strategies

9 Pediatric Family-Centered Rehabilitation 149
   Sylvie Naar-King and Jacobus Donders

10 Interventions to Support Families of Children with Traumatic 170
   Brain Injuries
   Shari L. Wade

11 Cognitive and Behavioral Rehabilitation 186
   Robert W. Butler

12 Students with Acquired Brain Injury: Identification, Accommodations, 208
   and Transitions in the Schools
   *Mary R. Hibbard, Tamar Martin, Joshua Cantor,
   and Alberto I. Moran*

13 Social Integration of Children with Physical Disabilities 234
   Pamela J. Thomas and Seth Warschausky

14 Empirically Based Interventions for Children with Autism 249
   *Elaine Clark, Lora Tuesday-Heathfield, Daniel Olympia,
   and William R. Jenson*

15 Systems Interventions for Comprehensive Care 269
   Janet E. Farmer and Elena Harlan Drewel

16 Cultural Perspectives in Pediatric Rehabilitation 289
   Ruben J. Echemendía and Michael Westerveld

17 Epilogue 309
   Ida Sue Baron

   Index 323

Part I

Overview

1

Introduction to Childhood Disability

JANET E. FARMER
KATHLEEN K. DEIDRICK

Children with neurodevelopmental disabilities are those with central nervous system impairments who have, or are at risk for, persistent limitations in everyday functioning and reduced participation in life activities (Mudrick, 2002; Spreen, Risser, & Edgell, 1995). The personal and economic costs associated with neurodevelopmental disabilities are often extraordinarily high. However, simply knowing that a child has a congenital or acquired neurological impairment, such as cerebral palsy or traumatic brain injury, provides limited information about the extent of disability or about the types of interventions and supports required to maximize daily functioning. The purpose of this chapter is to define this broad and heterogeneous group of children, to provide an overview of psychosocial aspects of functioning, and to highlight gaps in the psychological assessment and treatment of children with neurodevelopmental disorders.

CLASSIFICATION AND EPIDEMIOLOGY OF NEURODEVELOPMENTAL DISABILITIES

Many child health conditions involve neurological impairments that increase the likelihood of delayed and/or atypical development, including congenital anomalies, chronic diseases, and catastrophic injuries. A variety of approaches have been used to define, classify, and count the number of children with neurodevelopmental disabilities, but there is no universally accepted method for identifying this group. Traditionally, classification strategies have been based on: (1) disease category, (2) program eligibility requirements, and/or (3) functional status (Mudrick, 2002). For example, children have been categorized based on medical diagnosis using health condition codes (e.g., *Diagnostic and Statistical Manual of Mental Disorders*, fourth edition [American Psychiatric Association, 1994]; *International Classification of Diseases*, ninth revision, *Clinical Modification* [Medicode, 2000]). The following types of health conditions are commonly identified as neurodevelopmental disorders: epilepsy, cerebral palsy, mental retardation, disorders of attention and hyperactivity, specific learning disabilities, communication disorders, autism, sensory disturbances involving hearing and/or vision, and orthopedic conditions such as spina bifida (Capute & Accardo, 1996; Msall et al., 2003). Pediatric neuropsychologists and rehabilitation psychologists have called attention to the disabling neurobehavioral consequences of other brain-based conditions such as traumatic brain injury, brain tumors, low birthweight, hydrocephalus, meningitis, sickle cell disease, leukemia, and human immunodeficiency virus (Baron, Fennell, & Voeller, 1995; Spreen et al., 1995; Yeates, Ris, & Taylor, 2000). As shown in Table 1.1, these neurodevelopmental disorders may be subclassified based on etiological causes originating in the prenatal, perinatal, and postnatal periods (Luckasson et al., 2002). Such classifications are not always discrete, as in the case of disorders such as cerebral palsy and hearing impairment that are often related to prenatal causes but also may result from perinatal or postnatal insults.

Diagnostic and etiological classification systems demonstrate the range of neurodevelopmental disorders that may result in functional limitations during childhood, but they are inadequate for determining the actual prevalence of disability in children. As Mendola, Selevan, Gutter, and Rice (2002) point out, there is a spectrum of developmental consequences associated with neurological insults during childhood, ranging from mild to profound cognitive, sensory, motor, behavioral and/or emotional impairments. For this reason, children's service programs have devised a combination of diagnostic and performance criteria to identify disability and qualify children for supports. In school settings, the Individuals with Disabilities Education Act (IDEA; 1997) set forth 13 special education service categories. Table 1.2 depicts the prevalence of childhood disability defined in this way. Using a different approach, the federal Supplemental Security Income (SSI) financial assistance program developed eligibility criteria based on diagnosis, degree of functional impairment, and family income. To qualify as disabled under SSI, a child must have a physical and/or mental condition expected to last more than 12 months that results in marked and severe functional limitations in major life activities such as self-care, mobility, communication, and learning (Social Security Administration, 2001). Far

TABLE 1.1. Common Causes of Neurodevelopmental Disabilities

Prenatal	Perinatal	Postnatal

Genetic–metabolic disorders
  Chromosome abnormalities
  Fragile X
  Down syndrome
  Phenylketonuria (PKU)
  Hypothyroidism
  Autism
 	
Disruption of normal brain development
  Spina bifida
  Hydrocephalus
  Cerebral palsy
 	
Hearing impairment
 	
Environmental causes
  Fetal alcohol exposure
  Irradiation during pregnancy
	Intrauterine disorders
	  Chronic placental insufficiency
	
	Neonatal disorders
	  Prematurity and associated early medical risks such as
	  • periventricular hemorrhage and leukomalacia
	  • retinopathy
	  • respiratory distress syndrome
	
	Human immunodeficiency virus
		Traumatic brain injury
		
		Spinal cord injury
		
		Infection
		  Encephalitis
		  Meningitis
		
		Demyelinating and neurodegenerative disorders
		
		Seizure disorders
		
		Chronic illness with central nervous system effects
		  Sickle cell anemia
		  Acute lymphocytic leukemia
		  End-stage renal disease
		  Diabetes
		
		Lead poisoning
		
		Malnutrition

Note. Adapted from Luckasson et al. (2002). Copyright 2002 by the American Association on Mental Retardation. Adapted by permission.

fewer children meet these criteria compared to educational criteria. In 2000, 843,000 children under 18 qualified for SSI, with the most prevalent conditions being mental retardation (32.8%), other psychiatric disorders (29.2%), diseases of the nervous system and sense organs (11.7%), congenital anomalies (5.3%), and neoplasms (1.1%) (Social Security Administration, 2000).

In an effort to obtain a more standard estimate of childhood disability, researchers turned to the assessment of functional level in children regardless of diagnosis. These noncategorical studies often have utilized population-based national health surveys to determine the extent of activity limitations among children with special health care needs (CSHCN), a group broadly defined as those with chronic physical, developmental, behavioral or emotional conditions that require more health and related services than their peers (Bethell et al., 2002; Davidoff, 2004; Msall et al., 2003; Newacheck & Halfon, 1998; Newacheck et al., 1998; Stein & Silver, 1999). For example, using data from the 1992–1994 National Health Interview Survey on Disability, Newacheck and colleagues (1998) found that approximately 18% (12.6 million) of noninstitutionalized U.S. children un-

TABLE 1.2. Number and Percent of U.S. Children Receiving Special Education Services in 2000–2001 by Age and Disability

Educational diagnosis	Ages 3–5		Ages 6–21	
	Number	Percent	Number	Percent
Specific learning disabilities	20,022	3.3	2,887,217	50.0
Speech or language impairments	330,838	55.2	1,093,808	18.9
Mental retardation	25,640	4.3	612,978	10.6
Emotional disturbance	8,508	1.4	473,663	8.2
Multiple disabilities	12,662	2.1	122,559	2.1
Hearing impairments	8,259	1.4	70,767	1.2
Orthopedic impairments	10,683	1.8	73,057	1.3
Other health impairments	13,355	2.2	291,850	5.1
Visual impairments	3,487	0.6	25,975	0.4
Autism	15,590	2.6	78,749	1.4
Deafness–blindness	208	0.0	1,320	0.0
Traumatic brain injury	891	0.1	14,844	0.3
Developmental delay	149,535	24.9	28,935	0.5
All disabilities	599,678	100.0	5,775,722	100.0

Note. Data from U.S. Department of Education (2002).

der age 18 had a chronic health condition, and 6.5% (4.4 million) experienced limitations in their ability to engage in activities at home, at school, and in the community. Other noncategorical prevalence estimates have been slightly higher, with 7.9–14.8% of children under age 18 found to have significant functional limitations (Centers for Disease Control and Prevention, 1995; Mudrick, 2002; Stein & Silver, 1999). These studies show that disability is more likely among older children, boys, and those living in low-income families or single-parent homes. Communication (5.3%) and learning disorders (10.5%) occur more frequently than mobility (1.2%) and self-care (0.9%) limitations (Msall et al., 2003).

Noncategorical estimates help to define the scope of childhood disability, but this approach also has limitations, because functional outcomes vary substantially depending on the underlying health condition (Msall et al., 2003; Newacheck & Halfon, 1998). As shown in Table 1.3, Msall and colleagues (2003) found marked differences in everyday functioning when they compared children with various medical diagnoses. For instance, children with different neurodevelopmental diagnoses varied in the extent of functional disabilities in mobility, self-care, and communication. Nearly every child with mental retardation or autism spectrum disorder had a significant disability, while less than half of those with neurosensory or genetic disorders showed marked functional limitations.

None of these classification systems fully specify the extent of disability and variability in functioning among children with central nervous

TABLE 1.3. Disability Indicators in Relation to Medical Impairments in 43,000 Children Ages 5–17 Years

Health condition	N	Significant functional limitations	Mild functional limitations	No functional limitations	Special education needs	Limited or no school attendance	No school limitations
Neurodevelopmental	809.4	51.4%	9.5%	39.1%	34.5%	9.2%	56.4%
Neurosensory	508.8	46.0%	10.6%	43.6%	28.5%	10.0%	61.5%
MR and autism spectrum	112.7	98.2%	1.9%	0%	79.1%	6.7%	14.2%
Genetic	188.0	38.0%	11.0%	51.0%	24.1%	8.4%	67.7%
Physical	1,294.8	23.3%	8.8%	67.9%	12.1%	11.9%	76.0%
Behavioral/ADHD/LD	849.9	73.3%	14.6%	12.1%	33.4%	4.1%	62.5%
Asthma	928.2	14.5%	8.1%	77.4%	6.4%	18.1%	75.5%
Any medical impairments	3,882	38.0%	10.0%	52.0%	20.1%	11.1%	68.8%
None	37,418	4.7%	3.5%	91.7%	2.4%	0.7%	97.0%

Note. N represents weighted data from 1994–1995 National Health Interview Survey—Disability Supplement for Children. Significant functional limitations represents children with major or multiple limitations in mobility, self-care, communication, or learning. Neurodevelopmental includes diagnoses such as cerebral palsy, spina bifida, and epilepsy. Physical includes episodic, chronic, and life threatening illness and injuries. MR, mental retardation; ADHD, attention-deficit/hyperactivity disorder; LD, learning disability. Adapted from Msall et al. (2003). Reproduced with permission from *Pediatrics*, Vol. 111, Pages 548–553, Copyright 2003.

ystem impairments. An emerging solution to this problem is to utilize multidimensional classification systems. These systems are based on a conceptual framework of health and functioning that integrates medical components with personal, social, and environmental determinants of disability (Institute of Medicine, 1991; Luckasson et al., 2002; World Health Organization, 2001). Figure 1.1 illustrates the model proposed by the International Classification of Functioning, Disability, and Health (ICF; World Health Organization, 2001). The ICF considers three major dimensions of human functioning—body function/structure, activity level, and participation in social roles—and classifies level of disability based on ratings of impairments, activity limitations, and social disadvantage or lack of opportunity. It provides a common language for communication about health and functioning, and it offers a taxonomy for classification purposes.

To determine level of impairment in body function/structure, the ICF codes anatomical, physiological, and psychological integrity (e.g., cognitive status, mood). To assess activity level and opportunity for participation, there are indicators of capacity and performance. Capacity ratings reflect how well the person can execute a task or action under optimal conditions in nine life areas, ranging from basic skills, such as learning and communication, to activities that require composite skills, such as participating in

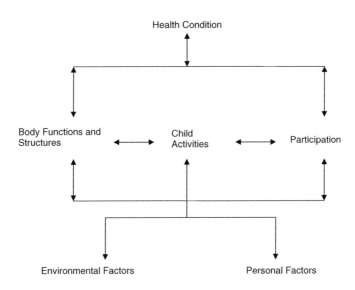

FIGURE 1.1. Conceptual model of factors that influence child outcome based on the *International Classification of Functioning, Disability, and Health* (World Health Organization, 2001).

school or working. Performance ratings examine how well the person can execute the same activities in his or her actual environment. The difference between performance and capacity ratings reflects the impact of social and contextual factors on functioning. Environmental factors such as family functioning, geographic location, financial assets, and access to health and educational services are reported separately. The model also allows for the inclusion of personal variables such as age, time since onset, and gender. Thus, the ICF can be used to obtain a fine-grained profile of the multiple factors that transact to influence functional outcomes in children, including physical and mental health, developmental level, and social and environmental milieu.

Much work remains to be done to establish adequate measurement tools for many of the ICF components for children, so applications of this approach to childhood disability are in the early stages of development (Simeonsson et al., 2003). Conceptually, the disability classification system recently designed for individuals with mental retardation (Luckasson et al., 2002) is more focused on children and families than the ICF, but it is also more limited in scope. Continued effort to refine these multidimensional approaches to disability classification in children is warranted. They appear to have the potential to improve surveillance of children with neurodevelopmental disorders, to promote better screening for early intervention, to increase understanding of risk factors that influence child outcomes, and to identify supports required to reduce disability and promote adaptive functioning (Luckasson et al., 2002; Simeonsson et al., 2003).

OVERVIEW OF PSYCHOSOCIAL ASPECTS OF CHILD FUNCTIONING

Psychosocial functioning is of critical importance to psychologists and other mental health professionals, forming the primary target of assessment and treatment. The following section reviews common areas of concern for children with neurodevelopmental disabilities, highlighting the relationships between neurological impairments, psychological adaptation, school and community participation, and family functioning over the course of development.

Emotional and Behavioral Functioning

Children with neurodevelopmental disabilities are at increased risk for problems with behavior and emotions when compared to healthy children and to children with non-neurological disabilities (e.g., asthma, cystic fibrosis) (Breslau, 1985; Howe, Feinstein, Reiss, Molock, & Berger, 1993). For example, early population-based studies of the residents of the Isle of

Wight (Graham & Rutter, 1968; Rutter, Graham, & Yule, 1970) indicated that children with a known lesion of the brain and/or seizure disorder (34.3%) were five times more likely than healthy controls (6.6%) and three times more likely than children with non-neurological chronic health conditions (11.5%) to exhibit some type of psychiatric difficulty. Similar findings are reported in a recent study of children recruited from outpatient medical clinics (Glazebrook, Hollis, Heussler, Goodman, & Coates, 2003), with children treated for neurological disabilities six times more likely to exhibit significant emotional and behavioral problems than children in the general population.

There is no specific pattern of emotional or behavioral difficulty common to all children with neurological impairments. Children may exhibit problems with mood, anxiety, obsessive–compulsive traits, withdrawal, acting-out behavior, inattention, and high activity level (Glazebrook et al., 2003; Howe et al., 1993). Psychological problems may be more persistent among children with neurological problems than among children in the general population, with some children exhibiting difficulties with emotions and behavior into their adolescent and adult years (Breslau & Marshall, 1985; Howlin & Udwin, 2002).

Several models describe the multiple biomedical, child, and family factors that place children with disabilities at risk for poor adjustment (Wallander, Thompson, & Alriksson-Schmidt, 2003). Risk for psychiatric disorder may be heightened for children with more severe neurological impairment, perhaps because compromised brain function and associated learning and communication problems make coping effectively more difficult (Graham & Rutter, 1968; Rutter et al., 1970; Witt, Riley, & Coiro, 2003). In addition, social factors such as socioeconomic status, home environment, family psychiatric history, and family functioning have a strong impact on psychological adjustment, with children who experience both neurological insult and environmental risks displaying the most difficulties (Graham & Rutter, 1968).

Social Adjustment

In the area of social behaviors, children with neurodevelopmental disabilities appear to be less socially competent, more isolated, and less liked by peers than nondisabled peers and peers with other, non-neurological health conditions (Breslau, 1985; La Greca, Bearman, & Moore, 2002; Nassau & Drotar, 1997). For example, in a population-based study by Marder, Wagner, and Sumi (2003), the special education students with the most problematic social adjustment were also the most likely to have neurodevelopmental diagnoses (e.g., autism or multiple disabilities) and cognitive, functional, and social skill impairments. Recent studies provide additional support for the link between neurological impairments, difficulties with cognitive and communicative skills, and reduced social functioning (Boni, Brown, Davis, Hsu, & Hopkins, 2001; Yeates et al., 2004).

Some children with neurologically based disorders are at risk for delinquent and antisocial behavior. In the Dunedin Longitudinal Study that followed a cohort of New Zealand infants through early adulthood, children were more likely to exhibit antisocial behavior during adulthood if there were early indicators of neurological impairment such as perinatal complications; abnormal neurological examinations at age 3; neuropsychological, motor, and language-processing weaknesses; symptoms of attention-deficit/hyperactivity disorder; and poor school achievement (Moffitt, 1993). The interaction between these neurocognitive weaknesses and a deficient home environment predisposed children to aggressive and antisocial behavior as adults (Moffitt & Caspi, 2001).

In contrast, other studies do not describe increased risk for antisocial or delinquent behavior among children with known neurodevelopmental disabilities (Howlin & Udwin, 2002). For example, a recent follow-up study of children born at very low birthweight reported unusually low involvement in criminal activity and substance abuse (Hack et al., 2002), as does a follow-up study of adults previously diagnosed with nonspecific developmental disabilities (Keogh, Bernheimer, & Guthrie, 2004). A longitudinal study of children receiving special education services offers some explanation for these observations (Marder et al., 2003). Adolescents in special education classes who exhibited severe functional impairments (e.g., autism, multiple disability, and some orthopedic impairments) were even less likely than children in the general population to get into trouble, presumably due to a corresponding reduction in the children's participation in social activities. In contrast, children who were less functionally impaired (e.g., learning disability, speech–language impairment, and emotional disturbance) were more likely to spend time with friends and also more likely to get into trouble. Some groups (e.g., those with emotional disturbance) exhibited even higher than expected rates of delinquent behavior, particularly if they displayed symptoms of attention-deficit/hyperactivity disorder. Thus, such behavioral outcomes appear to be the result of an interaction between type of condition, degree of impairment, and the social environment.

Educational and Vocational Outcomes

Compared to nondisabled peers, children with neurodevelopmental disabilities are at increased risk for poor educational outcomes due at least in part to underlying neuropsychological processing deficits (Goldstein & Reynolds, 1999; Yeates et al., 2000). Children with neurodevelopmental disabilities constitute a large proportion of children receiving special education services. In a population-wide study summarized in Table 1.3, children identified with a neurodevelopmental disorder were more likely to need or receive special education services than children who did not have a disability (Msall, Burant, Holding, Klein, & Hack, 2002). Within the neurodevelopmental group, those with mental retardation or autistic disorders were more likely to receive these services compared to those with neurosensory and genetic disorders.

As a result of health concerns and academic challenges, children with neurodevelopmental disabilities may also be more likely than peers to miss days of school (see Table 1.3) and less likely to receive a high school diploma (Blackorby, Edgar, & Kortering, 1991; Blackorby & Wagner, 1996; Msall et al., 2003; Newman, Davies-Mercier, & Marder, 2003; U.S. Department of Education, 2002). For example, in a national study of the transition from adolescence to adulthood, students receiving special education services were less likely to graduate from high school with a standard diploma than students in the general population (55.4 vs. 92.5%) (Wagner & Levine, 2003). Youth who graduated took longer to do so than is typical (Keogh et al., 2004), and they were less likely to attend postsecondary education than students in the general population (27 vs. 68%) (Blackorby & Wagner, 1996). The lack of postsecondary education in this population is of concern, because research suggests that additional years of training beyond high school can improve outcomes for children with disabilities (Blackorby & Wagner, 1996).

In addition to reduced educational outcomes, children with neurodevelopmental disabilities experience poorer vocational outcomes and less independence in adulthood relative to typically developing peers (Blackorby & Wagner, 1996; Keogh et al., 2004). Blackorby and Wagner (1996) found lower employment rates among former special education students than among regular education students (57 vs. 69% 3–5 years post high school). Furthermore, those with disabilities were less likely to be employed full time, to be engaged in competitive employment, and to be paid at a wage comparable to their nondisabled peers.

Type and severity of disability is closely related to employment status and wages received (Blackorby & Wagner, 1996; Wagner & Blackorby, 1996; Wells, Sandefur, & Hogan, 2003). More specifically, Blackorby and colleagues (1996) found that young adults with speech and learning disabilities were no less likely than adults without a disability to be employed (65 vs. 69%). In contrast, young adults diagnosed with multiple disabilities were unlikely to be employed (17%). Employment rates were also lower for women and minority students with disabilities. In addition, personal characteristics are increasingly identified as important determinants of outcome. For example, the recent literature emphasizes the role of the adult's self-determination in predicting employment outcomes, particularly for persons of higher intellect (Wehmeyer & Palmer, 2003).

Family Functioning

Many parents of children with neurodevelopmental disabilities successfully manage the demands of caring for their child, describing aspects of the experience as positive and meaningful (Hastings & Taunt, 2002). In contrast, a subgroup of parents experiences high levels of parenting stress, caregiving strain, and depression or other psychological problems (Wallander et al., 2003; Wamboldt & Wamboldt, 2000). For example, in response to a national survey, one-fifth of mothers reported high levels of strain related to caring for their child with a disability, and they were more likely than mothers of children without disabilities to endorse distress, depression, and physical health problems (Witt et al., 2003). Contrary to common belief, research suggests that parental distress may not be the direct result of the severity of the child's condition and/or associated impairments in adaptive behavior. Instead, theoretical models (e.g., the risk and resistance model; Wallander, Varni, Babani, Banis, & Wilcox, 1988) and available evidence suggest that a multitude of other interrelated child (e.g., maladaptive behaviors) and family factors (e.g., social support, other life stressors, role disruption, marital conflict, and coping appraisals) are associated with parental distress and unmet family needs (Cohen, 1999; Farmer, Marien, Clark, Sherman, & Selva, 2004; Hastings, 2002; Wallander et al., 2003; Wiegner & Donders, 2000).

The relationship between parent stress and child psychosocial adjustment is likely to be bidirectional (Cohen, 1999; Hastings, 2002). The poorly adapted child may be very difficult to manage, resulting in negative feelings and high levels of parent stress. The converse may also be true, with parent stress negatively affecting child well-being, perhaps through disrupted parenting strategies (Hastings, 2002). A longitudinal study of a mixed sample of children diagnosed with borderline intellectual functioning or mental retardation illustrated this point (Baker et al., 2003). Authors noted that child behavior problems at 36 months of age predicted parent stress when the child reached 48 months of age. However, the reverse was also observed, with parent stress predicting later child behavior problems.

Siblings may also experience distress related to having a brother or sister with a neurodevelopmental disability. Stressors may be direct, such as taking on caregiving duties for a sibling with a disability, or indirect, including coping with a stressed family environment (Cohen, 1999). Two recent meta-analyses suggested small but significant adverse effects of having a sibling with a chronic illness (Sharpe & Rossiter, 2002) or mental retardation (Rossiter & Sharpe, 2001). Specifically, the psychological well-being of the sibling was negatively impacted, with a somewhat larger increase in internalizing than in externalizing problems and a reduction in engagement in social activities. For siblings of children who were chronically ill, cognitive development was also negatively impacted (Sharpe & Rossiter, 2002). Psychosocial outcomes were poorer for children whose sibling required more intense and chronic care. Interestingly, these negative effects are reported by parents and other direct observers, but not by siblings themselves. Furthermore, the personal relationship between siblings was stronger in families where a brother or sister had a chronic illness or mental retardation (Rossiter & Sharpe, 2001; Sharpe & Rossiter, 2002). Factors promoting positive adjustment for siblings may include increased understanding of and better feelings about the disability, strong family functioning, positive maternal adjustment, social support, and more family financial resources (Williams et al., 2002).

The Role of Development

Disability in adults is a dynamic process, and functioning may vary over time depending on abilities, life circumstances, and level of supports (Institute of Medicine, 1991). This dynamic quality is even more apparent for children, since the developing central nervous system is in constant flux (Mendola et al., 2002; Simeonsson et al., 2003). Disruption in an early developmental stage may interfere with all subsequent stages and result in a cumulative impact on child functioning. Children are quite vulnerable to both biological and environmental disruptions in development. For instance, a child exposed prenatally to alcohol and born into a family that is unable to provide adequate care experiences a combination of risk factors. The initial neurotoxic effects of alcohol may be exacerbated by parental limitations that allow the emergence of disabling secondary conditions such as behavioral problems and poor school attendance (Luckasson et al., 2002; Mendola et al., 2002; Simeonsson, McMillen, & Huntington, 2002). Tasks demands also increase over time, and older children clearly are more likely to exhibit problems in functioning relative to their younger peers (Centers for Disease Control and Prevention, 1995; Stein & Silver, 1999; U.S. Department of Education, 2002).

On the other hand, early intervention during the course of development may be more effective in ameliorating problems or reducing their significance (Luckasson et al., 2002; Simeonsson et al., 2002). As a case in point, children with neurodevelopmental disabilities may experience problems with peer relationships that extend into adolescence and adulthood, culminating in a lack of friendships and isolation/loneliness (Howlin & Udwin, 2002; Keogh et al., 2004). However, supports that encourage positive social integration may buffer children from the psychological impact of managing a disability, help them engage in positive disability management activities and healthy behaviors, and promote sustained friendships as they emerge into adulthood (La Greca et al., 2002).

Measuring functioning and disability during development also presents a challenge, since children's abilities and environmental demands differ markedly over time as they grow from infancy to childhood to adolescence (Mendola et al., 2002; Simeonsson et al., 2003). At each developmental stage, the presenting problems may differ (e.g., incontinence in a young child with spina bifida vs. social isolation in an adolescent) and functional indicators typically change (e.g., caregiver–child interaction for an infant, play for a preschooler, classroom participation for an older child). Although measuring child functioning is essential, it is equally important to devise adequate measures of social and environmental factors that are often the target of interventions (e.g., parenting behaviors, educational and agency supports).

CONCLUSIONS

Disability during childhood is a fluid process that is multiply determined by the child's emerging capabilities, ever-changing environmental demands, and supports available to the child and family. Understanding the psychological and social aspects of childhood disability is critical for adequate treatment and prevention. Children may develop problems in psychosocial functioning due to factors associated with neurological compromise, including primary impairments (e.g., cognitive deficits leading to poor academic performance and/or social isolation) and secondary impairments resulting from a lack of appropriate supports (e.g., mood disorders, conduct problems). In addition, children's overall health and functioning may be influenced by contextual factors in the social environment that either buffer or exacerbate the disabling process. The multifaceted classification systems reviewed in this chapter (e.g., ICF) represent an attempt to capture and clearly delineate the psychosocial, as well as medical, aspects of disability.

The wide array of interrelated determinants of outcome suggests multiple possible points of entry for treatment and prevention. Interventions in this population might occur at the level of the child, focusing on remediation of medical problems, cognitive deficits, behavior problems, and social skills. Alternatively, broader contextual interventions might target families, schools, multidisciplinary teams, larger systems and public policy issues, and cultural issues. However, one of the major remaining questions in the field of neurodevelopmental disabilities is how to intervene most effectively to promote optimal child health and functioning. Psychologists, other health professionals, and educators routinely provide services to children with neurodevelopmental disorders in medical and community settings with limited guidance from the research literature (e.g., rehabilitation for children with traumatic brain injury; Chesnut et al., 1999). Although there are excellent resources on the cognitive or general psychological aspects of childhood disabilities (e.g., Yeates et al., 2000), few texts describe systematic and empirically supported intervention methods, especially as applied to the rehabilitation of these children. Furthermore, some literature addresses neuropsychological intervention, but it is typically dedicated either exclusively to adults (Eslinger, 2002) or focuses on a single condition (Semrud-Clikeman, 2001).

To fill this gap, the remainder of this book summarizes available evidence about the psychosocial aspects of the most common congenital and acquired disabilities in children, with an emphasis on empirically supported methods of assessment and intervention. The focus is on ways to promote child health and community functioning through interdisciplinary collaboration and family-centered care, while maintaining a long-term developmental perspective. Key themes may emerge related to the provision of medical, social, behavioral, and educational supports, since these appear to be primary determinants of functioning and disability during childhood (Luckasson et al., 2002). By providing a current reference on emerging best practices in the rehabilitation of children with neurodevelopmental disabilities, this book may also help to set an agenda for future research on strategies that maximize functioning and reduce disability.

REFERENCES

American Psychiatric Association. (1994). *Diagnostic and statistical manual of mental disorders* (4th ed.). Washington, DC: Author.

Baker, B. L., McIntyre, L. L., Blacher, J., Crnic, K., Edelbrock, C., & Low, C. (2003). Pre-school children with and without developmental delay: Behaviour problems and parenting stress over time. *Journal of Intellectual Disability Research, 47,* 217–230.

Baron, I. S., Fennell, E. B., & Voeller, K. K. S. (1995). *Pediatric neuropsychology in the medical setting.* London: Oxford University Press.

Bethell, C. D., Read, D., Stein, R. E., Blumberg, S. J., Wells, N., & Newacheck, P. W. (2002). Identifying children with special health care needs: Development and evaluation of a short screening instrument. *Ambulatory Pediatrics, 2,* 38–48.

Blackorby, J., Edgar, E., & Kortering, L. J. (1991). A third of our youth?: A look at the problem of high school dropout among students with mild handicaps. *Journal of Special Education, 25,* 102–113.

Blackorby, J., & Wagner, M. (1996). Longitudinal postschool outcomes of youth with disabilities: Findings from the National Longitudinal Transition Study. *Exceptional Children, 62,* 399–413.

Boni, L. C., Brown, R. T., Davis, P. C., Hsu, L., & Hopkins, K. (2001). Social information processing and magnetic resonance imaging in children with sickle cell disease. *Journal of Pediatric Psychology, 26,* 309–319.

Breslau, N. (1985). Psychiatric disorder in children with physical disabilities. *Journal of the American Academy of Child Psychiatry, 24,* 87–94.

Breslau, N., & Marshall, I. A. (1985). Psychological disturbance in children with physical disabilities: Continuity and change in a 5-year follow-up. *Journal of Abnormal Child Psychology, 13,* 199–215.

Capute, A. J., & Accardo, P. J. (Eds.). (1996). *Developmental disabilities in infancy and childhood: Vol. I. Neurodevelopmental diagnosis and treatment.* Baltimore: Brookes.

Centers for Disease Control and Prevention. (1995, August). Disabilities among children aged less than or equal to 17 years—United States, 1991–1992. *Morbidity and Mortality Weekly Report, 2.* Retrieved from www.cdc.gov/mmwr//index.html.

Chesnut, R. M., Carney, N., Maynard, H., Patterson, P., Mann, N. C., & Helfand, M. (1999). *Rehabilitation for traumatic brain injury in children and adolescents: Summary, evidence report/technology assessment* (Evidence Report No. 2, Contract 290-97-0018 to Oregon Health Sciences University). Rockville, MD: Agency for Health Care Policy and Research. Retrieved from www.ncbi.nlm.nih.gov/books/bv.fcgi?rid=hstat1.chapter.1280.

Cohen, M. S. (1999). Families coping with childhood chronic illness: A research review. *Families, Systems and Health, 17,* 149–164.

Davidoff, A. J. (2004). Identifying children with special health care needs in the National Health Interview Survey: A new resource for policy analysis. *Health Services Research, 39,* 53–71.

Eslinger, P. J. (Ed.). (2002). *Neuropsychological interventions: Clinical research and practice.* New York: Guilford Press.

Farmer, J. E., Marien, W. E., Clark, M. J., Sherman, A., & Selva, T. J. (2004). Primary care supports for children with chronic health conditions: Identifying and predicting unmet family needs. *Journal of Pediatric Psychology, 29,* 355–367.

Glazebrook, C., Hollis, C., Heussler, H., Goodman, R., & Coates, L. (2003). Detecting emotional and behavioral problems in pediatric clinics. *Child: Care, Health and Development, 29,* 141–149.

Goldstein, S., & Reynolds, C. R. (Eds.). (1999). *Handbook of neurodevelopmental and genetic disorders in children.* New York: Guilford Press.

Graham, P., & Rutter, M. (1968). Organic brain dysfunction and child psychiatric disorder. *British Medical Journal, 3,* 695–700.

Hack, M., Flannery, D. J., Schluchter, M., Cartar, L., Borawski, E., & Klein, N. (2002). Outcomes in young adulthood for very-low-birth-weight infants. *New England Journal of Medicine, 346,* 149–157.

Hastings, R. P. (2002). Parental stress and behaviour problems of children with developmental disability. *Journal of Intellectual and Developmental Disability, 27,* 149–160.

Hastings, R. P., & Taunt, H. M. (2002). Positive perceptions in families of children with developmental disabilities. *American Journal on Mental Retardation, 107,* 116–127.

Howe, G. W., Feinstein, C., Reiss, D., Molock, S., & Berger, K. (1993). Adolescent adjustment to chronic physical disorders: I. Comparing neurological and nonneurological conditions. *Journal of Child Psychology and Psychiatry and Allied Disciplines, 34,* 1153–1171.

Howlin, P., & Udwin, O. (Eds.). (2002). *Outcomes in neurodevelopmental and genetic disorders.* New York: Cambridge University Press.

Individuals with Disabilities Education Act. Amendments of 1997. Public Law 105-17.20 U.S.C. § 1400 et seq.

Institute of Medicine. (1991). *Disability in America: Toward a national agenda for prevention.* Washington, DC: National Academies Press.

Keogh, B. K., Bernheimer, L. P., & Guthrie, D. (2004). Children with developmental delays twenty years later: Where are they? How are they? *American Journal on Mental Retardation, 109,* 219–230.

La Greca, A. M., Bearman, K. J., & Moore, H. (2002). Peer relations of youth with pediatric conditions and health risks: Promoting social support and healthy lifestyles. *Journal of Developmental and Behavioral Pediatrics, 23,* 271–280.

Luckasson, R., Borthwick-Duffy, S., Buntinx, W. H. E., Coulter, D. L., Craig, E. M., Reeve, A., et al. (2002). *Mental retardation: Definition, classification, and systems of supports* (10th ed.). Washington, DC: American Association on Mental Retardation.

Marder, C., Wagner, M., & Sumi, C. (2003). The social adjustment of youth with disabilities. In M. Wagner, C. Marder, J. Blackorby, R. Cameto, L. Newman, P. Levine, & E. Davies-Mercier (Eds.), *The achievements of youth with disabilities during secondary school: A report from the National Longitudinal Transition Study–2 (NLTS2).* Menlo Park, CA: SRI International. Retrieved from www.nlts2.org/pdfs/achievements_ch5.pdf.

Medicode. (2000). *2001 Physician International Classification of Diseases, ninth revision, Clinical modification* (6th ed.). Salt Lake City, UT: Author.

Mendola, P., Selevan, S. G., Gutter, S., & Rice, D. (2002). Environmental factors associated with a spectrum of neurodevelopmental deficits. *Mental Retardation and Developmental Disabilities Research Reviews, 8,* 188–197.

Moffitt, T. E. (1993). The neuropsychology of conduct disorder. *Development and Psychopathology, 5,* 135–151.

Moffitt, T. E., & Caspi, A. (2001). Childhood predictors differentiate life-course persistent and adolescence-limited antisocial pathways among males and females. *Development and Psychopathology, 13,* 355–375.

Msall, M. E., Avery, R. C., Tremont, M. R., Lima, J. C., Rogers, M. L., & Hogan, D. P. (2003). Functional disability and school activity limitations in 41,300 school-age children: Relationship to medical impairments. *Pediatrics, 111,* 548–553.

Msall, M. E., Burant, C., Holding, P. A., Klein, N., & Hack, M. (2002). Sources of variability in sequelae of very low birth weight. *Pediatrics, 8,* 163–178.

Mudrick, N. R. (2002). The prevalence of disability among children: Paradigms and estimates. *Physical Medical Rehabilitation Clinics North American, 13,* 775–792.

Nassau, J. H., & Drotar, D. (1997). Social competence among children with central nervous system-related chronic health conditions: A review. *Journal of Pediatric Psychology, 22,* 771–793.

Newacheck, P. W., & Halfon, N. (1998). Prevalence and impact of disabling chronic conditions in childhood. *American Journal of Public Health, 88*, 610–617.

Newacheck, P. W., Strickland, B., Shonkoff, J. P., Perrin, J. M., McPherson, M., McManus, M., et al. (1998). An epidemiologic profile of children with special health care needs. *Pediatrics, 102*, 117–123.

Newman, L., Davies-Mercier, E., & Marder, C. (2003). School engagement of youth with disabilities. In M. Wagner, C. Marder, J. Blackorby, R. Cameto, L. Newman, P. Levine, & E. Davies-Mercier (Eds.), *The achievements of youth with disabilities during secondary school: A report from the National Longitudinal Transition Study–2 (NLTS2)*. Menlo Park, CA: SRI International. Retrieved from www.nlts2.org/pdfs/achievements_ch3.pdf.

Rossiter, L., & Sharpe, D. (2001). The siblings of individuals with mental retardation: A quantitative integration of the literature. *Journal of Child and Family Studies, 10*, 65–84.

Rutter, M., Graham, P., & Yule, W. (1970). *A neuropsychiatric study in childhood*. London: Spastics International Medical Publications.

Semrud-Clikeman, M. (2001). *Traumatic brain injury in children and adolescents: Assessment and intervention*. New York: Guilford Press.

Sharpe, D., & Rossiter, L. (2002). Siblings of children with a chronic illness: A meta-analysis. *Journal of Pediatric Psychology, 27*, 699–710.

Simeonsson, R. J., Leonardi, M., Lollar, D., Bjorck-Akesson, E., Hollenweger, J., & Martinuzzi, A. (2003). Applying the international classification of functioning, disability and health (ICF) to measure childhood disability. *Disability and Rehabilitation: An International Multidisciplinary Journal, 25*, 602–610.

Simeonsson, R. J., McMillen, J. S., & Huntington, G. S. (2002). Secondary conditions in children with disabilities: Spina bifida as a case example. *Mental Retardation and Developmental Disabilities Research Reviews, 8*, 198–205.

Social Security Administration. (2000). *Children Receiving SSI—December 2000*. Retrieved September 15, 2004, from www.ssa.gov/policy/docs/statcomps/ssi_children/2000/dec/chreport.pdf.

Social Security Administration. (2001). *Disability evaluation under Social Security* (No. 64–039). Washington, DC: Office of Disability, Social Security Administration.

Spreen, O., Risser, A. H., & Edgell, D. (1995). *Developmental neuropsychology*. London: Oxford University Press.

Stein, R. E., & Silver, E. J. (1999). Operationalizing a conceptually based noncategorical definition: A first look at US children with chronic conditions. *Archives of Pediatrics and Adolescent Medicine, 153*, 68–74.

U.S. Department of Education. (2002). *To assure the free appropriate education of all children with disabilities: Twenty-fourth annual report to Congress on the implementation of the Individuals with Disabilities Education Act*. Washington, DC: U.S. Government Printing Office. Retrieved from www.ed.gov/about/reports/annual/osep/2002/index.html.

Wagner, M., & Blackorby, J. (1996). Transition from high school to work or college: How special education students fare. *Future of Children, 6*, 103–120.

Wagner, M., & Levine, P. (2003). The schools attended by secondary school students with disabilities. In M. Wagner, L. Newman, R. Cameto, P. Levine, & C. Marder

(Eds.), *Going to school: Instructional contexts, programs, and participation of secondary school students with disabilities: A report from the National Longitudinal Transition Study–2 (NLTS2)*. Menlo Park, CA: SRI International. Retrieved from www.nlts2.org/pdfs/goschool_ch3.pdf.

Wallander, J. L., Thompson, R. J., Jr., & Alriksson-Schmidt, A. (2003). Psychosocial adjustment of children with chronic physical conditions. In M. C. Roberts (Ed.), *Handbook of pediatric psychology* (3rd ed., pp. 141–158). New York: Guilford Press.

Wallander, J. L., Varni, J. W., Babani, L., Banis, H. T., & Wilcox, K. T. (1988). Children with chronic physical disorders: Maternal reports of their psychological adjustment. *Journal of Pediatric Psychology, 13*, 197–212.

Wamboldt, M. Z., & Wamboldt, F. S. (2000). Role of the family in the onset and outcome of childhood disorders: Selected research findings. *Journal of the American Academy of Child and Adolescent Psychiatry, 39*, 1212–1219.

Wehmeyer, M. L., & Palmer, S. B. (2003). Adult outcomes for students with cognitive disabilities three-years after high school: The impact of self-determination. *Education and Training in Developmental Disabilities, 38*, 131–144.

Wells, T., Sandefur, G. D., & Hogan, D. P. (2003). What happens after the high school years among young persons with disabilities? *Social Forces, 82*, 803–832.

Wiegner, S., & Donders, J. (2000). Predictors of parental distress after congenital disabilities. *Journal of Developmental and Behavioral Pediatrics, 21*, 271–277.

Williams, P. D., Williams, A. R., Graff, J., Hanson, S., Stanton, A., Hafeman, C., et al. (2002). Interrelationships among variables affecting well siblings and mothers in families of children with a chronic illness or disability. *Journal of Behavioral Medicine, 25*, 411–424.

Witt, W. P., Riley, A. W., & Coiro, M. J. (2003). Childhood functional status, family stressors, and psychosocial adjustment among school-aged children with disabilities in the United States. *Archives of Pediatric and Adolescent Medicine, 157*, 687–695.

World Health Organization. (2001). *International classification of functioning, disability, and health: ICF*. Geneva, Switzerland: Author.

Yeates, K. O., Ris, M. D., & Taylor, H. G. (Eds.). (2000). *Pediatric neuropsychology: Research, theory, and practice*. New York: Guilford Press.

Yeates, K. O., Swift, E., Taylor, H. G., Wade, S. L., Drotar, D., Stancin, T., et al. (2004). Short- and long-term social outcomes following pediatric traumatic brain injury. *Journal of the International Neuropsychological Society, 10*, 412–426.

Part II

Psychological and Social Aspects of Childhood Disability

2

Traumatic Brain Injury

JACOBUS DONDERS

Traumatic brain injury (TBI) occurs when a child's brain is compromised as the direct or indirect result of acute external forces to the skull. Although many cases of childhood TBI are preventable (Rivara, 1995), it is a fairly common acquired condition, accounting for about 30% of all childhood injury deaths. This chapter reviews the most common and significant behavioral, cognitive, and psychosocial sequelae in survivors of pediatric TBI.

BACKGROUND INFORMATION

Epidemiology and Pathophysiology

Incidence statistics concerning pediatric TBI vary considerably across studies due to differences in definition and exclusion criteria. In a comprehensive review of various studies, Kraus (1995) estimated an average incidence of 180 per 100,000 children per year. Rates for boys tend to be about 1.3 to 2.0 times greater than those for girls (Rivara, 1994). Falls are a common cause in young children, and motor vehicle accidents account for the majority of severe injuries with increasing age (DiScala, Osberg, Gans, Chin, & Grant, 1991). Child abuse TBI affects primarily children under 3 years of age (Brown & Minns, 1993).

TBI causes brain impairment through both primary and secondary mechanisms. Primary injuries result from external accelerating or decelerating forces to the skull, including linear displacements that cause focal lesions, such as cortical contusions, and intracranial rotations that may result in diffuse lesions, such as axonal shearing. Focal prefrontal lesions, as well as involvement of the corpus callosum and other white matter regions, have been related to an increased risk for long-term psychological sequelae (Dennis, Guger, Roncadin, Barnes, & Schachar, 2001; DiStefano et al., 2000; Gerring et al., 2000; Levin et al., 2000a, 2004; Slomine et al., 2002; Verger et al., 2001).

Secondary or indirect injuries arise primarily as the result of disruption of cerebral circulation and cellular homeostasis, including cerebral ischemia and edema, as well as neurotoxicity that may result from a sudden sharp increase in excitatory amino acids (Downard et al., 2000; Hackbarth et al., 2002; Statler et al., 2001). Unless treated properly, these secondary lesions may be even more damaging in the long run than primary lesions (Geddes et al., 2001; Ruppel et al., 2001).

Most classifications of severity of TBI, such as the Glasgow Coma Scale (GCS; Teasdale & Jennett, 1974), were initially developed for use with adults, so caution is necessary when applying them to children. Focal neurological signs such as pupillary reflex abnormalities or intracranial lesions on neuroimaging are considered to be indicative of more serious injury, even when the GCS is in the "mild" (13–15) range (Prasad, Ewing-Cobbs, Swank, & Kramer, 2002; Williams, Levin, & Eisenberg, 1990; Woodward et al., 1999). Such cases can be considered "complicated mild" or "moderate" injuries. The time it takes children to follow verbal commands (equivalent to a score of 6 on the Motor subscale on the GCS) is a fairly reliable and commonly used indicator of length of coma (Massagli, Michaud, & Rivara, 1996).

Mild injuries that are not associated with prolonged coma, intracranial lesions, or focal neurological signs constitute the bulk (at least 80%) of cases of pediatric TBI. Although many of these children may have some cognitive inefficiencies and behavioral or mood instability within the first 1–3 months postinjury (Mittenberg, Wittner, & Miller, 1997; Yeates et al., 1999), the vast majority of children who sustain uncomplicated mild TBI have an essentially unremarkable long-term psychological recovery (Bijur & Haslum, 1995; Bijur, Haslum, & Golding, 1996; Fay et al., 1993; Light et al., 1998; Satz et al., 1997). In contrast, long-term behavioral, cognitive, and psychosocial sequelae are likely with moderate–severe injuries such as those associated with coma > 24 hours and/or lesions compromising the frontal–subcortical system. Persistent neurobehavioral symptoms after uncomplicated mild TBI are more likely to occur in children with premorbid neurological, psychiatric, or special education histories, or with family problems (Ponsford et al., 1999).

Common Cognitive Sequelae

Moderate–severe pediatric TBI can result in a wide range of cognitive sequelae and there is no unitary or invariant profile in this regard. In fact, various distinct subtypes of functioning have been described and related to injury characteristics (Donders & Warschausky, 1997). It is also important to realize that some commonly reported symptoms, such as difficulties with attention or executive skills, are not specific to TBI and may also occur with various other conditions such as attention-deficit/hyperactivity disorder (ADHD; Barkley, 1997; Bayliss & Roodenrys, 2000) or with anxiety disorder or depression (Livingston, Stark, Haak, & Jennings, 1996; Moradi, Doost, Taghavi, Yule, & Dalgeish, 1999). At the same time, some authors have suggested that moderate–severe TBI may result in "secondary" ADHD (Gerring et al., 2000). Review of prior academic records is typically essential to evaluate the degree of further deterioration in children with TBI who have prior complicating psychiatric or special education histories (Donders & Strom, 1997, 2000; Farmer et al., 2002).

With all of these reservations in mind, some cognitive sequelae can be identified that are relatively common after moderate–severe pediatric TBI. These children often demonstrate deficits on tasks requiring speed of information processing and/or learning and explicit recall of complex new information, whereas overlearned skills such as basic vocabulary or word recognition tend to be relatively preserved (Anderson, Catroppa, Rosenfeld, Haritou, & Morse, 2000; Catroppa & Anderson, 2002; Chapman et al., 1997; Donders, 1997; Farmer et al., 1999; Hoffman, Donders, & Thompson, 2000; Levin et al., 2000b; Roman et al., 1998; Tremont, Mittenberg, & Miller, 1999; Yeates et al., 2002). This does not mean that all language skills are typically normal. Children with moderate–severe TBI do tend to have difficulties with high-level organizational and abstraction aspects of verbal discourse (Chapman et al., 2001; Ewing-Cobbs, Brookshire, Scott, & Fletcher, 1998a), and with the pragmatic and inferential aspects of language (Barnes & Dennis, 2001; Dennis & Barnes, 2001; Dennis, Purvis, Barnes, Wilkinson, & Winner, 2001).

In order to illustrate the differential ways in which moderate–severe TBI can affect various cognitive areas, Figure 2.1 presents psychometric data from a consecutive series of children (62% boys, 82% Caucasian) between the ages of 9 and 16 years ($M = 13.93$, $SD = 2.34$) who all had sustained TBI associated with positive intracranial findings on neuroimaging. These children had all been referred for neuropsychological assessment at Mary Free Bed Rehabilitation Hospital in Grand Rapids, Michigan, over the course of approximately 7 years. Most injury circumstances involved motor vehicle accidents (62%). Children with complicating premorbid histories (e.g., learning disability, child abuse) were excluded. Data collection continued until there were 30 children in each of two groups: Children without prolonged coma responded to verbal commands within 24 hours (within 1 hour in 80% of the cases), whereas children with prolonged coma had a median duration of loss of consciousness of 3.5 days (range 1–25). The two groups did not differ significantly on any demographic background variables or in the relative frequencies of diffuse or focal cerebral lesions ($p > .10$ on all variables). All of these children were evaluated within 12 months after injury ($M = 2.32$, $SD = 1.61$) with the Wechsler Intelligence Scale for Children—Third Edition (WISC-III; Wechsler, 1991), the California Verbal Learning Test—Children's Version (CVLT-C; Delis, Kramer, Kaplan, & Ober, 1994), and the Children's Category Test—Level 2 (CCT; Boll, 1993). Although most of the children had taken additional psychometric tests, only these three instruments were routinely administered to all referred patients except when this was contraindicated by variables such as non-English language background or orthopedic injury to the dominant hand. Furthermore, age-based norms were available for all three tests for the entire age range of this sample. For reasons of convenience, all variables in Figure 2.1 were converted to standard scores ($M = 100$, $SD = 15$), with higher scores reflecting better performance.

Inspection of Figure 2.1 suggests that the performance of the group without prolonged coma was generally superior to that of the group with prolonged coma, $F (6, 53) = 3.68$, $p < .01$. This was, of course, not surpris-

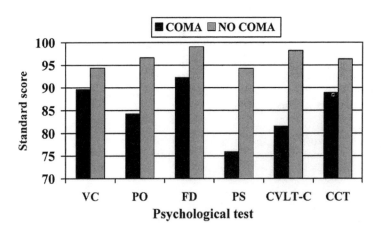

FIGURE 2.1. Neuropsychological test performance of children with ($N = 30$) and without ($N = 30$) duration of coma 24 hours. VC, verbal comprehension; PO, perceptual organization; FD, freedom from distractibility; PS, processing speed; CVLT-C, California Verbal Learning Test—Children's Version; CCT, Children's Category Test.

ing. However, the degree of the difference was not the same on all variables. For example, on the Verbal Comprehension index (based on tasks pertaining to overlearned language knowledge), the difference was less than one-third of a standard deviation, whereas on the Processing Speed index (based on tasks emphasizing rapid and accurate paper-and-pencil skills), the difference exceeded one standard deviation. Using a minimum level of alpha of .01 to balance the relative risks of type I and type II errors, group differences reached statistical significance only on the following three variables: Perceptual Organization, $F (1, 58) = 8.43$, $p < .01$, $\eta^2 = 0.13$; Processing Speed, $F (1, 58) = 23.01$, $p < .0001$, $\eta^2 = 0.28$, and the composite index of the CVLT-C, $F (1, 58) = 11.01$, $p < .01$, $\eta^2 = 0.16$. These three variables have in common that they either emphasize and reward fast performance (Perceptual Organization and Processing Speed) or require the learning of new information that is presented at a fairly rapid pace (CVLT-C). Even though the CCT also requires new learning, it does not make major demands on speed or memory, which probably makes it far less sensitive to the effect of injury severity. These findings are consistent with the broader literature suggesting that skills that require fast and efficient performance and/or memory for new information are relatively most sensitive to the effects of moderate–severe TBI (Yeates et al., 2002a).

PSYCHOSOCIAL OUTCOMES

Behavioral, Emotional, and Social Outcomes

There is no such thing as a "signature" psychosocial outcome profile in children with moderate–severe TBI, and the symptoms may cover a wide spectrum. Again, various distinct subtypes have been described in this regard (Butler, Rourke, Fuerst, & Fisk, 1997; Hayman-Abello, Rourke, & Fuerst, 2003). However, there is no doubt that moderate–severe TBI is a risk factor for a range of novel psychiatric disorders, and the most common and most disabling symptoms are affective instability and impaired social judgment (Bloom et al., 2001; Max et al., 1998b, 2000; Max, Robertson, & Lansing, 2001).

It has been reported that injury severity as well as postinjury level of perceived stress are contributing factors to new-onset mood and anxiety disorder after pediatric TBI (Luis & Mittenberg, 2002). Recent research also suggests that long-term behavior problems can be predicted by severity of TBI and socioeconomic disadvantage, as well as preinjury behavioral difficulties (Schwartz et al., 2003). However, children with moderate–severe TBI may demonstrate difficulties with social problem solving, even in the absence of overt psychiatric malfunction, and this can contribute to difficulties with peer integration (Bohnert, Parker, & Warschausky, 1997;

Janusz, Kirkwood, Yeates, & Taylor, 2002; Warschausky, Cohen, Parker, Levendosky, & Okun, 1997). This effect of social problem solving on psychosocial outcomes appears to be largely independent of contributions of cognitive dysfunction and impaired pragmatic language to such outcomes (Yeates et al., 2004).

It is important to realize that "real life" psychosocial outcomes are not always captured very well by the cognitive tests that are typically included in neuropsychological evaluations. In fact, it has been suggested that such assessments rely too much on tasks administered in an artificial, highly structured environment without distractions or other challenging variables (Silver, 2000). The recent introduction of instruments such as the Behavior Rating Inventory of Executive Function (BRIEF; Gioia, Isquith, Guy, & Kenworthy, 2000) that specifically address behavioral regulation, as well as metacognitive skills in day-to-day life, has been an encouraging development in this regard. The BRIEF appears to offer incremental information about the daily functioning of children with moderate–severe TBI, above and beyond what can be accounted for on the basis of laboratory tests alone (Mangeot, Armstrong, Colvin, Yeates, & Taylor, 2002; Vriezen & Pigott, 2002).

Academic Outcomes

Because of the significant cognitive deficits that may result from moderate–severe pediatric TBI, a considerable proportion of these children need special education services for extended periods of time (Arroyos-Jurado, Paulsen, Merrell, Lindgren, & Max, 2000; Clark, Russman, & Orme, 1999; Ewing-Cobbs et al., 1997b; Kinsella et al., 1997). In the United States, TBI is a federally recognized separate category of eligibility for special education services, but individual states vary considerably in the exact definition of what is considered TBI (e.g., some states include anoxic encephalopathies). Neuropsychological test scores, particularly those pertaining to new learning, such as performance on the CVLT-C when obtained within the first few months after injury, can add significantly to the accuracy of prediction of long-term special education placement, above and beyond the variance that can be explained by demographic or injury variables (Miller & Donders, 2003). At the same time, a considerable minority of children with residual sequelae of TBI who could profit from special education support do not always receive adequate services (Taylor et al., 2003). Hibbard, Martin, Cantor, and Moran (Chapter 12, this volume) provide further details about problems and prospects for transitioning children with TBI into the educational system.

Clear professional guidelines, knowledge of state and federal special education guidelines, and active parental involvement are often needed to make sure that children with moderate–severe TBI receive education and support in the least restrictive environment (Katsiyannis & Conderman, 1994). Parents typically need to request special education support services through an Individualized Educational Planning Committee. If they do not agree with the resulting recommendations regarding accommodations or placement, they can request a "due process" arbitration or mediation hearing (Lorber & Yurk, 1999; Savage, Lash, Bennett, & Navalta, 1995). Since the needs of children with moderate–severe TBI tend to change over the years, special education plans may need to be reviewed more frequently (Glang, Singer, & Todis, 1997; Semrud-Clikeman, 2001; Ylvisaker et al., 2001).

Family Outcomes

Pediatric TBI can lead to considerable disruption of family functioning, both in acute care, where parents often feel a need to be with their injured child constantly, and over subsequent years, when it is often up to parents to be persistent advocates for their children with academic and health care establishments. Several studies have suggested that substantial proportions of families of children with moderate–severe TBI continue to report high levels of stress associated with some aspects of the child's recovery and/or impact on the family several years later (Benn & McColl, 2004; Hawley, Ward, Magnay, & Long, 2003; Rivara et al., 1996; Wade, Taylor, Drotar, Stancin, & Yeates, 1998; Wade et al., 2001, 2002). These studies have indicated that open communication styles, lack of rigidity, and use of acceptance and humor as coping styles foster better family adjustment. Other studies have also emphasized the need for families to receive sufficient information about their child's TBI, as well as having a variety of treatment options (Hawley, 2003; Waaland, Burns, & Cockrell, 1993).

The research by Taylor and colleagues (2001) has suggested that there is a reciprocal influence in child and family adjustment after pediatric TBI: More child behavior problems at 6 months postinjury were associated with higher parental distress at 12 months, even after controlling for earlier family adjustment outcomes, whereas higher parental distress at 6 months was associated with more child behaviors at 12 months, even after controlling for earlier child behavioral outcomes. Child behavior problems after TBI may also negatively affect sibling relationships and may contribute to sibling behavior problems (Swift et al., 2003). Although siblings of children with TBI as a group do not necessarily demonstrate greater degrees of psychosocial adjustment than their own classmates, they do tend to have more symptoms of depression and lower self-concept when the child with TBI has worse functional outcome (McMahon, Noll, Michaud, & Johnson, 2001).

Developmental Change over Time

Many cognitive skills show partial recovery within the first year after moderate–severe TBI, with a subsequent relative plateau (Yeates et al., 2002a). The behavior problems of most children who have adjustment difficulties several years postinjury tend to be evident already within the first year after TBI (Max et al., 2000; Schwartz et al., 2003). In general, recovery may actually be more favorable for cognitive than for behavioral and psychosocial adjustment characteristics (Taylor et al., 2002). Particularly in terms of adaptive behavior and social integration, considerable sequelae of moderate–severe TBI have been described several years postinjury (Woodward et al., 1999). It is important to take a long-term developmental perspective in the evaluation of sequelae of moderate–severe TBI, because the full extent of the injury may not become apparent until years later, when the prefrontal systems of the brain mature and when environmental demands on the child increase in complexity (Fay et al., 1994; Gil, 2003; Max et al., 1998b).

There is no support for the common myth that recovery from pediatric TBI tends to be better with younger age of onset. In fact, considerable evidence suggests that moderate–severe TBI that is sustained early in life tends to interfere with vulnerable skills that are in a phase of rapid development and is therefore associated with an increased risk for long-term neurobehavioral deficits (Anderson et al., 1997; Chapman & McKinnon, 2000; Ewing-Cobbs et al., 1997a; Taylor & Alden, 1997; Woodward et al., 1999). A particularly concerning issue with very young children is child abuse TBI, which tends to result in more severe injuries and is associated with poorer cognitive and behavioral outcomes (Ewing-Cobbs et al., 1998c). Those children most at risk for child abuse TBI are infants in their first year of life, with higher incidences noted in boys, and children born to younger mothers and/or as the result of multiple births (Keenan et al., 2003).

Moderating Variables

Variables that specify the circumstances under which a particular condition results in specific outcomes are known as "moderators" (Holmbeck, 2002). In addition to age, several other demographic variables have been described as affecting the psychosocial outcomes after moderate–severe TBI. A number of studies have suggested that socioeconomic disadvantage is a risk variable with regard to psychosocial child outcome (Kirkwood et al., 2000; Max et al., 1998a). It is possible that socioeconomic disadvantage is associated with fewer health or community resources, but it must also be realized that studies involving extended follow-up of psychosocial functioning typically suffer from differential attrition, with proportionally more children lost from lower socioeconomic strata (Schwartz et al., 2003; Woodward et al., 1999). Similarly, although ethnic minority status has also been proposed as an additional risk factor for long-term family distress and burden, independent of socioeconomic status, this relationship is also affected by the fact that participation and attrition in such longitudinal research vary by ethnicity (Yeates et al., 2002b). Similarly, although ethnic minority status has been implicated as a risk factor for child abuse TBI, it is not clear to what extent this is due to overlap with other (e.g., socioeconomic) factors (Keenan et al., 2003; Sinal et al., 2000; Wagner, Sasser, Hammond, Wiercisiewski, & Alexander, 2000). When socioeconomic status, ethnicity, and injury severity are controlled, male gender may be associated with less favorable outcomes in some areas of cognitive functioning (Donders & Woodward, 2003), but there does not appear to be an effect of gender on social integration (Woodward et al., 1999).

A lower or complicated preinjury level of functioning (e.g., prior adjustment or learning problem) is clearly a risk factor with regard to worse psychosocial outcome, both for the child (Donders & Ballard, 1996; Ponsford et al., 1999; Schwartz et al., 2003; Woodward et al., 1999) and for the family (Rivara et al., 1996). A postinjury family environment characterized by low levels of stress and more adaptive interpersonal dynamics may act as a buffer regarding the impact of moderate–severe pediatric TBI (Anderson et al., 2001; Kinsella, Ong, Murtagh, Prior, & Sawyer, 1999; Max et al., 1999; Rivara et al., 1996; Yeates et al., 1997). Taylor and colleagues (2001, 2002) have demonstrated that the influences between child neurobehavioral problems and family adjustment are bidirectional in nature, and that the moderating effect of family characteristics is greater on psychosocial than on cognitive outcomes.

CLINICAL IMPLICATIONS

Neurobehavioral morbidity is common in survivors of moderate–severe TBI, particularly in terms of reduced speed of information processing, limited memory capacity, affective instability, and suboptimal social integration. A long-term developmental perspective is necessary in the follow-up of these children, because some deficits may not become fully manifest until several years after injuries sustained in early childhood. Expanded and more frequent monitoring within the school system is often needed (Hibbard et al., Chapter 12, this volume).

It is important for those engaging in neuropsychological assessment of children with moderate–severe TBI to avoid overreliance on measures of academic achievement and crystallized intelligence, and instead concentrate on measures that tap into speed of information processing and new learning. In addition, caution is needed with the interpretation of test results obtained under artificial and structured laboratory circumstances. Comparison with premorbid school records and supplementation with review of family history, as well as standardized rating scales of current daily functioning, is highly desirable. Practitioners also need to be aware of local guidelines and regulations for special education services for children with TBI.

It is important to review carefully premorbid characteristics of the child and the family, as well as the postinjury family environment, in the evaluation of outcome of moderate–severe pediatric TBI. In the long run, psychosocial sequelae may be more detrimental than cognitive deficits. Furthermore, the accumulating evidence for the moderating influence of family characteristics in the outcome of TBI suggests opportunities for psychotherapeutic intervention. Active involvement of the family throughout the rehabilitation process may facilitate child and family psychosocial outcomes (see Naar-King & Donders, Chapter 9, this volume).

FUTURE RESEARCH DIRECTIONS

There continue to be important goals for future research. Particularly with regard to TBI sustained early in life, longer term follow-up is needed to delineate predictors of variability in neurobehavioral recovery into the teen and adolescent years. Even some of the best studies have been limited to 4 or 5 years of follow-up, and more extended tracking of developmental changes and their interaction with family and other environmental characteristics is needed. Future research should also explore the possible contributions of functional neuroimaging in the evaluation of sequelae of TBI, because most studies to date have focused exclusively on structural imaging methods.

With regard to neuropsychological assessment, more research is needed to develop better age-based norms for some of the currently available tests. Greater evidence for the ecological and long-term predictive validity of those instruments is especially needed. In the assessment of sequelae of TBI, it is necessary but not sufficient to demonstrate that a particular test has sensitivity to injury severity. The more important thing is to determine the degree to which neuropsychological assessment, including formal measures of child psychosocial adjustment, adds to our understanding of the sequelae of TBI beyond what can already be ascertained on the basis of demographic and neurological variables. In other words, further evidence is needed with regard to the incremental value of neuropsychological tests.

Finally, more research is needed with regard to both the prevention and the effectiveness of treatment of pediatric TBI. With regard to the former, this may range from something as simple as clearer instructions concerning the installation of car seats for infants to the provision of community-based parental education programs for very young expecting parents. With regard to the latter, there is a need for more empirical evidence for the long-term benefits of individual or family psychotherapeutic interventions after pediatric TBI. Further research is also needed concerning exactly which acute care interventions are the most effective in not only saving lives but also with regard to matters such as preventing secondary neurological injuries, the degree to which family-centered approaches to rehabilitation facilitate better outcomes, and the effectiveness of cognitive and psychotherapeutic interventions for children with TBI and their families (see Butler, Chapter 11, and Wade, Chapter 10, this volume). In addition, more research is desirable to improve the identification of those children who are most likely to benefit from rehabilitative intervention with regard to their psychosocial adjustment.

ACKNOWLEDGMENT

Completion of this chapter was supported in part by a grant from the U.S. Department of Education National Institute on Disability and Rehabilitation Research (No. H188G000038).

REFERENCES

Anderson, V. A., Catroppa, C., Haritou, F., Morse, S., Pentland, L., Rosenfeld, J., et al. (2001). Predictors of acute child and family outcome following traumatic brain injury in children. *Pediatric Neurosurgery, 34*, 138–148.

Anderson, V. A., Catroppa, C., Rosenfeld, J., Haritou, F., & Morse, S. A. (2000). Recovery of memory function following traumatic brain injury in pre-school children. *Brain Injury, 14*, 679–692.

Anderson, V. A., Morse, S. A., Klug, G., Catroppa, C., Haritou, F., Rosenfeld, J., et al. (1997). Predicting recovery from head injury in young children: A prospective analysis. *Journal of the International Neuropsychological Society, 3*, 568–580.

Arroyos-Jurado, E., Paulsen, J. S., Merrell, K. W., Lindgren, S. D., & Max, J. E. (2000). Traumatic brain injury in school-age children: Academic and social outcome. *Journal of School Psychology, 38*, 571–587.

Barkley, R. A. (1997). Attention-deficit/hyperactivity disorder, self-regulation, and time: Toward a more comprehensive theory. *Journal of Developmental and Behavioral Pediatrics, 18*, 271–279.

Barnes, M. A., & Dennis, M. (2001). Knowledge-based inferencing after childhood head injury. *Brain and Language, 76*, 253–265.

Bayliss, D. M., & Roodenrys, S. (2000). Executive processing and attention deficit hy-

peractivity disorder: An application of the supervisory attentional system. *Developmental Neuropsychology, 17,* 161–180.
Benn, K. M., & McColl, M. A. (2004). Parental coping following childhood acquired brain injury. *Brain Injury, 18,* 239–255.
Bijur, P. E., & Haslum, M. (1995). Cognitive, behavioral, and motoric sequelae of mild head injury in a national birth cohort. In S. H. Brown & M. E. Michel (Eds.), *Traumatic head injury in children* (pp. 147–164). New York: Oxford University Press.
Bijur, P. E., Haslum, M., & Golding, J. (1996). Cognitive outcomes of multiple head injuries in children. *Journal of Developmental and Behavioral Pediatrics, 17,* 143–148.
Bloom, D. R., Levin, H. S., Ewing-Cobbs, L., Saunders, A. E., Song, J., Fletcher, J. M., et al. (2001). Lifetime and novel psychiatric disorders after pediatric traumatic brain injury. *Journal of the American Academy of Child and Adolescent Psychiatry, 40,* 572–279.
Bohnert, A. M., Parker, J. G., & Warschausky, S. A. (1997). Friendship and social adjustment of children following a traumatic brain injury: An exploratory investigation. *Developmental Neuropsychology, 13,* 477–486.
Boll, T. (1993). *Children's Category Test.* San Antonio, TX: Psychological Corporation.
Brown, J. K., & Minns, R. A. (1993). Non-accidental head injury, with particular reference to whiplash shaking injury and medicolegal aspects. *Developmental Medicine and Child Neurology, 35,* 849–869.
Butler, K., Rourke, B. P., Fuerst, D. R., & Fisk, J. L. (1997). A typology of psychosocial functioning in pediatric closed-head injury. *Child Neuropsychology, 3,* 98–133.
Catroppa, C., & Anderson, V. (2002). Recovery in memory function in the first year following TBI in children. *Brain Injury, 16,* 369–385.
Chapman, S. B., & McKinnon, L. (2000). Discussion of developmental plasticity: Factors affecting cognitive outcome after pediatric traumatic brain injury. *Journal of Communication Disorders, 33,* 333–344.
Chapman, S. B., McKinnon, L., Levin, H. S., Song, J., Meier, M. C., & Chiu, S. (2001). Longitudinal outcome of verbal discourse in children with traumatic brain injury: Three-year follow-up. *Journal of Head Trauma Rehabilitation, 16,* 441–455.
Chapman, S. B., Watkins, R., Gustafson, C., Moore, S., Levin, H. S., & Kufera, J. A. (1997). Narrative discourse in children with closed head injury, children with language impairment, and typically developing children. *American Journal of Speech and Language Pathology, 6,* 66–75.
Clark, E., Russman, S., & Orme, S. (1999). Traumatic brain injury: Effects on school functioning and intervention strategies. *School Psychology Review, 28,* 242–250.
Delis, D. C., Kramer, J. H., Kaplan, E., & Ober, B. A. (1994). *California Verbal Learning Test—Children's Version.* Austin, TX: Psychological Corporation.
Dennis, M., & Barnes, M. A. (2001). Comparison of literal, inferential, and intentional text comprehension in children with mild or severe closed head injury. *Journal of Head Trauma Rehabilitation, 16,* 456–468.
Dennis, M., Guger, S., Roncadin, C., Barnes, M., & Schachar, R. (2001). Attentional–

inhibitory control and social–behavioral regulation after childhood closed head injury: Do biological, developmental, and recovery variables predict outcome? *Journal of the International Neuropsychological Society, 7*, 683–692.

Dennis, M., Purvis, K., Barnes, M. A., Wilkinson, M., & Winner, E. (2001). Understanding literal truth, ironic criticism, and deceptive praise following childhood head injury. *Brain and Language, 78*, 1–16.

DiScala, J. A., Osberg, J. S., Gans, B., Chin, L. J., & Grant, C. C. (1991). Children with traumatic head injury: Morbidity and postacute management. *Archives of Physical Medicine and Rehabilitation, 72*, 662–666.

DiStefano, G., Bachevalier, J., Levin, H. S., Song, J. X., Scheibel, R. S., & Fletcher, J. M. (2000). Volume of focal brain lesions and hippocampal formation in relation to memory function after closed head injury in children. *Journal of Neurology, Neurosurgery, and Psychiatry, 69*, 210–216.

Donders, J. (1997). Sensitivity of the WISC-III to injury severity in children with traumatic head injury. *Assessment, 4*, 107–109.

Donders, J., & Ballard, E. (1996). Psychological adjustment characteristics of children before and after moderate to severe traumatic brain injury. *Journal of Head Trauma Rehabilitation, 11*, 67–73.

Donders, J., & Strom, D. (1997). The effect of traumatic brain injury on children with learning disability. *Pediatric Rehabilitation, 1*, 179–184.

Donders, J., & Strom, D. (2000). Neurobehavioral recovery after pediatric head trauma: Injury, pre-injury, and post-injury issues. *Journal of Head Trauma Rehabilitation, 15*, 792–803.

Donders, J., & Warschausky, S. (1997). WISC-III factor index score patterns after traumatic head injury in children. *Child Neuropsychology, 3*, 71–78.

Donders, J., & Woodward, H. (2003). Gender as a moderator of memory after traumatic brain injury in children. *Journal of Head Trauma Rehabilitation, 18*, 106–115.

Downard, C., Hulka, F., Mullins, R. J., Piatt, J., Chestnut, R., Quint, P., et al. (2000). Relationship of cerebral perfusion pressure and survival in pediatric brain-injured patients. *Journal of Trauma, 49*, 654–658.

Ewing-Cobbs, L., Brookshire, B., Scott, M. A., & Fletcher, J. M. (1998a). Children's narratives following traumatic brain injury: Linguistic structure, cohesion, and thematic recall. *Brain and Language, 61*, 395–419.

Ewing-Cobbs, L., Fletcher, J. M., Levin, H. S., Francis, D. J., Davidson, K., & Miner, M. E. (1997). Longitudinal neuropsychological outcome in infants and preschoolers with traumatic brain injury. *Journal of the International Neuropsychological Society, 3*, 581–591.

Ewing-Cobbs, L., Fletcher, J. M., Levin, H. S., Iovino, I., & Miner, M. E. (1998b). Academic achievement and academic placement following traumatic brain injury in children and adolescents: A two-year longitudinal study. *Journal of Clinical and Experimental Neuropsychology, 20*, 769–781.

Ewing-Cobbs, L., Kramer, L., Prasad, K., Canales, D. N., Louis, P. T., Fletcher, J. M., et al. (1998c). Neuroimaging, physical, and developmental findings after inflicted and noninflicted traumatic brain injury in young children. *Pediatrics, 102*, 300–307.

Farmer, J. E., Haut, J. S., Williams, J., Kapila, C., Johnstone, B., & Kirk, K. S. (1999).

Comprehensive assessment of memory functioning following traumatic brain injury in children. *Developmental Neuropsychology, 15*, 269–289.

Farmer, J. E., Kanne, S. M., Haut, J. S., Williams, J., Johnstone, B., & Kirk, K. (2002). Memory functioning following traumatic brain injury in children with premorbid learning problems. *Developmental Neuropsychology, 22*, 455–469.

Fay, G. C., Jaffe, K. M., Polissar, N. L., Liao, S., Martin, K. M., Shurtleff, H. A., et al. (1993). Mild pediatric traumatic brain injury: A cohort study. *Archives of Physical Medicine and Rehabilitation, 74*, 895–901.

Fay, G. C., Jaffe, K. M., Polissar, N. L., Liao, S., Rivara, J. B., & Martin, K. M. (1994). Outcome of pediatric traumatic brain injury at three years: A cohort study. *Archives of Physical Medicine and Rehabilitation, 75*, 733–741.

Geddes, J. F., Vowles, G. H., Hackshaw, A. K., Nickols, C. D., Scott, I. S., & Whitwell, H. L. (2001). Neuropathology of inflicted head injury in children: II. Microscopic brain injury in infants. *Brain, 124*, 1299–1306.

Gerring, J., Brady, K., Chen, A., Quinn, C., Herskovits, E., Bandeen-Roche, K., et al. (2000). Neuroimaging variables related to development of secondary attention deficit hyperactivity disorder after closed head injury in children and adolescents. *Brain Injury, 14*, 205–218.

Gil, A. M. (2003). Neurocognitive outcomes following pediatric brain injury: A developmental approach. *Journal of School Psychology, 41*, 337–353.

Gioia, G. A., Isquith, P. K., Guy, S. C., & Kenworthy, L. (2000). *Behavior Rating Inventory of Executive Function.* Odessa, FL: Psychological Assessment Resources.

Glang, A., Singer, G. H., & Todis, B. (1997). *Students with acquired brain injury: The school's response.* Baltimore: Brookes.

Hackbarth, R. M., Rzeszutko, K. M., Sturm, G., Donders, J., Kuldanek, A. S., & Sanfilippo, D. J. (2002). Survival and functional outcome in pediatric traumatic brain injury: A retrospective review and analysis of predictive factors. *Critical Care Medicine, 30*, 1630–1635.

Hawley, C. A. (2003). Reported problems and their resolution following mild, moderate and severe traumatic brain injury amongst children and adolescents in the UK. *Brain Injury, 17*, 105–129.

Hawley, C. A., Ward, A. B., Magnay, A. R., & Long, J. (2003). Parental stress and burden following traumatic brain injury amongst children and adolescents. *Brain Injury, 17*, 1–23.

Hayman-Abello, S. E., Rourke, B. P., & Fuerst, D. R. (2003). Psychosocial status after pediatric traumatic brain injury: A subtype analysis using the Child Behavior Checklist. *Journal of the International Neuropsychological Society, 9*, 887–898.

Hoffman, N., Donders, J., & Thompson, E. H. (2000). Novel learning abilities after traumatic head injury in children. *Archives of Clinical Neuropsychology, 15*, 47–58.

Holmbeck, G. N. (2002). Post-hoc probing of significant moderational and mediational effects in studies of pediatric populations. *Journal of Pediatric Psychology, 27*, 87–96.

Janusz, J. A., Kirkwood, M. W., Yeates, K. O., & Taylor, H. G. (2002). Social problem-solving skills in children with traumatic brain injury: Long-term outcomes and prediction of social competence. *Child Neuropsychology, 8*, 179–194.

Katsiyannis, A., & Conderman, G. (1994). Serving individuals with traumatic brain injury: A national survey. *Remedial and Special Education, 15*, 319–325.

Keenan, H. T., Runyan, D. K., Marshall, S. W., Nocera, M. A., Merten, D. F., & Sinal, S. H. (2003). A population-based study of inflicted traumatic brain injury in young children. *Journal of the American Medical Association, 290*, 621–626.

Kinsella, G., Ong, B., Murtagh, D., Prior, M., & Sawyer, M. (1999). The role of the family for behavioral outcome in children and adolescents following traumatic brain injury. *Journal of Consulting and Clinical Psychology, 67*, 116–123.

Kinsella, G. J., Prior, M., Sawyer, M., Ong, B., Murtagh, D., Eisenjaher, R., et al. (1997). Predictors and indicators of academic outcome in children 2 years following traumatic brain injury. *Journal of the International Neuropsychological Society, 3*, 608–616.

Kirkwood, M., Janusz, J., Yeates, K. O., Taylor, H. G., Wade, S. L., Stancin, T., et al. (2000). Prevalence and correlates of depressive symptoms following traumatic brain injury in children. *Child Neuropsychology, 6*, 195–208.

Kraus, J. F. (1995). Epidemiological features of brain injury in children: Occurrence, children at risk, causes, and manner of injury, severity, and outcomes. In S. H. Broman & M. E. Michel (Eds.), *Traumatic head injury in children* (pp. 22–39). New York: Oxford University Press.

Levin, H. S., Benavidez, D. A., Verger-Maestre, K., Perachio, N., Song, J., Mendelsohn, D. B., et al. (2000a). Reduction of corpus callosum growth after severe traumatic brain injury in children. *Neurology, 54*, 647–653.

Levin, H. S., Song, J., Scheibel, R. S., Fletcher, J. M., Harward, H. N., & Chapman, S. B. (2000b). Dissociation of frequency and recency processing from list recall after severe closed head injury in children and adolescents. *Journal of Clinical and Experimental Neuropsychology, 22*, 1–15.

Levin, H. S., Zhang, L., Dennis, M., Ewing-Cobbs, L., Schachar, R., Max, J., et al. (2004). Psychosocial outcome of TBI in children with unilateral frontal lesions. *Journal of the International Neuropsychological Society, 10*, 305–316.

Light, R., Asarnow, R., Satz, P., Zaucha, K., McCleary, C., & Lewis, R. (1998). Mild closed-head injury in children and adolescents: Behavior problems and academic outcomes. *Journal of Consulting and Clinical Psychology, 66*, 1023–1029.

Livingston, R. B., Stark, K. D., Haak, R. A., & Jennings, E. (1996). Neuropsychological profiles of children with depressive and anxiety disorders. *Child Neuropsychology, 2*, 48–62.

Lorber, R., & Yurk, H. (1999). Special pediatric issues: Neuropsychological applications and consultations in schools. In J. Sweet (Ed.), *Forensic neuropsychology: Fundamentals and practice* (pp. 369–418). Lisse, The Netherlands: Swets & Zeitlinger.

Luis, C. A., & Mittenberg, W. (2002). Mood and anxiety disorders following pediatric traumatic brain injury: A prospective study. *Journal of Clinical and Experimental Neuropsychology, 24*, 270–279.

Mangeot, S., Armstrong, K., Colvin, A. N., Yeates, K. O., & Taylor, H. G. (2002). Long-term executive function deficits in children with traumatic brain injuries: Assessment using the Behavior Rating Inventory of Executive Function (BRIEF). *Child Neuropsychology, 8*, 271–284.

Massagli, T. L., Michaud, L. J., & Rivara, F. P. (1996). Association between injury indices and outcome after severe traumatic brain injury in children. *Archives of Physical Medicine and Rehabilitation, 77,* 125–132.

Max, J. E., Castillo, C. S., Bokura, H., Robin, D. A., Lindgren, S. D., Smith, W. L., et al. (1998a). Oppositional defiant disorder symptomatology after traumatic brain injury: A prospective study. *Journal of Nervous and Mental Disease, 186,* 325–332.

Max, J. E., Koele, S. L., Castillo, C. C., Lindgren, S. D., Arndt, S., Bokura, H., et al. (2000). Personality change disorder in children and adolescents following traumatic brain injury. *Journal of the International Neuropsychological Society, 6,* 279–289.

Max, J. E., Koele, S. L., Smith, W. L., Sato, Y., Lindgren, S. D., Robin, D. A., et al. (1998b). Psychiatric disorders in children and adolescents after severe traumatic brain injury: A controlled study. *Journal of the American Academy of Child and Adolescent Psychiatry, 37,* 832–840.

Max, J. E., Roberts, M. A., Koele, S. L., Lindgren, S. D., Robin, D. A., Arndt, S., et al. (1999). Cognitive outcome in children and adolescents following severe traumatic brain injury: Influence of psychosocial, psychiatric, and injury-related variables. *Journal of the International Neuropsychological Society, 5,* 58–68.

Max, J. E., Robertson, B. A. M., & Lansing, A. E. (2001). The phenomenology of personality change due to traumatic brain injury in children and adolescents. *Journal of Neuropsychiatry and Clinical Neurosciences, 13,* 161–170.

McMahon, M. A., Noll, R. B., Michaud, L. J., & Johnson, J. C. (2001). Sibling adjustment of pediatric traumatic brain injury: A case-controlled study. *Journal of Head Trauma Rehabilitation, 16,* 587–594.

Miller, L. J., & Donders, J. (2003). Prediction of educational outcome after pediatric traumatic brain injury. *Rehabilitation Psychology, 48,* 237–241.

Mittenberg, W., Wittner, M. S., & Miller, L. J. (1997). Postconcussion syndrome occurs in children. *Neuropsychology, 11,* 447–452.

Moradi, A. R., Doost, H. T. N., Taghavi, M. R., Yule, W., & Dalgeish, T. (1999). Everyday memory deficits in children and adolescents with PTSD: Performance on the Rivermead Behavioural Memory Test. *Journal of Child Psychology and Psychiatry and Allied Disciplines, 40,* 357–361.

Ponsford, J., Willmott, C., Cameron, P., Ayton, G., Nelms, R., Curran, C., et al. (1999). Cognitive and behavioral outcome following mild traumatic head injury in children. *Journal of Head Trauma Rehabilitation, 14,* 360–372.

Prasad, M. R., Ewing-Cobbs, L., Swank, P. R., & Kramer, L. (2002). Predictors of outcome following traumatic brain injury in young children. *Pediatric Neurosurgery, 36,* 64–74.

Rivara, F. P. (1994). Epidemiology and prevention of pediatric traumatic brain injury. *Pediatric Annals, 23,* 12–17.

Rivara, F. P. (1995). Developmental and behavioral issues in childhood injury prevention. *Journal of Developmental and Behavioral Pediatrics, 16,* 362–370.

Rivara, J. B., Jaffe, K. M., Polissar, N. L., Fay, G. C., Liao, S., & Martin, K. M. (1996). Predictors of family functioning and change 3 years after traumatic brain injury in children. *Archives of Physical Medicine and Rehabilitation, 77,* 754–764.

Roman, M. J., Delis, D. C., Willerman, L., Magulac, M., Demadura, T. L., De La Pena, J. J., et al. (1998). Impact of pediatric traumatic brain injury on compo-

nents of verbal memory. *Journal of Clinical and Experimental Neuropsychology, 20*, 245–258.
Ruppel, R. A., Kochanek, P. M., Adelson, P. D., Rose, M. E., Wisniewki, S. R., Bell, M. J., et al. (2001). Excitatory amino acid concentrations in ventricular cerebrospinal fluid after severe traumatic brain injury in infants and children: The role of child abuse. *Journal of Pediatrics, 138*, 1–3.
Satz, P., Zaucha, K., McCleary, C., Light, R., Asarnow, R., & Becker, D. (1997). Mild head injury in children and adolescents: A review of studies (1970–1995). *Psychological Bulletin, 122*, 107–131.
Savage, R. C., Lash, M., Bennett, K., & Navalta, C. (1995). Special education for students with brain injury. *TBI Challenge, 3*(2), 3–7.
Schwartz, L., Taylor, H. G., Drotar, D., Yeates, K. O., Wade, S. L., & Stancin, T. (2003). Long-term behavior problems following pediatric traumatic brain injury: Prevalence, predictors, and correlates. *Journal of Pediatric Psychology, 28*, 251–263.
Semrud-Clikeman, M. (2001). *Traumatic brain injury in children and adolescents: Assessment and intervention.* New York: Guilford Press.
Silver, C. H. (2000). Ecological validity of neuropsychological assessment in childhood traumatic brain injury. *Journal of Head Trauma Rehabilitation, 15*, 973–988.
Sinal, S., Petree, A., Herman-Giddens, M., Rogers, M., Enand, C., & DuRant, R. (2000). Is race or ethnicity a predictive factor in shaken baby syndrome? *Child Abuse and Neglect, 24*, 1241–1246.
Slomine, B. S., Gerring, J. P., Grados, M. A., Vasa, R., Brady, K. D., Christensen, J. R., et al. (2002). Performance on measures of executive function following pediatric traumatic brain injury. *Brain Injury, 16*, 759–772.
Statler, K. D., Jenkins, L. W., Dixon, C. E., Clark, R. S. B., Marion, D. W., & Kochanek, P. M. (2001). The simple model versus the super model: Translating experimental traumatic brain injury research to the bedside. *Journal of Neurotrauma, 18*, 1195–1206.
Swift, E. E., Taylor, H. G., Kaugars, A. S., Drotar, D., Yeates, K. O., Wade, S. L., et al. (2003). Sibling relationship and behavior after pediatric traumatic brain injury. *Journal of Developmental and Behavioral Pediatrics, 24*, 24–31.
Taylor, H. G., & Alden, J. (1997). Age-related differences in outcomes following childhood brain insults: An introduction and overview. *Journal of the International Neuropsychological Society, 3*, 555–567.
Taylor, H. G., Yeates, K. O., Wade, S. L., Drotar, D., Stancin, T., & Burant, C. (2001). Bidirectional child–family influences on outcomes of traumatic brain injury in children. *Journal of the International Neuropsychological Society, 7*, 755–767.
Taylor, H. G., Yeates, K. O., Wade, S. L., Drotar, D., Stancin, T., & Minich, N. (2002). A prospective study of short- and long-term outcomes after traumatic brain injury in children: Behavior and achievement. *Neuropsychology, 16*, 15–27.
Taylor, H. G., Yeates, K. O., Wade, S. L., Drotar, D., Stancin, T., & Montpetite, M. (2003). Long-term educational interventions after traumatic brain injury in children. *Rehabilitation Psychology, 48*, 227–236.
Teasdale, G., & Jennett, B. (1974). Assessment of coma and impaired consciousness: A practical scale. *Lancet, 2*, 81–84.

Tremont, G., Mittenberg, W., & Miller, L. J. (1999). Acute intellectual effects of pediatric head trauma. *Child Neuropsychology, 5*, 104–114.

Verger, K., Junqué, C., Levin, H. S., Jurado, M. A., Pérez-Gómez, M., Bartrés-Faz, D., et al. (2001). Correlation of atrophy measures on MRI with neuropsychological sequelae in children and adolescents with traumatic brain injury. *Brain Injury, 15*, 211–221.

Vriezen, E. R., & Pigott, S. E. (2002). The relationship between parental report on the BRIEF and performance-based measures of executive function in children with moderate to severe traumatic brain injury. *Child Neuropsychology, 8*, 296–303.

Waaland, P. K., Burns, C., & Cockrell, J. (1993). Evaluation of needs of high- and low-income families following pediatric traumatic brain injury. *Brain Injury, 7*, 135–146.

Wade, S. L., Borawski, E. A., Taylor, H. G., Yeates, K. O., & Stancin, T. (2001). The relationship of caregiver coping to family outcomes during the initial year following pediatric traumatic injury. *Journal of Consulting and Clinical Psychology, 69*, 406–415.

Wade, S. L., Taylor, H. G., Drotar, D., Stancin, T., & Yeates, K. O. (1998). Family burden and adaptation during the initial year following traumatic brain injury in children. *Pediatrics, 102*, 110–116.

Wade, S. L., Taylor, H. G., Drotar, D., Stancin, T., Yeates, K. O., & Minich, N. M. (2002). A prospective study of long-term caregiver and family adaptation following brain injury in children. *Journal of Head Trauma Rehabilitation, 17*, 96–111.

Wagner, A. K., Sasser, H. C., Hammond, F. M., Wiercisiewki, D., & Alexander, J. (2000). Intentional traumatic brain injury: Epidemiology, risk factors, and associations with injury severity and mortality. *Journal of Trauma, 49*, 404–410.

Warschausky, S., Cohen, E. H., Parker, J. G., Levendosky, A. A., & Okun, A. (1997). Social problem-solving skills of children with traumatic brain injury. *Pediatric Rehabilitation, 1*, 77–81.

Wechsler, D. (1991). *Wechsler Intelligence Scale for Children—Third Edition*. San Antonio, TX: Psychological Corporation.

Williams, D. H., Levin, H. S., & Eisenberg, H. M. (1990). Mild head injury classification. *Neurosurgery, 27*, 422–428.

Woodward, H., Winterhalter, K., Donders, J., Hackbarth, R., Kuldanek, A., & Sanfilippo, D. (1999). Prediction of neurobehavioral outcome 1–5 years post pediatric traumatic head injury. *Journal of Head Trauma Rehabilitation, 14*, 351–359.

Yeates, K. O., Luria, J., Bartkowski, H., Rusin, J., Martin, L., & Bigler, E. D. (1999). Postconcussive symptoms in children with mild closed head injuries. *Journal of Head Trauma Rehabilitation, 14*, 337–350.

Yeates, K. O., Swift, E., Taylor, H. G., Wade, S. L., Drotar, D., Stancin, T., et al. (2004). Short- and long-term social outcomes following pediatric traumatic brain injury. *Journal of the International Neuropsychological Society, 10*, 412–426.

Yeates, K. O., Taylor, H. G., Drotar, D., Wade, S. L., Klein, S., Stancin, T., & Schatschneider, C. (1997). Preinjury family environment as a determinant of recovery from traumatic brain injuries in school-age children. *Journal of the International Neuropsychological Society, 3*, 617–630.

Yeates, K. O., Taylor, H. G., Wade, S. L., Drotar, D., Stancin, T., & Minich, N. (2002a). A prospective study of short- and long-term neuropsychological outcomes after traumatic brain injury in children. *Neuropsychology, 16*, 514–523.

Yeates, K. O., Taylor, H. G., Woodrome, S. E., Wade, S. L., Stancin, T., & Drotar, D. (2002b). Race as a moderator of parent and family outcomes following pediatric traumatic brain injury. *Journal of Pediatric Psychology, 27*, 393–403.

Ylvisaker, M., Todis, B., Glang, A., Urbanczyk, B., Franklin, C., De Pompei, R., et al. (2001). Educating students with TBI: Themes and recommendations. *Journal of Head Trauma Rehabilitation, 16*, 76–93.

3

Spinal Cord Injury

CAROLINE J. ANDERSON
LAWRENCE C. VOGEL

Spinal cord injuries (SCIs) are devastating events that are particularly tragic when they affect children or adolescents who have barely had an opportunity to experience life (Betz & Mulcahey, 1996; Massagli, 2000; Vogel, Betz, & Mulcahey, 1997; Vogel, 1997; Vogel & Anderson, 2003; Vogel, Hickey, Klaas, & Anderson, 2004). The most prominent manifestations of SCIs are paralysis, loss of sensation, and bladder, bowel, and sexual dysfunction (Lin, 2003; Kirshblum, Campagnolo, & DeLisa, 2002). The extent of paralysis, loss of voluntary muscle movement, and loss of sensation is determined by the location of the spinal cord damage. Damage to the cervical spinal cord results in tetraplegia, with limited motor function and sensation in both the upper and lower extremities. Damage to the thoracic, lumbar, or sacral segments of the spinal cord results in paraplegia or loss of motor function and sensation in the lower extremities. SCIs may be further categorized as a specific neurological level and the degree of completeness. The neurological level is the most caudal segment of the spinal cord with normal motor and sensory function. An SCI is considered to be complete if there is an absence of sensory and motor function in the lowest sacral segments. In contrast, an SCI may be incomplete, with varying degrees of preservation of sensory and motor function below the zone of the SCI (American Spinal Injury Association, 2000).

The impairments associated with an SCI have different consequences at the various levels of an individual's functioning, ranging from activities of daily living to participation in community activities. Loss of motor function may limit the ability to manipulate objects with one's fingers or the ability to walk or drive. Loss of sensation places a child at risk of pressure ulcers or thermal skin injury. Bladder and bowel dysfunction are manifested by loss of the normal control of initiating or postponing micturition or defecation. This may result in urinary or fecal incontinence and places children at risk of urinary tract infections and constipation. The extent and specifics of sexual dysfunction depend upon the level of an SCI, whether it is a complete lesion or not, and whether the patient is spastic. Some of the issues related to sexuality that should be considered include sexual development, the onset or resumption of menses, sexual performance, and fertility.

Approximately 20% of all SCIs that occur annually in the United States affect children and adolescents (Price, Makintubee, Herndon, & Istre, 1994). Although males more commonly sustain SCI than females during adolescence, the preponderance of males becomes less marked as age of injury decreases, with females equaling males in those 5 years of age and younger (DeVivo & Vogel, 2004). The severity of the neurological injury also varies as a function of age, with younger children more likely having paraplegia or complete injuries. Among individuals who were 12 years or younger when injured, approximately two-thirds had paraplegia, and a similar proportion had complete lesions (DeVivo & Vogel, 2004). In contrast, the neurological severity in adolescents with SCI is similar to the adult SCI population, with approximately 50% having paraplegia and 50% having complete injuries. Life expectancy for children and adolescents with SCI is somewhat less than that in the general population and is a function of neurological level and degree of completeness. The less severe the SCI, in respect to both level and category, the longer the expected survival. In comparison to the general population, life expectancy ranges from 67–69% for individuals with the most severe injuries to 92–93% for those with the least severe injuries (DeVivo, 2002).

Motor vehicle crashes are the most common cause of SCI in children and adolescents. Violence is a significant cause of SCI throughout childhood and adolescence, and is especially prominent in African Americans and Hispanics, and in those injured after 5 years of age. Sports are a more common cause of SCI in adolescents compared to younger children or adults, whereas medical/surgical causes are more common among those injured younger than 5 years. Last, compared to adult etiology, falls are a less common etiology of SCI in both children and adolescents (DeVivo & Vogel, 2004).

Unique etiologies of SCI in children and adolescents include birth injuries, lap-belt injuries, child abuse, and transverse myelitis. Additionally, children with skeletal dysplasias, juvenile rheumatoid arthritis, and Down syndrome are susceptible to cervical SCI. Lap-belt injuries primarily occur in children weighing between 40 and 60 pounds, when the lap belt is positioned above the pelvic brim, resulting in flexion–distraction forces in the midlumbar spine (Apple & Murray, 1996). Three components of lap-belt injuries are abdominal wall bruising due to the lap belt, intra-abdominal injuries, and an SCI. In order to reduce the incidence of lap-belt injuries, children who weigh more than 40 pounds and who are 4–8 years of age should travel in motor vehicles with approved belt-positioning booster seats (Centers for Disease Control and Prevention, 2000).

Distinctive anatomical and physiological features of children and adolescents, along with growth and development, are responsible for unique manifestations, consequences, and complications of SCI in the pediatric population. SCI without radiographic abnormality (SCIWORA), lap-belt injuries, birth injuries, and delayed onset of neurological deficits are relatively unique to pediatric SCI and are a result of sustaining an SCI at a young age. Although plain radiographs and computerized tomography are normal, magnetic resonance imaging (MRI) abnormalities are present in approximately two-thirds of individuals with SCIWORA (Pang, 1996). SCIWORA occurs in 64% of children who sustain an SCI at 5 years of age or younger, 33% of those 6–12 years old, and 20–22% of adolescents (DeVivo & Vogel, 2004).

Impairments associated with an SCI have varying consequences and implications for management because of growth and developmental changes inherent in children and adolescents and the age when the child is injured. At one extreme is a child who is injured at birth, where the SCI has an impact on physiological, physical, and psychosocial development throughout the individual's lifespan. As a result of muscle paralysis, the child is at high risk of developing orthopedic complications, such as scoliosis and hip dislocation. Impaired mobility may affect the infant's and toddler's exploration of their environment, which is so vital to their development. By 9–15 months of age, infants can begin standing in a variety of standers or parapodia. Toddlers and young children with paraplegia can progress to ambulation using different orthotics, such as reciprocating gait orthoses (RGOs) or knee–ankle–foot orthoses (KAFOs), whereas those with tetraplegia may continue using standing devices or parapodia. In the absence of urological complications, diapers are used for management of the neurogenic bladder and bowel in an infant or toddler. Generally, intermittent catheterization and a bowel program are initiated at about 3 years of age, when children normally begin potty training. By 5–7 years of age, most children are cognitively capable of beginning a self-catheterization program.

In contrast to SCIs acquired at birth, injuries sustained during adolescence result in dramatic lifestyle changes that have different implications. The major issues that adolescents face include psychosocial and sexual problems, and continued participation in school and in their communities

(Mulcahey, 1992; Geller & Greydanus, 1979; Bloom & Joseph, 2003). Although the initial goal of all adolescents who sustain an SCI is to walk, the majority of adolescents will at most utilize braces for ambulation selectively, primarily in a therapeutic setting. Because adolescents want ready and comprehensive access to community activities, lightweight or power wheelchairs and adapted motor vehicles are important. Although individuals of all ages with an SCI are at risk of many complications such as pressure ulcers, depression, and urinary tract infections, the tumultuous nature of adolescents may make them more vulnerable to SCI-related complications.

An additional complication of SCI can be a concomitant head injury (Davidoff, Morris, Roth, & Bleiberg, 1985). Because a variety of measures are used to assess traumatic brain injury (TBI) in patients with SCIs, estimates of the frequency of TBI vary widely, and the difficulty of making an unequivocal diagnosis is recognized (Davidoff, Roth, & Richards, 1992; Richards et al., 1991) If a brain injury is serious and obvious, it can have a major impact on the ability of the individual to participate in rehabilitation. A complex mild brain injury in a young child is often difficult to assess, and the brain injury may not appear to impact functioning significantly (Rivara et al., 1993). Mild brain injury in adults who sustain an SCI can often be described by individuals or their families in subtle terms such as "harder to concentrate," "memory is not quite as good," or "just not as sharp." For children, a mild head injury is much more difficult to diagnose, because most of those children will not have had any premorbid cognitive testing and will not be aware of subtle changes or possible learning disabilities (Miles & Cawley, 1996). If there have been physical signs of brain injury or loss of consciousness, parents, teachers, and health care professionals need to keep that issue in mind regarding learning or behavioral problems.

EMOTIONAL, BEHAVIORAL, AND SOCIAL ISSUES

Although SCIs may be diagnosed at the time of birth, the great majority of injuries to children or adolescents occur suddenly in individuals who have been developing normally and fully participating in life. To be faced with an abrupt, severe, and typically permanent change in function is emotionally devastating for most patients and their families (Warschausky, Engel, Kewman, & Nelson, 1996; Anderson, 1997, 2003). The youngest children may not grasp the situation, but may nevertheless be upset by hospital procedures, surgeries, unfamiliar environments, different schedules, limitations to their functioning, and the therapy requirements of rehabilitation (Johnson, Berry, Goldeen, & Wicker, 1991). They may also be affected by the stress and grief that their parents are feeling (Aitken et al., 2005). Older children and many parents may have some familiarity with the notion of an SCI and paralysis, but few will be aware of all of the associated issues such as needing to catheterize, performing bowel programs, doing pressure reliefs, and considering the impact of the SCI on sexual functioning and fertility (Vogel & Anderson, 2003). From this perspective, it is clear that patients and families not only have to deal with the initial shock of the diagnosis of SCI but also, as they obtain more complete information, the news seems to get worse, not better. Adding to the stress is the requirement for patients and parents to learn an extensive amount of new information about the care required for an SCI and then, in most instances, patients and/or their parents will actually need to learn how to perform the care themselves. Both for parents and for older children and adolescents, the fact that parents are dealing with bowel and bladder care may feel like regressing to the time when the patients were babies. The acute hospitalization and the initial rehabilitation process are truly periods that can be emotionally overwhelming.

At one time, it was popular to assume that most adults who sustained an SCI would go through a series of stages of emotional adjustment, including denial, anger, and depression (Hammell, 1992; Trieschmann, 1988). However, there is no empirical support for these theories, and it is more common now to consider each person individually, taking into account variations in personalities, styles of coping, and support available (Trieschmann, 1988; Stiens, Bergman, & Formal, 1997; Fichtenbaum & Kirshblum, 2002; Moverman, 2003). For children or adolescents and their parents, the initial adjustment to injury is made even more complicated by the developmental issues that vary with the age of the child. Infants and preschoolers tend to focus on the present and are most comforted by family. During initial rehabilitation, recreation and play activities provided can be very helpful (Johnson & Klaas, 2000). Adapted toys are especially important for children with tetraplegia. School-age children, who typically have developed the independence to toilet, dress, feed, and bathe themselves, may feel frustrated after injury by the difficulties of trying to do self-care and needing the help of others. Many will verbalize that they want to walk and return to their activities of bike riding, playing sports, running, and skating. Since most children of this age are very social, they will fear being left out of neighborhood and school activities with their friends. Even the younger school-age children can grasp the concept that their disability is permanent, although they may continue to make statements about being able to walk when they "get better." Other concerns of this age group are often fears that others will make fun of them, stare, ask what is wrong, and refuse to include them in play activities.

Adolescence is the most common age for pediatric-onset SCI and is arguably the most difficult age at which to sustain an injury (Bloom & Joseph, 2003; Rutledge & Dick, 1983; Kennedy, Gorsuch, & Marsh, 1995). Adolescents are at a stage of increasing independence from parents, often affiliating more with peers than with family. Appearance, popularity, fitting in, and self-esteem are particularly important (Mulcahey, 1992). There is an increasing awareness and interest in sexuality. In addition, especially older teens are beginning to formulate plans for careers, independent living, and adult identities. An injury that occurs in adolescence almost always forces teens to become more dependent on parents and to spend more time with them than with peers during initial rehabilitation. Teens may react to their loss of independence by showing anger toward staff and parents. Other behaviors are typical of attempts to avoid dealing with the situation: sleeping, placing blankets over their heads so they cannot see or be seen, refusing therapy, and refusing to go out into the community (Perilstein & Williams, 1996). Depression and even suicidal ideation may occur. Finally, at a developmental stage when privacy and sexuality are important issues, catheterization, bowel programs, and showers that are performed by parents or staff adds to a teen's feeling of degradation. In addition, some adolescents are noncompliant with their care (Grossman & Merenda, 2004).

In treating children and adolescents, family-centered care is a goal and, in the case of traumatic SCI, parents and family members typically need at least as much support as the patient (Boyer, Ware, Knolls, & Kafkalas, 2003; Engel, Brooks, &Warschausky, 2003). It is common for parents to feel guilty that they were not able to protect their son or daughter from injury. Additionally, it is not unusual for parents or other family members to be involved to some extent in causing the injury; for example, a parent might have been driving a car when it crashed, or a child might have fallen from a bed in the presence of a parent. At times, blame may be placed on a family member by others. During initial rehabilitation, parents often have to leave their jobs for several weeks, endure financial worries, and find ways to meet the needs of the rest of their children. The sources of stress are immense. Individual and family counseling can be important, but help with resources, education, and mentors is equally important as family members begin to gain control of their life again. The family's initial expectation may be that the child, regardless of age at injury, may never be able to live independently, have a job, become financially independent, or have a family of his or her own as an adult. Allaying those fears is important not only for the family members' peace of mind but also to ensure that parents continue to raise their child with the same expectations they had prior to injury.

In summary, the initial emotional response to SCI in the patient and/or family may be depression, anxiety, fear, and anger, but these emotions will not necessarily occur. In addition, posttraumatic stress symptoms may be evident, and this has been found in adult-onset SCI as well (Radnitz et al., 1995; Butt, 1998). In children and adults ages 11–24 years with SCI, 25% were reported to have some symptoms of posttraumatic stress (Boyer, Knolls, Kafkalas, & Tollen, 2000). Among the common symptoms are flashbacks or re-experiencing an event, such as a car crash, that caused the injury, and avoidance of discussions, pictures, or individuals that might be associated with the traumatic event.

Finally, an uncommon behavioral complication of SCI, self-injurious behavior, may be a result of dysesthesia, and may be responsive to treatment with anticonvulsants (Vogel & Anderson, 2002).

Each individual patient and his or her parents need to be carefully evaluated for emotional status and needs throughout acute hospitalization, rehabilitation, and follow-up. It is known that children and adolescents with physical disabilities are at risk for overall adjustment problems (Lavigne & Faier-Routman, 1992). It is also known that there are relationships between the way family members respond and the adjustment of the patient (Warschausky, Majchrzak, Lifford, Dixon, & Tate, 2004; Elliott, Shewchuk, & Richards, 1999). Individual, group, or family counseling may be recommended. Regular SCI team meetings enable the observations of all team members to add to a composite view of additional support and interventions that might be helpful. Medication, especially for depression, may be warranted.

Planning for discharge begins at the time the patient first enters the rehabilitation program, and both parents and patients often feel resistant to ordering wheelchairs and building ramps, and to making other modifications to homes and vehicles. These activities are stark reminders that the injury may have a permanent impact. Similarly, patients and families may be resistant to being discharged from the hospital, because they felt they would "walk out of here" and have difficulty accepting that they are wheelchair users. Support from all SCI team members is needed to help families through this process. It is helpful to have regularly scheduled goal conferences at which patient, family, and all staff working with the patient can set goals, assess progress, and develop an organized plan leading to discharge (Beck & Spoltore, 1996).

SCHOOL ISSUES

One of the most important issues in discharge planning is to help the patient and family prepare for the child's return to school (Dudgeon, Massagli, & Ross, 1997; Beck & Spoltore, 1996). Often patient and parents are reluctant to consider that the child could ever go to school in a wheelchair, using adaptive equipment or needing to catheterize. Compared to the relative freedom and normalcy of the child or adolescent's previous experiences at school, it can be very intimidating to think of returning to school after an injury. In addition, parents may worry that the child will not receive adequate attention for his or her medical needs in school. Children and adolescents with new injuries may feel negatively about suddenly having to take accessible busses. They may also worry about how their teachers and classmates will react (Mulcahey, 1992).

SCI in children and young adolescents is relatively rare, and most schools will be unfamiliar with the condition. Even schools that are well-prepared to educate children with physical disabilities may need to be taught the important medical issues related to SCI. Furthermore, school principals and staff may adopt the approach that the patient does not have to return to school for the rest of the year because "we will pass them anyway." This approach does not help the patient educationally, emotionally, or socially. Our clinical experience has been that returning to school almost immediately after discharge is apt to result in a happier, healthier, and more social child or adolescent. Typically, if the return to school is delayed, it becomes more and more difficult to transition back to school.

From the time the patient is admitted for initial rehabilitation, work should begin on the school issue. The importance of returning to school will be discussed with the patient and family and the school will be contacted. The ideal plan is for the child or adolescent to return to his or her previous school. Accessibility will need to be addressed, although most larger or newer schools will not find this to be a problem. Individuals with higher levels of tetraplegia may need aides to help with feeding, toileting, writing, and participating in activities. Almost all patients, those with tetraplegia or paraplegia, will need to catheterize either by themselves or with assistance. Having privacy for this process is an important issue. Although most older school-age children and adolescents should be able to be responsible for remembering to catheterize, younger children and some of the less mature older ones may need guidance. In addition, school staff need to be aware of the important medical complications that might arise, such as overheating. The fact that most of the children and adolescents with SCI have a loss of sensation is also an important issue, so staff may remind them that they need to sit on cushions, perform pressure reliefs, and avoid heat sources or sunburns. A pamphlet that provides basic information about SCI for school staff is helpful, but direct contact with school staff is also highly recommended to discuss the individual patient's needs.

For elementary school children, three additional issues commonly arise about school. The first is the activity of the child on the playground and during recess. Although teachers may be tempted to encourage the child to stay in the classroom and play games or read books, the best solution from a psychological perspective is to have accessible playgrounds or encourage activities that the child might be able to participate in, such as ball games for those with paraplegia. The second problem area for many children with SCI is physical education. Again, the best solution is thoughtful programming that will include the child with an SCI in many of the games and activities. Finally, a common problem in many schools is the issue of field trips. Sometimes all of the children in the class ride on a regular school bus, while a child with SCI rides alone on an accessible bus, isolating that child from peers. Since much of the fun and interest of field trips is socializing on the bus, having all of the children together on an accessible bus is a better solution. For high school students, there may be similar problems with band trips, away games, and any other activities that students typically attend on a school bus. To facilitate the participation of teens with SCIs in all of the typical high school activities, such as dances or football games, special efforts should be made to assure accessibility. Adolescents are especially sensitive to relationships with peers (Perilstein & Williams, 1996; Mulcahey, 1992).

FAMILY

Following initial rehabilitation, the child or adolescent with an SCI typically returns home to live with family. The family home and vehicles will need to be accessible, and this may require either major or minor changes. Changes in family dynamics may be even more striking. This is often an issue for families with children who have either traumatic injuries or chronic disabilities (Johnson & Kastner, 2005; Boyer et al., 2003; Warschausky et al., 1996). In cases where both parents were working prior to injury, one may stay home to help with SCI care. Particularly when the individual with an SCI has tetraplegia and limited function, parents may be doing care that is physically difficult, such as lifting, turning, bathing, and feeding. It is not unusual for family members to come back for their first clinic visit after discharge and report how exhausted they are. To prevent pressure sores, some higher level patients have to be turned in the middle of the night, and some may need nighttime catheterizations. This results in a lack of sleep in caregivers. In addition, parents may suddenly feel that their own mobility is limited by the need to stay home and care for their child or be there to ensure the child's safety. This can be especially difficult for single parents. Much of the stress for the caregivers depends on the physical needs of the child or adolescent and the number of supportive adults available to help, whether a spouse, grandparents or other relatives, friends, neighbors, or paid assistants.

Another stressor for parents is the change in role relative to their child. This is particularly true for parents of adolescents. Parents will often say, "I don't want to be my child's nurse, I want to be his [her] mother." Just at the point when the teen was becoming independent of parents, he or she is suddenly dependent, and this can be tough transition for both teen and parents. The SCI can also produce changes in the dynamics of a marital relationship, particularly when it is also associated with one or the other spouse spending major amounts of time in caregiving, or when there is a loss of a job and financial stress.

Siblings are not immune to the impact of the SCI. Traumatic injuries in children, as well as chronic disabilities of children, change the family dynamics and affect the siblings (Faux, 1993; Coleby, 1995). Typically, over the period of the initial hospitalization and rehabilitation, brothers and sisters will be worried and dealing with much of the same emotional trauma as the patient and parents. Some may begin to feel resentful of the time, attention, and gifts given to the injured sibling. Others may feel guilty because of some real or imagined way in which they might have contributed to or prevented the injury. Siblings also have to adjust to changes in their parents' roles when the patient returns home, changes in the activities that they may have done with their sibling, and restrictions on some of the activities that the whole family may have enjoyed together. Siblings who are old enough will also be expected to help out as needed. Some siblings who are still able to participate in activities, such as sports, that the sibling with the SCI can no longer do, will feel reluctant to continue, because it would seem unfair.

DEVELOPMENTAL CHANGES OVER TIME

Childhood and adolescence are periods of rapid development of knowledge and skills. As a result, rehabilitation and habilitation for SCI varies substantially with age at injury. In addition, after children sustain an injury, their needs and abilities continue to change as they grow and develop. For this reason, when patients return to the outpatient clinic for periodic assessment over the years, they are seen by all members of the SCI team, including psychologists, social workers, recreation therapists, and child life specialists. There are several goals. The first is to ensure that the patient develops increasing knowledge and skill regarding SCI and independence. This is a dynamic process in which the parent gradually decreases responsibility for care as the child becomes more mature. This is a more complicated process than it seems, because health care for SCI is critical. As is typical of any 8-year-old, a child with SCI may be able to catheterize and know that he or she should, but may forget or simply decide not to do it. Similarly, he or she may decide to ignore pressure reliefs. At the same time, parents can appreciate the importance of these issues for their child's health and may be reluctant to turn responsibility over to the child. It is always tricky to obtain the right balance, and parents often need to be vigilant and provide a safety net as the child gradually takes on the responsibility for care. The SCI team provides guidance and encouragement (Blomquist, Brown, Peersen, & Presler, 1998).

The second issue of importance related to development is to ensure that the child with an SCI keeps up with peers in all aspects of community participation as he or she grows. For example, although it varies from community to community, it may be common for children from 4 to 10 years of age to attend birthday parties of classmates. If the child with an SCI is not invited because parents are nervous or houses are inaccessible, it becomes an issue of social isolation and poor self-esteem. Similarly, issues arise for all of the activities of childhood and adolescence, whether it is scouting, band, camps, park district programs, or sports. Research has shown that children and adolescents with SCI spend more hours per day on activities such as listening to music, using a computer, and watching television than is typical for the able-bodied pediatric population (Johnson, Klaas, Vogel, & McDonald, 2004). The SCI team needs to assess community participation at each clinic visit to provide guidance and suggestions. This may include resources for specialized camps or recreation programs, but it may also be a matter of just making parents aware that participation is important for all children and adolescents regardless of their injury.

A third issue related to development is preparation for adult employment. Parents, consciously or unconsciously, help prepare their children for employment by encouraging them to do chores and neighborhood jobs such as paper routes or babysitting, and then to take part-time jobs as adolescents. Yet many parents of children who have sustained an SCI may be so focused on all of the care and therapy issues that chores or jobs are lost in the background. As a result, adolescents with SCI, like those with other disabilities, have typically had far less exposure to work experiences than their peers and are transitioning to adulthood with a disadvantage (Anderson & Vogel, 2000; Pless, Cripps, Davies, & Wadsworth, 1989). This is another area that the SCI team can address in clinic visits over the years to help parents and patients gradually prepare for transition to adulthood.

Another topic that needs to be addressed as the patient grows and develops is sexuality. As noted earlier, the topic should be initiated at the time of injury, regardless of the age of the child, so that parents can raise the child with the knowledge that sexuality is a developmental process for a child with SCI, just as it is for any child. However, as children reach ages 8–12, when sexuality programs are typically initiated in schools, they may have questions about how their SCI affects sexual function or menstruation (Yarkony & Anderson, 1996; Anderson, 1997). These topics need to be initiated by the SCI team, and parents need to be knowledgeable so they can educate their children. In adolescence, patients may have specific questions about erection, ejaculation, fertility, birth control, and pregnancy. Recommendations in this area have changed substantially in the past decade and probably will continue to change. For example, the risk of latex allergies has to be discussed in relationship to condoms, and the introduction of medications for erectile dysfunction is of interest to males with SCIs (Elliott, 2003). Although females with SCIs can become pregnant, males with SCIs may have problems with fertility, and the myriad fertility clinics and procedures are of interest to them if they wish to consider having a family (Elliott, 2003).

RISK FACTORS FOR POOR PSYCHOSOCIAL OUTCOMES

There is a paucity of research on pediatric-onset SCI and little empirical information about risk factors for poorer outcomes in the years following injury. Our observations indicate, however, that smaller, more rural communities may provide more support for families with a new SCI. This often takes the form of fund-raisers, community help with house modifications, and neighborly support for the family. In contrast, large cities may provide less of that support but more opportunities for wheelchair recreational activities and jobs. Larger cities also provide greater access to other individuals with SCIs who can be mentors, and closer access to specialized SCI care. Our clinical observations also indicate that individuals who may get large monetary settlements, from car crashes, for example, may have money to build new accessible housing and obtain vehicles that make their lives easier and more pleasant. It is not necessarily the case that large settlements actually increase the likelihood of happier or more successful adult lives. There are also clinical examples in our practice of risk-taking adolescents who may have been involved in drugs, drinking, and wild activities and continued with those activities following their injury. For others who had a similar background, the injuries changed their lives and led to improved social awareness and more responsible behavior. All of these issues need to be addressed with substantial research efforts.

Long-term outcomes for individuals with pediatric-onset SCI have received research attention. Among those in young adulthood, longer duration of injury has been found to be associated with higher quality of life (Putzke, Richards, & Dowler, 2000). Also, individuals who sustain SCIs as children or adolescents have higher education levels than their noninjured peers when they are age 24 years and older (Vogel, Klaas, Lubicky, & Anderson, 1998). In contrast, their levels of employment, marriage, independent living, and income are substantially below the level of their peers, as indicated by U.S. census data for the same age range (Anderson & Vogel,

2002; Anderson, Krajci, & Vogel, 2003). Similarly, compared to community controls of the same gender and age, adults with pediatric-onset SCI are less satisfied with their lives, less employed, less likely to live independently, and less likely to be married or have children (Anderson, Vogel, Betz, & Willis, 2004). Level and severity of injury are, for the most part, not as strongly associated with life satisfaction as are functional independence and community participation (Anderson et al., 2002). Medical complications and use of street drugs are also associated with less life satisfaction (Anderson, Krajci, & Vogel, 2002). Among several medical complications, those with the greatest impact on outcomes were pressure ulcers, severe urinary tract infections, and spasticity (Vogel, Krajci, & Anderson, 2002). Although younger age at injury is also associated with greater life satisfaction in individuals with pediatric-onset SCI, age at injury within this population is not strongly associated with most outcomes (Anderson et al., 2004). Nevertheless, the employment rate of adults with pediatric-onset SCI is about 50%, excluding students and homemakers (Anderson & Vogel, 2002). This is a lower employment rate than the general population of the same age, but it is a higher employment rate than is typically reported for some groups with primarily adult-onset SCI (Castle, 1994; Engel, Murphy, Athanasou, & Hickey, 1998; Krause, Sternberg, Maides, & Lottes, 1998).

Adults with pediatric-onset SCI were asked to rate their satisfaction with seven different domains of their life. They reported being least satisfied with income, job opportunities, dating and sexual experiences. They were most satisfied with transportation in the community, educational achievements, and social and recreational opportunities (Anderson & Vogel, 2003).

IMPLICATIONS FOR TREATMENT

Although children and adolescents who sustain an SCI and their parents are understandably devastated at the time of injury, there is ample evidence that an SCI does not have to prevent patients from having full, satisfying lives, with opportunities to succeed in almost all endeavors. For the SCI health care team, a number of strategies are key components to helping the patient and family to succeed. The first is that patients and families must have the expectation, from the time of injury, that patients can become independent, self-sufficient, employed, and married adults with satisfying recreation and leisure activities. The second strategy is to ensure over the years that the child or adolescent is keeping up with activities similar to those of peers in their community. This includes school, social, recreational, and job-preparation activities (Anderson & Vogel, 2000). The third strategy is to help the patient benefit from a team approach. For example, if fishing is an important interest and activity of the adolescent, the recreational therapist and occupational therapist may work together to devise an adapted pole that will work for the patient. The fourth strategy is to take advantage of new technologies and treatments that will increase an individual's independence. This includes environmental adaptations such as switches to control speaker phones and power chairs. It also includes surgeries, such as tendon transfers that can improve an individual's hand function (James, 1996; Mulcahey, 1996), or the Mitrofanoff procedure that may enable an individual to catheterize independently through a stoma rather than to require assistance to be transferred to a bed and catheterized by an attendant or family member (Pontari et al., 2000; Chaviano, Matkov, Anderson, McGovern, & Vogel, 2000; Spoltore et al., 2000).

The fifth strategy for improving psychosocial outcomes in pediatric-onset SCI is to have a carefully devised program for ensuring that responsibility for the care of the child is systematically transferred from parent to child as the child develops (Klaas & Hickey, 2001). Part of this process is to ensure that medical complications are minimized. Complications such as pressure ulcers or bladder accidents can have a devastating impact on a child's social activities and life satisfaction (Vogel et al., 2002). The ultimate goal is to help the individual with an SCI to prepare throughout childhood and adolescence to transition to adulthood totally prepared for a healthy, satisfying adult life (Blomquist, Brown, Peersen, & Presler, 1998; Anderson, Johnson, Klaas, & Vogel, 1998).

RESEARCH

From a psychosocial perspective, the paucity of research in pediatric-onset SCI is frustrating. Because the incidence is low and most hospitals or rehabilitation centers will see many more adult-onset than pediatric-onset SCIs, research on this population is necessarily difficult. One would like to have more data, for example, on the impact of returning to school following injury and its effect on adjustment, of rural versus urban settings, of multidisciplinary SCI team care compared with local hospital and pediatrician care, of the roles of social and family support, and the impact of special recreation and specialized camps on outcomes. One research goal would certainly be to develop pediatric-outcome measures similar to those used by the SCI Model Systems programs to provide benchmarks of success.

Not specific to pediatric-onset SCI but common to all SCI are the issues of preventing, curing, and ameliorating SCI. The work of the Christopher Reeve Foundation, the Miami Project, and the research done by scientists throughout the world on stem cells, neuron regeneration, and activity-based therapy are the basic science that we all hope will result in the eventual cure for SCI (Schwab, 2002; Young, 1996; Fawcett, 2002; McDonald et al., 2002).

REFERENCES

Aitken, M. E., Korchbandi, P., Parnell, D., Parker, J. G., Stefans, V., Thompkins, E., & Schulz, E. G. (2005). Experiences from the development of a comprehensive family support program for pediatric trauma and rehabilitation patients. *Archives of Physical Medicine and Rehabilitation, 86,* 175–179.

American Spinal Injury Association, International Medical Society of Paraplegia. (2000). *International standards for neurological classification of spinal cord injury.* Chicago: American Spinal Injury Association.

Anderson, C. J. (1997). Psychosocial and sexuality issues in pediatric spinal cord injury. *Topics in Spinal Cord Injury Rehabilitation, 5,* 70–78.

Anderson, C. J. (2003). Pediatric-onset spinal cord injury: Psychosocial issues. *SCI Nursing, 20,* 212–213.

Anderson, C. J., Johnson, K. A., Klaas, S. J., & Vogel, L. C. (1998). Pediatric spinal cord injury: Transition to adulthood. *Journal of Vocational Rehabilitation, 10,* 103–113.

Anderson, C. J., Krajci, K. A., & Vogel, L. C. (2002). Life satisfaction in adults with pediatric-onset spinal cord injuries. *Journal of Spinal Cord Medicine, 25,* 184–190.

Anderson, C. J., Krajci, K. A., & Vogel, L. C. (2003). Community integration among adults who sustained spinal cord injuries sustained as children or adolescents. *Developmental Medicine and Child Neurology, 45,* 129–134.

Anderson, C. J., & Vogel, L. C. (2000). Work experience in adolescents with spinal cord injuries. *Developmental Medicine and Child Neurology, 42,* 515–517.

Anderson, C. J., & Vogel, L. C. (2002). Employment outcomes of adults who sustained spinal cord injuries as children or adolescents. *Archives of Physical Medicine and Rehabilitation, 83,* 791–801.

Anderson, C. J., & Vogel, L. C. (2003). Domain-specific satisfaction in adults with pediatric-onset spinal cord injuries. *Spinal Cord, 41,* 684–691.

Anderson, C. J., Vogel, L. C., Betz, R. R., & Willis, K. (2004). Overview of adult outcomes in pediatric-onset spinal cord injuries: Implications for transition to adulthood. *Spinal Cord Medicine, 27,* S98–S106.

Apple, D. F., & Murray, H. H. (1996). Lap belt injuries in children. In R. R. Betz & M. J. Mulcahey (Eds.), *The child with a spinal cord injury* (pp. 169–177). Rosemont, IL: American Academy of Orthopaedic Surgeons.

Beck, T., & Spoltore, T. (1996). Processes involved in discharge planning. In R. R. Betz & M. J. Mulcahey (Eds.), *The child with a spinal cord injury* (pp. 557–566). Rosemont, IL: American Academy of Orthopaedic Surgeons.

Betz, R. R., & Mulcahey, M. J. (Ed.). (1996). *The child with a spinal cord injury.* Rosemont, IL: American Academy of Orthopaedic Surgeons.

Blomquist, K. B., Brown, G., Peersen, A., & Presler, E. P. (1998). Transition to independence: Challenges for young people with disabilities and their caregivers. *Orthopaedic Nursing, 17,* 27–35.

Bloom, L., & Joseph, M. (2003). The effect of spinal cord injury in adolescence. *SCI Psychosocial Process, 16,* 237–243.

Boyer, B. A., Knolls, M. L., Kafkalas, C. M., & Tollen, L. G. (2000). Prevalence of posttraumatic stress disorder in patients with pediatric spinal cord injury: relationship to functional independence. *Topics in Spinal Cord Injury Rehabilitation,* 6(Suppl.), 125–133.

Boyer, B. A., Ware, C. J., Knolls, M. L., & Kafkalas, C. M. (2003). Posttraumatic stress among families experiencing pediatric spinal cord injury: A replication. *SCI Psychosocial Process, 16,* 244–252.

Butt, L. (1998). Post-traumatic stress disorder and spinal cord injury: Part 1. *SCI Psychosocial Process, 11,* 48–51.

Castle, R. (1994). An investigation into the employment and occupation of patients with a spinal cord injury. *Paraplegia, 32,* 182–187.

Centers for Disease Control and Prevention. (2000). Motor-vehicle occupant fatalities and restraint use among children aged 4–8 Years—United States, 1994–1998. *Morbidity and Mortality Weekly Reports, 49,* 135–137.

Chaviano, A. H., Matkov, T. G., Anderson, C. J., McGovern, P. A., & Vogel, L. C. (2000). Mitrofanoff continent catheterizable stoma for pediatric patients with spinal cord injury. *Topics in Spinal Cord Injury Rehabilitation,* 6(Suppl.), 30–35.

Coleby, M. (1995). The school-aged siblings of children with disabilities. *Developmental Medicine and Child Neurology, 37,* 415–426.

Davidoff, G., Morris, J., Roth, E., & Bleiberg, J. (1985). Cognitive dysfunction and mild closed head injury in traumatic spinal cord injury. *Archives of Physical Medicine and Rehabilitation, 66,* 489–491.

Davidoff, G. N., Roth, E. J., & Richards, J. S. (1992). Cognitive deficits in spinal cord injury: Epidemiology and outcome. *Archives of Physical Medicine and Rehabilitation, 73,* 275–284.

DeVivo, M. J. (2002). Epidemiology of traumatic spinal cord injury. In S. Kirshblum, D. I. Campagnolo, & J. A. DeLisa (Eds.), *Spinal cord medicine* (pp. 69–81). Philadelphia: Lippincott Williams & Wilkins.

DeVivo, M. J., & Vogel, L. C. (2004). Epidemiology of spinal cord injuries in children and adolescents. *Journal of Spinal Cord Medicine, 27,* S4–S10.

Dudgeon, B. J., Massagli, T. S., & Ross, B. W. (1997). Educational participation of children with spinal cord injury. *American Journal of Occupational Therapy, 51,* 553–561.

Elliot, S. (2003). Sexual dysfunction and infertility in men with spinal cord disorders. In V. Lin (Ed.), *Spinal cord medicine* (pp. 349–365). New York: Demos.

Elliot, T. R., Shewchuk, R. M., & Richards, J. S. (1999). Caregiver social problem-solving abilities and family member adjustment to recent-onset physical disability. *Rehabilitation Psychology, 44,* 104–123.

Engel, L., Brooks, M., & Warschausky, S. (2003). Meeting the psychosocial needs of ventilator assisted children: A social work and nursing collaboration. *SCI Psychosocial Process, 16,* 230–236.

Engel, S., Murphy, G. S., Athanasou, J. A., & Hickey, L. (1998). Employment outcomes following spinal cord injury. *International Journal of Rehabilitation Research, 21,* 223–229.

Faux, S. A. (1993). Siblings of children with chronic physical and cognitive disabilities. *Journal of Pediatric Nursing, 8,* 305–316.

Fawcett, J. (2002). Repair of spinal cord injuries: Where are we, where are we going? *Spinal Cord, 40,* 615–623.

Fitchtenbaum, J., & Kirshblum, S. (2002). Psychologic adaptation to spinal cord injury. In S. Kirshblum, D. Campangnolo, & J. Delisa (Eds.), *Spinal cord medicine* (pp. 299–311). Philadelphia: Lippincott Williams & Wilkins.

Geller, B., & Greydanus, D. E. (1979). Psychological management of acute paraplegia in adolescence. *Pediatrics, 63,* 562–564.

Grossman, M. B., & Merenda, L. A. (2004). Strategies for coping with the noncompliant adolescent spinal cord injury patient. *SCI Nursing, 21,* 35–37.

Hammell, K. R. (1992) Psychological and sociological theories concerning adjustment to traumatic spinal cord injury: The implications for rehabilitation. *Paraplegia, 30,* 317–326.

James, M. A. (1996). Surgical treatment of the upper extremity: Indications, patient assessment, and procedures. In R. R. Betz & M. J. Mulcahey (Eds.), *The child with a spinal cord injury* (pp. 393–403). Rosemont, IL: American Academy of Orthopaedic Surgeons.

Johnson, C. P., & Kastner, T. A. (2005). Helping families raise children with special health care needs at home. *Pediatrics, 115,* 507–511.

Johnson, K. A., & Klaas, S. J. (2000). Recreation involvement and play in pediatric spinal cord injury. *Topics in Spinal Cord Injury Rehabilitation, 6*(Suppl.), 105–109.

Johnson, K. A., Klaas, S. J., Vogel, L. C., & McDonald, C. (2004). Leisure characteristics of the pediatric spinal cord injury population. *Journal of Spinal Cord Medicine, 27,* S107–S109.

Johnson, K. M., Berry, E. T., Goldeen, R. A., & Wicker, E. (1991). Growing up with a spinal cord injury. *SCI Nursing, 8,* 11–19.

Kennedy, P., Gorsuch, N., & Marsh, N. (1995). Childhood onset of spinal cord injury: Self-esteem and self-perception. *British Journal of Clinical Psychology, 34,* 581–588.

Kirshblum, S., Campagnolo, D. I., & DeLisa, J. A. (Eds.). (2002). *Spinal cord medicine.* Philadelphia: Lippincott Williams & Wilkins.

Klaas, S., & Hickey, K. (2001). Transition to adult care. *SCI Nursing, 21,* 158–160.

Krause, J. S., Sternberg, M., Maides, J., & Lottes, S. (1998). Employment after spinal cord injury: Differences related to geographic region, gender, and race. *Archives of Physical Medicine and Rehabilitation, 79,* 615–624.

Lavigne, J. V., & Faier-Routman, J. (1992). Psychological adjustment to pediatric physical disorders: A meta-analytic review. *Journal of Pediatric Psychology, 17,* 133–157.

Lin, V. (Ed.). (2003). *Spinal cord medicine.* New York: Demos.

Massagli, T. L. (2000). Medical and rehabilitation issues in the care of children with spinal cord injury. *Physical Medicine and Rehabilitation Clinics of North America, 11,* 169–182.

McDonald, J. W., Becker, D., Sadowsky, C. L., Jane, J. A., Conturo, T. E., & Schultz,

L. M. (2002). Late recovery following spinal cord injury. *Journal of Neurosurgery: Spine, 97*(2). Retrieved July 29, 2004, from www.thejns-net.org.html.

Miles, M. A., & Cawley, M. F. (1996). Dual diagnosis: Spinal cord injury and traumatic brain injury. In R. R. Betz & M. J. Mulcahey (Eds.), *The child with a spinal cord injury* (pp. 761–771). Rosemont, IL: American Academy of Orthopaedic Surgeons.

Moverman, R. A. (2003). Psychosocial factors in spinal cord injury. In V. Lin (Ed.), *Spinal cord medicine* (pp. 931–939). New York: Demos.

Mulcahey, M. J. (1992). Returning to school after a spinal cord injury: Perspectives from four adolescents. *American Journal of Occupational Therapy, 46*, 305–332.

Mulcahey, M. J. (1996). Rehabilitation and outcomes of upper extremity tendon transfer surgery. In R. R. Betz & M. J. Mulcahey (Eds.), *The child with a spinal cord injury* (pp. 419–448). Rosemont, IL: American Academy of Orthopaedic Surgeons.

Pang, D. (1996). Spinal cord injury without radiographic abnormality (SCIWORA) in children. In R. R. Betz & M. J. Mulcahey (Eds.), *The child with a spinal cord injury* (pp. 139–160). Rosemont, IL: American Academy of Orthopaedic Surgeons.

Perilstein, B., & Williams, D. (1996). Perspectives on adolescent spinal cord injury. In R. R. Betz & M. J. Mulcahey (Eds.), *The child with a spinal cord injury* (pp. 591–599). Rosemont, IL: American Academy of Orthopaedic Surgeons.

Pless, I. B., Cripps, H. A., Davies, J. M., & Wadsworth, M. E. (1989). Chronic physical illness childhood: Psychological and social effects in adolescence and adult life. *Developmental Medicine and Child Neurology, 31*, 746–755.

Pontari, M. A., Weibel, B., Morales, V., Dean, G., Gaughan, J., & Betz, R. R. (2000). Improved quality of life after continent urinary diverson in pediatric patients with tetraplegia after spinal cord injury. *Topics in Spinal Cord Injury Rehabilitation, 6*(Suppl.), 25–29.

Price, C., Makintubee, S., Herndon, W., & Istre, G. R. (1994). Epidemiology of traumatic spinal cord injury and acute hospitalization and rehabilitation charges for SCIs in Oklahoma, 1988–1990. *American Journal of Epidemiology, 139*, 37–47.

Putzke, J. D., Richards, J. S., & Dowler, R. N. (2000). Quality of life after spinal cord injury: Developmental issues in late adolescence and young adulthood. *Topics in Spinal Cord Rehabilitation, 6*(Suppl.), 155–169.

Radnitz, C. L., Schlein, I. S., Walczak, S., Broderick, C. P., Binks, M., Trich, D. D., et al. (1995). The prevalence of posttraumatic stress disorder in veterans with spinal cord injury. *SCI Psychosocial Process, 8*, 145–149.

Richards, J. S., Osuna, F. J., Jaworski, T. M., Novack, T. A. S., Leli, D. A., & Boll, T. J. (1991). The effectiveness of different methods of defining traumatic brain injury in predicting postdischarge adjustment in a spinal cord injury population. *Archives of Physical Medicine and Rehabilitation, 72*, 275–279.

Rivara, J. B., Jaffe, K. M., Fay, G. C., Polissar, N. L., Martin, K. M., Shurtleff, H. A., & Liao, S. (1993). Family functioning and injury severity as predictors of child functioning one year following traumatic brain injury. *Archives of Physical Medicine and Rehabilitation, 74*, 1047–1055.

Rutledge, D. N., & Dick, G. (1983). Spinal cord injury in adolescence. *Rehabilitation Nursing, 8*, 18–21.
Schwab, M. E. (2002). Repairing the injured spinal cord. *Science, 295*, 1029–1031.
Spoltore, T., Mulcahey, M. J., Johnston, T., Kelly, K., Morales, V., & Rebuck, C. (2000). Innovative programs for children and adolescents with spinal cord injury. *Orthopaedic Nursing, 19*, 55–63.
Stiens, S. A., Bergman, S. B., & Formal, C. S. (1997). Spinal cord injury rehabilitation: 4. Individual experience, personal adaptation, and social perspectives. *Archives of Physical Medicine and Rehabilitation, 78*, S65–S72.
Trieschmann, R. B. (1988). *Spinal cord injuries: Psychological, social, and vocational rehabilitation*. New York: Demos.
Vogel, L. C. (Ed.). (1997). Pediatric issues. *Topics in Spinal Cord Injury Rehabilitation, 3*(2), 1–84.
Vogel, L. C., & Anderson, C. J. (2002). Self-injurious behavior in children and adolescents with spinal cord injuries. *Spinal Cord, 40*, 666–668.
Vogel, L. C., & Anderson, C. J. (2003). Spinal cord injuries in children and adolescents: A review. *Journal of Spinal Cord Medicine, 26*, 193–203.
Vogel, L. C., Betz, R. R., & Mulcahey, M. J. (1997). The child with a spinal cord injury. *Developmental Medicine Child Neurology, 39*, 202–207.
Vogel, L. C., Hickey, K. J., Klaas, S. J., & Anderson, C. J. (2004). Unique issues in pediatric spinal cord injury. *Orthopaedic Nursing, 23*, 300–308.
Vogel, L. C., Klaas, S. J., Lubicky, J. P., & Anderson, C. J. (1998). Long-term outcomes and life satisfaction of adults with pediatric spinal cord injuries. *Archives of Physical Medicine and Rehabilitation, 79*, 1496–1503.
Vogel, L. C., Krajci K. A., & Anderson, C. J. (2002). Adults with pediatric-onset spinal cord injuries: Part 3. Impact of medical complications. *Journal of Spinal Cord Medicine, 25*, 297–305.
Warschausky, S., Engel, L., Kewman, D., & Nelson, V. S. (1996). Psychosocial factors in rehabilitation of the child with a spinal cord injury. In R. R. Betz & M. J. Mulcahey (Eds.), *The child with a spinal cord injury* (pp. 471–478). Rosemont, IL: American Academy of Orthopaedic Surgeons.
Warschausky, S., Majchrzak, N. E., Lifford, M., Dixon, P., & Tate, D. (2004). Associations between family and child adjustment following traumatic injury of the brain versus spine. *SCI Psychosocial Process, 17*, 97–105.
Yarkony, G. M., & Anderson, C. J. (1996). Sexuality. In R. R. Betz & M. J. Mulcahey (Eds.), *The child with a spinal cord injury* (pp. 625–637). Rosemont, IL: American Academy of Orthopaedic Surgeons.
Young, W. (1996). Spinal cord regeneration. *Science, 273*, 451.

4

Early Medical Risks and Disability

GLEN P. AYLWARD

Risk in infancy refers to factors that increase the potential for negative developmental outcomes. There are three categories of risk: established, medical/biological, and environmental (Tjossem, 1976). Established risks are medical conditions of a known etiology whose compromised developmental outcome is well documented (e.g., genetic disorders such as Down syndrome or Tay–Sachs, HIV in infancy). Medical/biological risks include exposure to potentially noxious prenatal, perinatal, or postnatal events such as low birth weight (LBW), intraventricular hemorrhage (IVH), or asphyxia/hypoxic–ischemic encephalopathy (HIE). Environmental risks involve the quality of the caregiver–infant interaction, opportunities for developmental stimulation, and health care. Low socioeconomic status, poverty, and poor social support are additional environmental risks.

Because relationships between social class, perinatal complications, and cognitive development are complex and interrelated, many children are at both biological and environmental risk, this combination being referred to as "double jeopardy" or "double hazard" (Escalona, 1982; Parker, Greer, & Zuckerman, 1988). In these cases, nonoptimal biological and environmental risks work synergistically to affect negatively later function (Aylward, 1990, 1992). While medical/biological factors appear to determine the presence or absence of a developmental problem, environmental risk may influence the degree (Hunt, Cooper, & Tooley, 1988). This assumption is not accurate if the degree of biological risk is severe, thereby placing a ceiling on the child's developmental potential (Hack, Taylor, Klein, & Minich, 2000).

The focus of this chapter is on infants falling into the medical/biological risk category of being born prematurely, because this group is at increased risk for later cognitive, neuropsychological, behavioral, and school problems (Aylward, 2002a). Infants born at < 37 weeks' gestation comprise approximately 11–12% of live births, while infants born at LBW (< 2,500 grams) account for 7.4–7.6% (Paneth, 1995).

Improved survival rates of infants born at LBW (< 2,500 grams [5.5 pounds]), very low birth weight (VLBW; < 1,500 grams [3.3 pounds]), and extremely low birth weight (ELBW; < 1,000 grams [2.2 pounds]) have resulted in increased interest in developmental outcomes. This improvement in survival rates is attributable to increased use of antenatal steroids, more aggressive approaches to delivery room resuscitation, and surfactant replacement (Hack & Fanaroff, 1999). However, infants born between 501 and 1,500 grams contribute disproportionately to perinatal mortality and morbidity rates. Hence, there is concern that the increased survival of infants exposed to medical/biological risks and the concomitant potential for central nervous system insult will produce a greater prevalence of neurodevelopmental morbidity, particularly in cognitive and neuropsychological outcomes (Bregman, 1998).

The primary emphasis in outcome studies has been on the incidence of major disabilities: moderate–severe mental retardation, sensorineural hearing loss/blindness, cerebral palsy, and epilepsy. Babies born at LBW have a 6–8% incidence of these major handicaps, those born at VLBW have a 14–17% incidence, while babies of ELBW have a 20–25% rate, this increasing with lower birth weights (Bennett & Scott, 1997; Halsey, Collin, & Anderson, 1996; Hack, Taylor, & Klein, 1995). In comparison, major handicaps occur in 5% of infants born full-term. These rates of handicap have remained constant over the last decade. However, the nature of impairment is changing, with significant problems frequently found in "nondisabled" survivors. These high prevalence/low severity dysfunctions (Aylward, 2002a, 2003) are increasing and include learning disabilities, borderline mental retardation, attention-deficit/hyperactivity disorders, specific neuropsychological deficits (e.g., visual motor integration, executive function), and behavior problems. These dysfunctions occur in as many as 50–70% of infants born at VLBW, with an inverse birth weight gradient again being found (O'Callaghan et al., 1996; Goyen, Lui, & Woods, 1998; Taylor, Klein, Minich, & Hack, 2000). More than 50% of children born at VLBW will require special education services, 20% or more will need a self-contained learning disabilities placement, and 16–20% will repeat at least one grade (vs. 7.8% of the general population).

The situation is compounded by the fact that the social, ethnic, and educational backgrounds of mothers also influence the prevalence of these disabilities (reflecting environmental risk). While major disabilities are often identified during infancy, high prevalence/low severity dysfunctions become more obvious as the child grows older (i.e., school age). Moreover, predictors of these more subtle problems cannot be identified during infancy or preschool age. It is extremely difficult to determine early on whether identified problems are indicative of recovery or "catch-up" from the negative effects of extremely low gestational age and birth weight (reflecting a maturational lag), or the emergence of a more permanent handicap. This difficulty is due to continued cortical development, as well as to increased demands for performance in areas previously not emphasized. Subsequent outcome is the result of an interchange between normal developmental processes, recovery–reorganization of neurodevelopmental function in response to varying central nervous system insults, improvement in physical status, and environmental influences (Aylward, 1997a, 1997b).

Multiple factors are associated with a biological risk condition such as ELBW: (1) severity of neonatal course (admission status, birth weight, gestational age, days in hospital, other conditions); (2) sociodemographic factors (socioeconomic status [SES], social support, race); (3) subsequent illness (hospitalizations, need for oxygen); (4) maternal physical and mental health; and (5) environmental exposures to positive and negative experiences (early intervention, lead, smoking in household). Chronic lung disease, recurrent apnea and bradycardia, transient hypothyroxemia of prematurity (decreased thyroid hormone), hyperbilirubinemia, medications, and stress from hospitalization are additional considerations that have an impact on central nervous system integrity (Perlman, 2003). There are multiple outcome areas of concern such as neurodevelopmental–neurological, cognitive, behavioral, health-related quality of life (HRQL), functional outcomes, and social issues; however, the current discussion is restricted to cognitive, neuropsychological, and behavioral outcomes.

PATHOGENESIS

Developmental Disruptions

It is difficult to separate out biological risk that arises solely as a consequence of preterm birth from the specific effects attributable to perinatal insults such as IVH or HIE. These latter insults may be better considered as moderators of prematurity per se. Even in the absence of identifiable, nonoptimal central nervous system events, preterm birth is characterized by a failure of brain structures to proceed in a predictable temporal and spatial sequence of development. More specifically, there is a disruption of organizational events. Being born LBW or smaller also has an effect on biosynthesis of neurotransmitters such as dopamine and developmental regulation of specific neuroreceptor populations.

Most likely, a gradient exists in which disruption in corticogenesis and connectivity is inversely related to birth weight and/or gestational age (particularly in infants at < 33 weeks gestational age), even in the absence of other concomitant biomedical risks. This may be related to birth and insults occurring during several critical periods of brain development, such as (1) migration (3–5 months' gestational age); (2) organization/differentiation (6 months' gestation–3rd postnatal year); and (3) myelination (6th month gestational age onward). Many of these critical periods extend over the infant's hospital course (Geidd, 1997). Other developmental concerns that place the infant at risk are listed in Table 4.1.

Brain Insult

Factors that produce injury to the infant's brain are also listed in Table 4.1. Damage to oligodendrocytes (cells that produce myelin) will disrupt myelination and allow abnormal spread of signals from one axon to others; astroglyosis (damage to structural cells surrounding neurons) will have an impact as well.

Maternal infections such as chorioamnionitis place the infant at increased risk for neurodevelopmental impairment due to the circulation of proinflammatory cytokines and their damaging effect on oligodendrocytes (Grether & Nelson, 1997; Leviton & Gilles, 1996). Even in full-term babies, there is a 9-fold increase in the incidence of cerebral palsy in the presence of intrauterine infection, and a 19-fold increase in spastic quadraparesis (Grether & Nelson, 1997; Wilson-Costello et al., 1998). Hypoxia (reduced oxygenation of brain tissue) and ischemia (reduction of cerebral blood flow) combine to produce HIE (Biagas, 1999). A neurotoxic cascade occurs in which there is a massive glutamate (excitotoxic amino acid) release that binds to postsynaptic receptors, causing depolarization and an influx of calcium, producing what is sometimes termed "death by calcium." As a result, two types of cell death occur: (1) necrosis (rapid cell death, with the cell bursting and causing inflammatory injury to adjacent cells), and (2) apoptosis (cell death in which there is slow shrinkage and less secondary inflammation). Necrosis occurs with focal cerebral injury, while apoptosis occurs more distant to the site of injury. For example, after HIE, distant neurons in the hippocampus can survive initially, but then undergo delayed cell death via apoptosis. Therefore, hypoxic–ischemic brain damage is an evolving process that begins during the insult and extends into the recovery period (Biagas, 1999). Reperfusion after HIE produces secondary injury (see Table 4.1).

In full-term infants, HIE produces cell death in the cerebral cortex, diencephalon, brain stem, and cerebellum. Injury to the basal ganglia and thalamus also occurs. Moderate and severe HIE in term infants is associ-

TABLE 4.1. Factors Influencing the Brain Development of Infants Born Prematurely

Developmental disruptions

1. Ineffective blood–brain barrier < 27 weeks' gestational age due to immaturity of cells.
2. Disruption of myelination due to oligodendrocyte and precursor cells being in stages of migration and proliferation.
3. Absence of developmentally regulated endogenous protective factors to protect neurons and oligodendrocytes against cell death (neurotrophins, oligotrophins).
4. Disturbance of other organizational events: establishment of subplate neurons, alignment–orientation–layering of cortical neurons, synaptogenesis, cell death/pruning, proliferation of glial cells.

Brain insult

1. Maternal infections (e.g., chorioamnionitis).
2. Hypoxia–ischemia.
3. Reperfusion (free radicals, nitric oxide, granulocytes).
4. Biochemical events.

Note. Data from Biagas (1999); Dammann and Leviton (1999, 2000); Grether and Nelson (1997); Leviton and Gilles (1996); Perlman (2003); Volpe (1996, 2001); and Wilson-Costello et al. (1998).

ated with a high incidence of cognitive and motor dysfunction, including microcephaly, mental retardation, epilepsy, and cerebral palsy.

With infants born preterm, HIE causes cell death deeper within the brain, typically in the white matter behind and to the side of the lateral ventricles, due to damage to the highly vulnerable oligodendroglial precursor cells (Volpe, 2001). This is termed periventricular leukomalacia (PVL). There is less effect on gray matter in preterm than in full-term infants, and this insult is more often associated with spasticity, neurosensory, and motor problems than with cognitive deficits per se. Infants born prematurely are more susceptible to PVL because of the incomplete state of development of the vascular supply to the cerebral white matter, and a maturation-dependent impairment in regulation of cerebral blood flow.

Periventricular/intraventricular hemorrhage (PVH/IVH), caused by HIE, respiratory distress, or circulatory problems, involves bleeding into the subependymal germinal matrix (site of cell proliferation); this occurs in 20–25% of infants < 32 weeks' gestational age, with higher percentages found in babies of lower gestational ages. IVH is graded (I–IV), based on the amount of blood in the ventricles and the degree of distention, with grades III and IV being considered severe. Grading is an area of continued debate (Leviton, Kuban, & Paneth, 2004). Grade IV includes intracerebral involvement or other parenchymal lesions and is thought to not be on a continuum, reflecting periventricular hemorrhagic infarction (PVI; Volpe, 2001). The risk of later disability increases in relation to the grade of IVH: 5–10%

with Grade I; 15–20% with Grade II, 35–55% with Grade III, and > 90% with Grade IV (Volpe, 2001).

Specific Areas of Injury

The subplate neuron layer is a transient structure located beneath the cortical plate that peaks in activity between 22 and 36 weeks of gestation (Perlman, 2001, 2003). This structure is important in cerebral organization; it is where growing axons (afferents) from the thalamus and other distant cortical sites "wait," because their ultimate neuronal targets in the cortical plate have not yet developed. Subplate neurons also guide descending axon projections from the cortex to subcortical targets (thalamus, corpus callosum). This area is particularly vulnerable to the negative effects of glutamate (Perlman, 2003).

The basal ganglia, particularly the striatum, are components of the feedback loop that modulates cortical function, and disruption of cortico–striatal–thalamic pathways would have a major, negative impact on neurobehavioral functions such as modulation of attention and regulation of behavior (Isaacs et al., 2000). The basal ganglia components are particularly susceptible to the excitotoxic effects of glutamate, and damage also affects the dopaminergic system, having cognitive and motor ramifications (see Perlman, 2003). The hippocampus is particularly vulnerable to hypoxia and is sensitive to the effects of hypothyroxemia of prematurity (thyroid hormone is important for neurogenesis, axon and dendritic formation) and glucocorticoids (e.g., dexamethasone used in the treatment of chronic lung disease). Both the basal ganglia and hippocampus are highly susceptible to neuronal injury from excess bilirubin (hyperbilirubinemia), particularly in the presence of glutamate, which apparently exacerbates the negative effects in a synergistic manner.

While the functional significance of abnormalities in brain structures is unclear, several possibilities exist. Disruptions in white matter involve myelinization and dendritic connections, and would have an impact on cortical and subcortical units. There is also the suggestion of reduced gray matter volume, which would have an impact on cognitive functions (Nosarti et al., 2002). Reduced size of the posterior body of the corpus callosum (due to its proximity to periventricular arterial border zones) may be related to IQ deficits due to poor hemispheric interaction and disrupted linkage of the occipital and inferior temporal cortices (Fearon et al., 2004; Geidd, Blumenthal, & Jeffries, 1999). Functional magnetic resonance imaging (MRI) in adolescents has also shown that damage to the corpus callosum is associated with aberrant patterns of cortical activation to visual and auditory tasks (Santhouse, Ffytche, & Howard, 2002). Neonatal ultrasounds may not be sensitive enough to detect subtle injury to gray or white matter in infants born prematurely; this injury becomes more apparent on MRI performed in adolescence (Stewart et al., 1999). Babies born preterm, without early brain injury such as IVH, have smaller volumes than controls with respect to cortical gray matter, and in brain structures such as the basal ganglia, corpus callosum, amygdala, and hippocampus (Fearon et al., 2004; Peterson et al., 2000). A 46% increase in total ventricular volume and a 17% reduction in posterior corpus callosum volume have been found in MRIs of adults born at VLBW (Fearon et al., 2004).

Disruption of circuits connecting frontal, striatal, and thalamic regions (due to disruption of the subplate neuronal layer) may be associated with dysregulation of attention and arousal, due to disruption of the regulatory feedback loop (causing an attention-deficit/hyperactivity disorder [ADHD] or problems with executive function), while reduced hippocampal volume is associated with memory deficits and weakness in numeracy (Isaacs et al., 2000). Cerebellar volume reduction has been reported, which is associated with poorer cognitive performance in adolescence (Allin, Matsumoto, & Santhouse, 2001).

Summary

When considering infants born at medical/biological risk, it is better to shift conceptually from an emphasis on static, focal damage to consideration of diffuse, more subtle insult that occurs in conjunction with neural developmental processes (Ewings-Cobbs, Barnes, & Fletcher, 2003). "Recovery" (restoration of functions that were previously acquired), should be conceptually differentiated from "reorganization" (shifting of function to a different area of the brain). While reorganization is typically the primary process in established risk and congenital disorders, *both* recovery and reorganization will occur in those born preterm—with reorganization due to disruption in normal developmental processes, and recovery due to the effects of central nervous system insults. The impact of each varies depending on the infant's age and developmental level, as well as when the event was experienced (Ewing-Cobbs et al., 2003; Goldman-Rakic, 1994). This would partially explain the wide variation in outcomes.

SPECIFIC OUTCOMES

Implementation of effective intervention programs for infants born prematurely and provision of information to families require better understanding of potential cognitive strengths and deficits. Moreover, identification of the *nature* of cognitive deficits associated with prematurity will provide some indication of the compromised, underlying neural systems, which, in turn, could drive medical interventions (Anderson & Doyle, 2004).

The absence of definitive trends in outcome is attributable to problems in follow-up of infants born preterm. These fall into four broad areas: (1) conceptualization/design issues, (2) subject populations, (3) procedural issues, and (4) measurement–outcome (Aylward, 2002b; Aylward, Pfeiffer, Wright, & Verhulst, 1989). Lack of uniformity in sample selection criteria, consideration of both birth weight and gestational age, commingling infants born average for gestational age (AGA) and those small for gestational age (SGA; < 3rd percentile), method and length of follow-up, loss to follow-up, and use of various outcome measures and different diagnostic criteria all influence outcome statistics (Aylward, 2002b). As a result, the following discussion reflects general trends.

Intelligence Quotients

In a meta-analysis conducted 15 years ago, a 5–7 point mean difference was found between more than 4,000 infants born LBW and 1,568 term controls, favoring the latter (Aylward et al., 1989). More recent comparisons of those born at VLBW or ELBW and controls, adjusting for race, SES, and excluding participants with severe handicaps, reveal a 0.3 to 0.6 standard deviation (SD) decrease in IQ in those born prematurely. This translates to a 3.8–9.8 point decrement, although some studies report 12–17 point differences (Breslau, DelDotto, & Brown, 1994; Bhutta, Cleves, Casey, Craddock, & Arand, 2002; Halsey et al., 1996; Whitfield, Eckstein-Grunau, & Holst, 1997). Higher percentages of borderline IQ have been reported in the ELBW population, with the prevalence ranging from 13 to 15%, with some estimates being as high as 37% (Vohr et al., 2000; Whitfield et al., 1997). In a recent sibling control study, Kilbride, Thurstad, and Daily (2004) reported a 10-point difference between children born at ELBW and their siblings. The mean IQ was related to preterm–full-term status, and 84% of those born at ELBW had a lower IQ than their full-term siblings.

A gradient exists whereby heavier birth weights are associated with higher IQ scores; more than double the number of infants born at LBW and smaller subsequently have IQ scores that are 1 or more standard deviations below the mean, when compared to those born full-term. This same gradient is evident within the VLBW population at school age (Halsey et al., 1996; Saigal, Hoult, Streinder, Stoskopf, & Rosenbaum, 2000; Taylor, Klein, & Hack, 2000). Stated differently, the likelihood of an IQ less than 70 in one sample was 9.54 times greater in the < 750 grams group and 2.15 times greater in those born 750–1,499 grams than in term controls (Hack et al., 2000). Children born at VLBW who demonstrated suspect IQ findings at age 3 years (scores > 1 SD below average, or major discrepancies among scores) had later school-age IQ scores 12 to 14 points lower than either infants born at VLBW who did not have suspect findings at age 3, or full-term controls (Dewey, Crawford, Creighton, & Sauve, 1999).

Therefore, in children born at VLBW or below who do not have major handicaps, mean group IQs fall in the borderline to average range, with the majority of studies suggesting low average scores to be the mode (Aylward, 2002a; Bhutta et al., 2002). Scores are generally 8–11 points lower than in full-term counterparts (Bhutta et al., 2002). Nonetheless, this places infants born VLBW and smaller at distinct disadvantage when they have to compete with classmates whose IQs are average or above.

These differences exist regardless of urban or suburban environment (a proxy for SES), although the discrepancy among those born at LBW in urban and suburban households was much greater than that among children of normal birth weight living in each environment (15 points vs. 6 points; Breslau, Johnson, & Lucia, 2001). Kilbride et al. (2004) suggest that high SES modifies the impact of preterm status on cognitive but not motor scores, with mean scores in children from high SES households being 12 points greater than in those from low SES environments, independent of gestational age. IQs of term children from low SES circumstances did not differ statistically from children born at ELBW in high SES (87 vs. 91); high SES term children were most discrepant from those in the low SES ELBW group (101 vs. 80). However, SES exerts less of an impact on IQ in the smaller ELBW infants (Hack et al., 2000), suggesting that a ceiling effect occurs in which the impact of biological risk overrides moderating environmental influences (Aylward, 2002a).

Academic Achievement

More than one-half of children born at VLBW and 60–70% of those born at ELBW require special assistance in school. By middle school-age, ELBW children are three to five times more likely to have a learning problem in reading, spelling, mathematics, or writing (O'Callaghan et al., 1996), with mathematics and broad reading being most disrupted (Johnson & Breslau, 2000; Saigal et al., 2000). These rates are independent of IQ scores. Levels of LBW are not as strongly related to reading as to math (Taylor, Barant, Holding, Klein, & Hack, 2002), with one study suggesting that the effect of LBW accounted for a 0.4 standard deviation decrease in math and a 0.25 standard deviation decrement in reading (Breslau et al., 2001). By adolescence, there is an 8- to 10-fold increase in the use of remedial education resources or special arrangements in comparison to term controls (Taylor, Klein, Schatschneider, & Hack, 1998; Taylor et al., 2002; Saigal et al., 2000).

Many children born preterm also display later nonverbal learning disabilities (NVLDs; Fletcher et al., 1992). Here, verbal cognitive skills are better developed than nonverbal abilities (e.g., Verbal IQ/Performance IQ discrepancies). Visual motor integrative abilities, visual perception, mathematics, spatial skills, and fine motor speed are affected. In addition, verbal abstracting, reading comprehension, written output, and social skills are areas of deficit. The effects of this type of disorder are on a continuum with executive function disorders and can be extremely devastating in terms of academics, as well as social interactions.

Environment also has a moderating effect on learning disorders, because there is a smaller percentage of children born at VLBW from high-SES families in special education than in former VLBW infants from low SES families. Recent data suggest that biomedical and environmental risks are related to both educable mental handicap and specific learning impairment (Resnick et al., 1998). Most likely, the combined effects of lower SES, lower cognitive abilities, and behavioral issues inhibit adjustment to formal education, where complex concepts require problem solving at a more advanced level. Neuropsychological functioning may mediate the relationship between birth weight and achievement (Taylor et al., 2002). Heredity also plays a part in the prevalence of learning disorders; in a recent study, 23% of neonatal intensive care unit (NICU) graduates had strong heredity for deficits in reading and/or writing skills (Jennische & Sedin, 2001). Gender is also a consideration in learning disorders, with males (but not females) having a three- to sixfold increase when compared to controls (Johnson & Breslau, 2000). Therefore, while the spectrum of learning problems does not necessarily differ from the general school population, the prevalence of these disorders in increased fourfold. Moreover the potential combination of learning disorder, lower IQ, and other neuropsychological deficits (discussed later) place the child born prematurely at significant disadvantage.

Language

Many language functions are reasonably normal in children born at LBW, particularly vocabulary, receptive language, verbal fluency, and memory for prose (Frisk & Whyte, 1994; Jennische & Sedin, 2001; Ment et al., 2003; Taylor et al., 2002). However, more complex verbal processes (understanding of syntax, abstract verbal skills, verb production, mean length of utterance, auditory discrimination, imitation of articulatory patterns, following complex instructions, and language processing and reasoning) have been found to be deficient in children born preterm when compared to normal birth weight peers (Breslau et al., 1996; Le Normand & Cohen, 1999; Luciana, Lindeke, Mills, & Nelson, 1999). This is particularly true for males and those born 32 weeks gestational age. While these types of verbal problems are subtle, they are critically important in social and academic endeavors. Language is particularly susceptible to negative environmental influences; this requires consideration of the child's environment whenever this domain of function is assessed. Moreover, 11% of children born preterm in one study were found to have a positive family history of delayed speech and language, again raising the heritibility issue (Luciana et al., 1999). Executive function may mediate strategies for verbal memory and semantic clustering, and speech–language disabilities in children born at LBW are often associated with other disabilities (e.g., hearing or cognitive) (Jennische & Sedin, 2001).

Neuropsychological Outcomes

Visual–Motor Skills

Visual–motor function has multiple components: visual–motor control, visual perception, paper-and-pencil coordination, visual–fine motor function, visual–motor integration, eye–hand coordination, fine motor skills, and fine motor speed. The majority of children born ELBW and VLBW manifest some type of visual–motor problem (Anderson & Doyle, 2004; Dewey et al., 1999; Goyen et al., 1998; Mutch et al., 1993; Saigal, Rosenbaum, Szatmari, & Hoult, 1992; Waber & McCormick, 1995; Whitfield et al., 1997). Copying, perceptual matching, spatial processing, finger tapping, pegboard performance, visual memory, spatial organization, and visual-sequential memory are affected. Perceptual planning at age 11 has also been found to be impaired, again, on an inverse gradient (Taylor et al., 2002). These problems often exist in children whose IQs are in the normal range. Motor and visual–motor functioning deficits were found at school age in children born at VLBW who were developing normally at age 3 (Dewey et al., 1999). Visual–perceptual and visual–motor integration problems are estimated to be in the 11–20% range, while fine motor problems are as high as 71% (Goyen et al., 1998).

Visual–motor problems also have an impact on academic performance, particularly with regard to computational mathematics, written language, and orthographic reading problems. However, when visual–motor tasks such as the Rey–Osterrieth Complex Figure are employed, the cognitive and metacognitive abilities that the child possesses also have a major impact on the type of breakdown in visual–spatial function that is observed (Waber & McCormick, 1995). Visual–motor integrative and visual–perceptual problems are more strongly related to biological risk than are environmental influences (Aylward, 2002a).

Executive Function

Executive function (EF) refers to coordination of interrelated processes and involves purposeful, goal-directed behavior that is critical in cognitive, behavioral, emotional, and social functions. Deficits in EF have been noted in children born prematurely and include problems in conceptual reasoning, verbal working memory, spatial conceptualization, planning, and inhibition (Harvey, O'Callaghan, & Mohay, 1999; Luciana et al., 1999). Anderson and Doyle (2004) report executive dysfunction (ED) in a large cohort of children born at ELBW, when compared to controls born at normal birth weight. Essentially, there was a gradient of dysfunction, with children born at 23–25 weeks having more problems than those born at 26–27 weeks' gestational age. On the Behavior Rating Inventory of Executive Function (BRIEF; Gioia, Isquith, Guy, & Kenworthy, 2000), children born at ELBW, when compared to NBW controls, were two to three times more likely to have trouble starting activities, displaying flexibility in generating ideas and strategies for problem solving, holding information in short-term (working) memory, planning a sequence of actions in advance, and organizing information (Anderson & Doyle, 2004). Problems with behavioral regulation were not as prominent as those involving metacognition. While these deficits are subtle, they have a substantial impact on cognitive, social, and academic functioning. Deficits in EF also have generalized effects on IQ, as well as on the child's knowledge acquisition and fluid intelligence.

ADHD/Behavioral Issues

Symptoms suggestive of ADHD are reported to occur 2.6–4.0 times more frequently in children born at VLBW–ELBW than in controls, with some estimates indicating almost a sixfold increase. Furthermore, 9–10% of adolescents born at ELBW are reported to have ADHD (Botting, Powls, Cooke & Marlow, 1997; Breslau, 1995; Levy-Shiff, Einat, Mogilner, Lerman, & Krikler, 1994; Lou, 1996; Szatmari, Saigal, Rosenbaum, Campbell, & King, 1990; Saigal, Stoskopf, Streiner, & Burrows, 2001; Taylor, Hack, & Klein, 1998). Therefore, of those born at LBW and below, 20–30% have symptoms of ADHD. In addition, conduct disorders, shyness, unassertiveness, withdrawn behavior, anxiety, depression, and social skills deficits occur more frequently in those born at LBW than in normal birth weight peers (Botting et al., 1997; Whitaker, Van Rossen, & Feldman, 1997). It is assumed that behavioral, ADHD, and other concerns surface as the result of the mediating effect of both neuromotor and cognitive deficits that arise as sequelae of prematurity. Interestingly, there are fewer comorbid disruptive behavior disorders (conduct, oppositional), suggesting a "purer" or more biologically determined form of ADHD (Szatmari et al., 1990).

As indicated earlier, the relationship among neuropsychological function and other outcomes such as academic achievement is complex. Taylor et al. (2002) proposed a model in which biological and social risks influence neuropsychological skills, and these skills in turn influence achievement outcomes. Structural equation modeling revealed the strongest path between birth weight and a perceptual planning neuropsychological factor, while SES was more strongly linked to verbal working memory. These neuropsychological constructs in turn had different influences on achievement outcomes. Most intriguing is the finding that academic achievement is multiply determined, and disabilities in reading and mathematics may be indicative of deficits in any of several neuropsychological processes.

IMPLICATIONS

The spectrum of sequelae found in children born at biomedical risk and free of major handicaps does not differ dramatically from the array of problems found in the general school-age population. However, there is a disproportionately greater incidence and complexity of these problems and more specific profiles of deficits (Aylward, 2002a). Debate continues regarding whether deficits in children born at LBW and below are global or specific (Taylor et al., 2002). As indicated throughout this chapter, a direct pathway from a biomedical risk condition such as LBW to later outcome is often precluded because of mediators and moderators, where environmental, genetic, and neuroanatomical (due to disruptions and insult) influences intermingle. While some deficits have more direct linkage (e.g., visual–motor integration), others, such as IQ, academic achievement, and language, do not. Further compounding this issue is the interrelatedness of outcome constructs such as EF, attention, academic achievement, and IQ.

Assessment

Proper assessment is critical to evaluate areas of function that have an increased probability of problems. In both research and clinical practice, assessment must extend beyond traditional IQ and achievement testing. Global scores simply will not identify subtle problems that can interfere with a child's learning and development. Based on data reflecting areas having a higher probability of deficit, more specific tests or rating scales that measure the following areas should also be considered: (1) EFs (planning, organization, monitoring, inhibition, working memory) and attention; (2) language (phonological awareness, syntax, verbal fluency, comprehension of instructions, higher order abstracting functions); (3) sensory–motor functions (visual–motor precision, fine motor speed); (4) visual–spatial processes (design copying, visual closure, visual–spatial planning); (5) memory and learning (list learning, delayed recall, narrative memory, assessment of semantic–strategic and rote–episodic verbal and visual functions); and (6) behavioral adjustment (ADHD, internalizing and externalizing problems) (for specific instruments, see Aylward, 2002a; Vohr, Wright, Hack, Aylward, & Hirtz, 2004).

Developmental Course

Early indicators of later, high prevalence/low severity dysfunctions need to be identified during infancy or early childhood, so that timely interventions can be initiated. Continuity in function over infancy does exist in areas such as motor, verbal, and cognitive processes (Aylward, 2004); what is necessary is to make the connection from early functional abilities to later school age outcomes. Mild to moderate disabilities are identified at older ages, suggesting a frequent worsening of outcome over time. It is likely that these problems existed previously in a "silent period" but become more evident when demands for higher order skills cannot be met because of underlying cognitive or neuropsychological deficiencies. Subsequently, these children are less likely to take advantage of educational opportunities because of deficits in basic skills, or increasing frustration and loss of motivation, further setting a downward spiral.

Family Functioning

Families of children exposed to early medical risks face a series of hurdles. The first is viability, with survival being the parents' primary focus; possible neurodevelopmental sequelae are not a prime concern at that time. The next potential stress point emerges during infancy, when most major disabilities become obvious. A subsequent hurdle occurs at early school age, when high prevalence/low severity dysfunctions are identifiable. Arguably, later deficits are less severe, but unless the family is informed, these still could be devastating. Therefore, the clinician needs to be well versed in outcomes and the complex interrelationships biomedical and environmental factors have on these outcomes. Serial evaluations are essential to document the continuing transaction between the child and the environment. Anticipatory guidance is necessary, with the goal being to develop a balance between awareness of problematic indicators yet avoid hypervigilance.

Future Research

Prediction of later outcome will improve with the combined use of brain imaging techniques, functional magnetic resonance imaging (fMRI) of brain activity, biochemical markers (inflammatory cytokines), serial neurodevelopmental assessments with refined evaluation techniques, and use of approaches such as structural equation modeling, path analysis, and growth curve analysis to clarify longitudinal relationships among biomedical and background variables. While group data are informative, interindividual differences in the child and the environment make each case unique.

REFERENCES

Allin, M., Matsumoto, H., & Santhouse, A. M. (2001). Cognitive and motor function and the size of the cerebellum in adolescents born very preterm. *Brain, 124,* 60–66.

Anderson, P. J., & Doyle, L. W. (2004). Executive functioning in school-aged children who were born very preterm or with extremely low birth weight. *Pediatrics, 114,* 50–57.

Aylward, G. P. (1990). Environmental influences on the developmental outcome of children at risk. *Infants and Young Children, 2,* 1–9.

Aylward, G. P. (1992). The relationship between environmental risk and developmental outcome. *Journal of Developmental and Behavioral Pediatrics, 13,* 222–229.

Aylward, G. P. (1997a). *Infant and early childhood neuropsychology.* New York: Plenum Press.

Aylward, G. P. (1997b). Conceptual issues in developmental screening and assessment. *Journal of Developmental and Behavioral Pediatrics, 18,* 340–349.

Aylward, G. P. (2002a). Cognitive and neuropsychological outcomes: More than IQ scores. *Mental Retardation and Developmental Disabilities Research Reviews, 8,* 234–240.

Aylward, G. P. (2002b). Methodological issues in outcome studies of at-risk infants. *Journal of Pediatric Psychology, 27,* 37–45.

Aylward, G. P. (2003). Cognitive function in preterm infants: No simple answers. *Journal of the American Medical Association, 289,* 752–753.

Aylward, G. P. (2004). Prediction of function from infancy to early childhood: Implications for pediatric psychology. *Journal of Pediatric Psychology, 29,* 555–564.

Aylward, G., Pfeiffer, S. I., Wright, A., & Verhulst, S. J. (1989). Outcome studies of low birth weight infants published in the last decade: A meta-analysis. *Journal of Pediatrics, 115,* 515–520.

Bennett, F. C., & Scott, D. T. (1997). Long-term perspective on premature infant outcome and contemporary intervention issues. *Seminars in Perinatology, 21,* 190–201.

Bhutta, A. T., Cleves, M. A., Casey, P. H., Craddock, M., & Arand, K. (2002). Cognitive and behavioral outcomes of school-aged children who were born preterm. *Journal of the American Medical Association, 288,* 728–737.

Biagas, K. (1999). Hypoxic–ischemic brain injury: Advancements in the understanding of mechanisms and potential areas of therapy. *Current Opinions in Pediatrics, 11,* 223–228.

Botting, N., Powls, A., Cooke, R. W. I., & Marlow, N. (1997). Attention deficit hyperactivity disorders and other psychiatric outcomes in very low birth weight children at 12 years. *Journal of Child Psychology and Psychiatry, 38,* 931–941.

Bregman, J. (1998). Developmental outcome in very low birth weight infants: Current status and future trends. *Pediatric Clinics of North America, 45,* 673–690.

Breslau, N. (1995). Psychiatric sequelae of low birth weight. *Epidemiologic Reviews, 17,* 96–106.

Breslau, N., Chilcoat, H. D., & Del Dotto, J. E. (1996). Low birthweight and neurocognitive status at six years of age. *Biological Psychiatry, 40,* 379–387.

Breslau, N., DelDotto, J. E., & Brown, G. (1994). A gradient relationship between low birth weight and IQ at age 6 years. *Archives of Pediatric and Adolescent Medicine, 148,* 377–383.

Breslau, N., Johnson, E. O., & Lucia, V. C. (2001). Academic achievement of low birthweight children at age 11: The role of cognitive abilities at school entry. *Journal of Abnormal Child Psychology, 27,* 273–279.

Dammann, O., & Leviton, A. (1999). Brain damage in preterm newborns: Might enhancement of developmentally regulated endogenous protection open a door for prevention? *Pediatrics, 104,* 541–550.

Dammann, O., & Leviton, A. (2000). Brain damage in preterm newborns: Biological response modification as a strategy to reduce disabilities. *Journal of Pediatrics, 136,* 433–438.

Dewey, D., Crawford, S. G., Creighton, D. E., & Sauve, R. S. (1999). Long-term neuropsychological outcomes in very low birth weight children free of sensorineural impairments. *Journal of Clinical and Experimental Neuropsychology, 21,* 851–865.

Escalona, S. K. (1982). Babies at double hazard: Early development of infants at biologic and social risk. *Pediatrics, 70,* 670–676.

Ewing-Cobbs, L., Barnes, M. A., & Fletcher, J. M. (2003). Early brain injury in children: Development and reorganization of cognitive function. *Developmental Neuropsychology, 24,* 669–704.

Fearon, P., O'Connell, P., Frangou, S., Aquino, P., Nosarti, C., Allin, M., et al. (2004). Brain volumes in adult survivors of very low birth weight: A sibling controlled study. *Pediatrics, 114,* 367–371.

Fletcher, J. M., Francis, D. J., Thompson, N. M., Brookshire, B. L., Bohan, T. P., Landry, S. H., et al. (1992). Verbal and nonverbal skill discrepancies in hydrocephalic children. *Journal of Clinical and Experimental Neuropsychology, 14,* 593–609.

Frisk, V., & Whyte, H. (1994). The long-term consequences of periventricular brain damage on language and verbal memory. *Developmental Neuropsychology, 10,* 313–333.

Geidd, J. N. (1997). Normal development. *Neuroimaging: Child and Adolescent Psychiatric Clinics of North America, 6,* 265–282.

Geidd, J. N., Blumenthal, J., & Jeffries, N. O. (1999). Development of the human corpus callosum during childhood and adolescence: A longitudinal MRI study. *Progress in Neuropsychopharmacological and Biological Psychiatry, 23,* 571–588.

Gioia, G., Isquith, P., Guy, S., & Kenworthy, L. (2000). *BRIEF—Behavior Rating*

Inventory of Executive Function manual. Odessa, FL: Psychological Assessment Resources.

Goldman-Rakic, P. S. (1994). Specification of higher cortical functions. In S. H. Broman & J. Grafman (Eds.), *Atypical cognitive deficits in developmental disorders: Implications for brain function* (pp. 3–17). Hillsdale, NJ: Erlbaum.

Goyen, T., Lui, K., & Woods, R. (1998). Visual–motor, visual–perceptual, and fine-motor outcomes in very-low-birthweight children at 5 years. *Developmental Medicine and Child Neurology, 40,* 76–81.

Grether, J. K., & Nelson, K. B. (1997). Maternal infection and cerebral palsy in infants of normal birth weight. *Journal of the American Medical Association, 278,* 207–211.

Hack, M., & Fanaroff, A. A. (1999). Outcomes of children of extremely low birthweight and gestational age in the 1990s. *Early Human Development, 53,* 193–218.

Hack, M., Taylor, H. G., & Klein, N. (1995). Long term developmental outcome of low birthweight infants. In *The future of children: Low birth weight* (Vol. 5, pp. 176–196). Los Altos, CA: Packard Foundation.

Hack, M., Taylor, H. G., Klein, N., & Minich, N. M. (2000). Functional limitations and special health care needs of 10– to 14–year-old children weighing less than 750 grams at birth. *Pediatrics, 106,* 554–559.

Halsey, C. L., Collin, M. F., & Anderson, C. L. (1996). Extremely low-birth-weight children and their peers. *Archives of Pediatric and Adolescent Medicine, 150,* 790–794.

Harvey, J., O'Callaghan, M., & Mohay, H. (1999). Executive function of children with extremely low birth weight: A case control study. *Developmental Medicine and Child Neurology, 41,* 292–297.

Hunt, J. V., Cooper, B. A., & Tooley, W. H. (1988). Very low birth weight infants at 8 and 11 years of age: Role of neonatal illness and family status. *Pediatrics, 82,* 596–603.

Isaacs, E. B., Lucas, A., Chong, W. K., Wood, S. J., Johnson, C. L., & Marshall, C. (2000). Hippocampal volume and everyday memory in children of very low birth weight. *Pediatric Research, 47,* 713–720.

Jennische, M., & Sedin, M. (2001). Linguistic skills at 6½ years of age in children who required neonatal intensive care in 1986–1989. *Acta Pediatrica, 90,* 199–212.

Johnson, E. O., & Breslau, N. (2000). Increased risk of learning disabilities in low birthweight boys at age 11 years. *Biological Psychiatry, 47,* 490–500.

Kilbride, H. W., Thurstad, K., & Daily, D. K. (2004). Preschool outcome of less than 801–gram preterm infants compared with full-term siblings. *Pediatrics, 13,* 742–747.

LeNormand, M. T., & Cohen, H. (1999). The delayed emergence of lexical morphology in preterm children: The case of verbs. *Journal of Neurolinguistics, 12,* 235–246.

Leviton, A., & Gilles, F. (1996). Ventriculomegaly, delayed myelination, white matter hypoplasia, and "periventricular" leukomalacia: How are they related? *Pediatric Neurology, 15,* 121–136.

Leviton, A., Kuban, K., & Paneth, N. S. (2004). Grading intraventricular hemorrhage with no grades. *Pediatrics, 113*, 930–931.

Levy-Shiff, R., Einat, G., Mogilner, M. B., Lerman, M., & Krikler, R. (1994). Biological and environmental correlates of developmental outcome of prematurely born infants in early adolescence. *Journal of Pediatric Psychology, 19*, 63–78.

Lou, H. C. (1996). Etiology and pathogenesis of attention deficit hyperactivity disorder: Significance of prematurity and perinatal hypoxic–hemodynamic encephalopathy. *Acta Pediatrica, 85*, 1266–1271.

Luciana, M., Lindeke, L., Mills, M., & Nelson, C. (1999). Neurobehavioral evidence of white matter deficits in school-aged children with histories of prematurity. *Developmental Medicine and Child Neurology, 41*, 521–533.

Ment, L. R., Vohr, B., Allan, W., Kutz, K. H., Schneider, K. C., Westerveld, M., et al. (2003). Change in cognitive function over time in very low-birth-weight infants. *Journal of the American Medical Association, 289*, 705–711.

Mutch, L., Leyland, A., & McGee, A. (1993). Patterns of neuropsychological function in a low birthweight population. *Developmental Medicine and Child Neurology, 35*, 943–956.

Nosarti, C., Al-Asady, M. H., Frangou, S., Stewart, A. L., Rifkin, L., & Murray, R. M. (2002). Adolescents who were born very preterm have decreased brain volumes. *Brain, 125*, 1616–1623.

O'Callaghan, M. J., Burns, Y. R., Gray, P. H., Harvey, J. M., Mohay, H., Roger, Y. M., et al. (1996). School performance of ELBW children: A controlled study. *Developmental Medicine and Child Neurology, 38*, 917–926.

Paneth, N. S. (1995). The problem of low birth weight. In *The future of children: Low birthweight* (pp. 11–34). Los Altos, CA: Packard Foundation.

Parker, S., Greer, S., & Zuckerman, B. (1988). Double jeopardy: The impact of poverty on early child development. *Pediatric Clinics of North America, 35*, 1227–1240.

Perlman, J. M. (2001). Neurobehavioral deficits in premature graduates of intensive care—Potential medical and neonatal environmental risk factors. *Pediatrics, 108*, 1339–1348.

Perlman, J. M. (2003). The genesis of cognitive and behavioral deficits in premature graduates of intensive care. *Minerva Pediatrica, 55*, 89–101.

Peterson, B. S., Vohr, B., Staib, L. H., Cannestracis, C. J., Dohlberg, B. A., & Schneider, K. C. (2000). Regional brain volume abnormalities and long-term cognitive outcome in preterm infants. *Journal of the American Medical Association, 284*, 1939–1947.

Resnick, M. B., Gomatam, S. V., Carter, R. L., Ariet, M., Roth, J., Kilgore, K. L., et al. (1998). Educational disabilities of neonatal intensive care graduates. *Pediatrics, 102*, 308–316.

Saigal, S., Hoult, L. A., Streinder, D. L., Stoskopf, B. L., & Rosenbaum, P. L. (2000). School difficulties in adolescence in a regional cohort of children who were extremely low birth-weight. *Pediatrics, 105*, 325–331.

Saigal, S., Rosenbaum, P., Szatmari, P., & Hoult, L. (1992). Non-right handedness among ELBW and term children at eight years in relation to cognitive function

and school performance. *Developmental Medicine and Child Neurology, 34,* 925–933.
Saigal, S., Stoskopf, B. L., Streiner, D. L., & Burrows, E. (2001). Physical growth and current health status of infants who were of extremely low birth weight and controls at adolescence. *Pediatrics, 108,* 407–415.
Santhouse, A. M., Ffytche, D. H., & Howard, R. J. (2002). The functional significance of perinatal corpus callosum damage: An fMRI study in young adults. *Brain, 125,* 1782–1792.
Stewart, A. L., Rifkin, L., Amess, P. N., Kirkbride, V., Townsend, J. P., Miller, D. H., et al. (1999). Brain structure and neurocognitive and behavioral function in adolescents who were born very preterm. *Lancet, 353,* 1653–1657.
Szatmari, P., Saigal, S., Rosenbaum, P., Campbell, D., & King, S. (1990). Psychiatric disorders at five years among children with birthweights less than 1000g: A regional perspective. *Developmental Medicine and Child Neurology, 32,* 954–962.
Taylor, H. G., Burant, C. J., Holding, P. A., Klein, N., & Hack, M. (2002). Sources of variability in sequelae of very low birth weight. *Child Neuropsychology, 8,* 163–178.
Taylor, H. G., Hack, M., & Klein, N. K. (1998). Attention deficits in children with < 750 gram birth weight. *Developmental Neuropsychology, 4,* 21–34.
Taylor, H. G., Klein, N., & Hack, M. (2000). School-age consequences of birth weight less than 750 g.: A review and update. *Developmental Neuropsychology, 17,* 289–321.
Taylor, H. G., Klein, N., Minich, N. M., & Hack, M. (2000). Middle school age outcomes in children with very low birthweight. *Child Development, 71,* 1495–1511.
Taylor, H. G., Klein, N., Schatschneider, C., & Hack, M. (1998). Predictors of early school age outcomes in very low birth weight children. *Journal of Developmental and Behavioral Pediatrics, 19,* 235–243.
Tjossem, T. (1976). *Intervention strategies for high risk infants and young children.* Baltimore: University Park Press.
Vohr, B., Wright, L. L., Duscik, A. M., Mele, L., Verter, J., & Steichen, J. J. (2000). Neurodevelopmental and functional outcomes of extremely low birth weight infants in the National Institute of Child Health and Human Development Neonatal Research Network, 1993–1994. *Pediatrics, 105,* 1216–1226.
Vohr, B., Wright, L. L., Hack, M., Aylward, G. P., & Hirtz, D. (2004). Follow-up care of high risk infants, *Pediatrics, 114*(Suppl.), 1377–1394.
Volpe, J. J. (1996). Subplate neurons, missing link in brain injury of the premature infant? *Pediatrics, 97,* 112–113.
Volpe, J. J. (2001). Neurobiology of periventricular leukomalacia in the premature infant. *Pediatric Research, 50,* 553–562.
Waber, D. P., & McCormick, M. C. (1995). Late neuropsychological outcomes in preterm infants of normal IQ: Selective vulnerability of the visual system. *Journal of Pediatric Psychology, 20,* 721–735.
Whitaker, A. H., Van Rossen, R., & Feldman, J. F. (1997). Psychiatric outcomes in

low-birth weight children at age 6 years: Relation to neonatal cranial ultrasound abnormalities. *Archives of General Psychiatry, 54*, 847–856.

Whitfield, M. F., Eckstein-Grunau, R. V., & Holsti, L. (1997). Extremely premature (800g) school children: Multiple areas of hidden disability. *Archives of Diseases in Children, 77*, F85–F90.

Wilson-Costello, D., Borawski, E., Friedman, H., Redline, R., Fanaroff, A. A., & Hack, M. (1998). Perinatal correlates of cerebral palsy and other neurologic impairment among very low birth weight children. *Pediatrics, 102*, 315–322.

5

Physical Impairments and Disability

SETH WARSCHAUSKY

Neurodevelopmental diagnoses include congenital conditions associated with significant physical impairment and varying degrees of cognitive impairment. Two of the most common groupings of such conditions are cerebral palsy and spina bifida. Both groupings involve chronic conditions, but there is increasing knowledge about developmental changes in functional status, as well as specific changes associated with complications and comorbidities such as contractures, epilepsy, and hydrocephalus. In addition, there has been a significant increase in our understanding of the multifactorial nature of key predictors of psychological and social health in these populations. In contrast, there is a relative paucity of understanding of both the psychosocial and neurocognitive profiles of the subgroups of these populations with the most significant physical impairments, due in part to the continued lack of accessibility of both clinical and research assessment instruments.

CEREBRAL PALSY

Cerebral Palsy (CP) is an umbrella term applied to a group of non-progressive disorders of movement and posture caused by static defects in the immature, developing brain (Bax, 1964; Mutch, Alberman, Hadberg, Kodama, & Perat, 1992). Approximately 90% of CP is congenital, stemming from pre- or perinatal brain injury. Acquired CP stems from injury in the first few months of life; there is not a consensus for the upper age limit at which an injury would result in a CP diagnosis. There are no recent prevalence data for cerebral palsy in North America; therefore, the current estimates of 0.1–0.24% of live births typically are derived from other countries (Blair, 2001; Hagberg, Hagberg, Beckung, & Uvebrant, 2001; Nelson, 2002). There has been no change in the occurrence of CP in term and near-term (TNT) births over the past two decades, but there is some evidence of generally increased prevalence. Approximately 50% of children with CP have normal birth weights (Nelson, 2002). Among low-birth-weight children, the reliability of dichotomous judgments of presence or absence of CP has been questionable (Paneth et al., 2003). In contrast, when detailed information regarding motoric functioning is available, clinicians have demonstrated good-to-excellent ability to identify those with disabling CP, nondisabling CP, or no CP. Paneth et al. have recommended including levels of motor function in future CP prevalence literature. At this point, the most widely used functional level classification system is the Gross Motor Function Classification System (GMFCS; Palisano, Rosenbaum, Walter, Russell, Wood, & Galuppi, 1997).

There are persisting misconceptions regarding the multiple etiologies for CP. Asphyxia accounts for only 6% of spastic CP in infants of normal birth weight, but even in this subgroup, other factors such as intrauterine infection and maternal coagulation disorders are noted (Nelson & Grether, 1997). Similarly, in preterm infants with periventricular leukomalacia or ventricular dilatation due to white matter atrophy, only 6% showed metabolic acidosis, an indicator of hypoxia. A tight nuchal cord has been associated with specific risk for spastic tetraplegic CP (Nelson & Grether, 1998). Regarding stroke, in placentas of children with CP reviewed for litigation, thrombi were the most frequent type of lesion, and these can embolize, reaching the fetal brain (Kraus, 1997). Studies of hemiplegic CP show frequent evidence of cerebral infarction (Uvebrant, 1988).

Little is known about the role of intrauterine infection in CP in the TNT population. There is some indication of increased risk for CP, with evidence of histological chorionitis and some indirect evidence that maternal fever in labor or other signs of infection constitute risk, but more research is needed. At this point, with TNT newborns, the best predictor of CP is encephalopathy (Nelson, 2002). In preterm infants with periventricular leukomalacia or ventricular dilatation due to white matter atrophy, culture-positive neonatal infection was associated with white matter injury but histological chorioamnionitis was not (Graham, Holcroft, Rai, Donohue, & Allen, 2004).

Low birth weight clearly is associated with risk for CP. The prevalence of CP in children with very low birth weight (VLBW; < 1,500 grams) is 8%, or 40 times the prevalence rates noted in infants of normal birth weight (Escobar, Littenberg, & Petitti, 1991). Among children with CP, approximately 20% had VLBW compared with < 1% of the general population (Surman, Newkick, & Johnson, 2003). During the 1970s and 1980s, increases in CP rates among VLBW infants were reported, probably associated with increasing survival rates.

Multiple births are associated with increased risk of CP. It is not clear whether a premature twin is at greater risk than a premature singleton. In TNT twins or triplets, the major determinant of CP is death of a co-twin or co-triplet (Pharoah, Price, & Plomin, 2002). In general, there is not a significant difference in same- and different-sex twin CP risk, used as an estimate of the monozygotic–dizygotic distinction. However, when one twin dies, the survivor is at greater risk if it is of the same sex. It is not rare to note a "vanishing" twin with ultrasound, and it may be that many singleton cases of CP involve unrecognized death of a twin (Pharoah, 2001).

Pathophysiology: Type and Spasticity Pattern

The "Swedish" classification divides CP into spastic, ataxic, dyskinetic, and mixed types. The majority of children with CP exhibit spasticity (88%), and a large percentage (40%) exhibit mixed movement disorders. A significant percentage of children with CP are diagnosed as such by age 1 but no longer exhibit significant motoric symptoms by age 7; this includes virtually 100% of those with a monoparesis, approximately 75% with ataxic or dyskinetic symptoms, and 67% with spastic diplegia. Dyskinetic and spastic CPs tend to include different neuropathologies with more homogeneous basal ganglia lesions in the former and cortical, basal ganglia, and white matter lesions in the latter. Among children with bilateral lesions of the thalamus and basal ganglia, severity of magnetic resonance imaging (MRI) lesion patterns have been associated with type of CP (Krageloh-Mann et al., 2002). In this sample of children, all of whom exhibited CP, pure dyskinetic CP was only seen with mild MRI lesion patterns, involving only the nucleus lentiformis and ventrolateral thalamus. Dyskinetic–spastic CP was associated with intermediate MRI lesions, and pure spastic CP, with the more severe lesions. In addition, the children with intermediate and severe lesions exhibited reduced head growth associated with microcephaly.

Epilepsy

Epilepsy is common among children with CP and constitutes a critical risk factor for lower cognitive status. In the general population, the risk of epilepsy, defined as two or more seizures, is approximately 0.5% (Cowan, Bodensteiner, Leviton, & Doherty, 1989); in contrast, CP epilepsy estimates vary from 15 to 60%, depending upon the type of CP and origin of the sample (Carlsson, Hagberg, & Olsson, 2003). In Sweden, 38% of a 7-year cohort of 146 children with CP had epilepsy. Of those with epilepsy, 91% had developed the condition by age 6. White matter damage did not specifically increase risk of seizures within the sample, but central nervous system malformations, infections, and gray matter damage were associated with risk. All children in the Swedish sample with tetraplegic CP had a comorbid seizure disorder, compared to approximately one-third in other types of CP. Earlier onset of epilepsy was noted with tetraplegic CP. Partial seizures were most common, but 47% had had at least one episode of status epilepticus.

Neuropsychology

Given the heterogeneity of CP, a complex set of neuropsychological studies apply; thus, this topic could best be described as the neuropsychologies of the cerebral palsies. For example, the literature on neuropsychological outcomes from VLBW could be applicable to approximately 50% of the population with CP. The recent literature on cognitive and general developmental correlates of neuropathology associated with periventricular leukomalacia has been of increasing value both in understanding specific risks and needs associated with CPs and the more general concern with effects of early brain damage. Higher grades (III and IV) of periventricular leukomalacia, indicating greater parenchymal abnormalities, have been associated with higher risk for motoric and cognitive impairments (Serdaroglu, Telgul, Kitis, Sedaroglu, & Gokben, 2004). Approximately 50% of the Serdaroglu et al. (2004) sample with periventricular leukomalacia grade IV exhibited tetraplegic CP. Thinning of the corpus callosum and cortical atrophy were associated with significantly poorer developmental outcomes.

At this point, however, surprisingly little is known about multifactorial predictors of specific neuropsychological profiles associated with the CPs. There is high risk for mental retardation, in the range of 30–77%; however, there is long-standing concern that traditional cognitive measures are not accessible to children with significant communicative and motoric impairments (Allen, 1958; Byrne, Dywan, & Connolly, 1995; Sabbadini, Bonanni, Carolesimo, & Caltagirone, 2001; Tracht, 1948). There is some evidence that the risk of IQ < 70 is similar in children with dyskinetic, mixed, and spastic bilateral CP (Krageloh-Mann et al., 1993; Hagberg, Hagberg, & Olow, 1975). It is not unusual for intelligence to be underestimated in children with dyskinetic conditions. Children with hemiplegic or diplegic conditions tend to have better cognitive outcomes.

Neuropsychological knowledge derived from the typically developing population does not always apply to children with CP. For example, in typically developing children, articulation rate is associated with memory span (Hulme, Thomson, Muir, & Lawrence, 1984). In contrast, White, Craft,

Hale, and Park (1994) showed that in children with CP, there is a dissociation between articulation rate and memory span, suggesting that normal speech rates are not necessary for development of normal covert rehearsal rates.

A number of studies have examined specific neuropsychological risks associated with subtypes of CP. In children with spastic diplegia, there is specific risk for visuoperceptual impairments associated with evidence of perventricular leukomalacia (Ito et al., 1996). In children with diplegic CP, however, it is not clear to what extent noted visuoperceptual impairments have a multifactorial etiology that also includes the developmental effects of sensory vision loss, motoric impairments, oculomotor abnormalities, and impairments in anticipatory saccadic movement (Fedrizzi et al., 1998). Although there is preliminary evidence to suggest that children with dyskinetic or spastic CPs exhibit similar nonverbal reasoning, the dyskinetic subtype may be at lower risk for impairments in specific domains including auditory comprehension, visuospatial ability, aspects of memory, and verbal working memory (Pueyo, Junque, & Ventrell, 2003).

In one of the few studies to address executive functions, Christ, White, Brunstrom, and Abrams (2003) examined inhibitory control in relatively high-functioning children with bilateral spastic CP associated with periventricular leukomalacia and therefore possible damage to white matter tracts connecting prefrontal to posterior regions. As is typically the case in such studies of CP, no neuroimaging data were obtained. The associations between intellect and inhibitory control were not significant. The children with CP exhibited significantly impaired inhibitory control, in addition to processing speed impairments.

There has been specific interest in hemiplegic CP in the study of neuropsychological effects of early lateralized lesions; again, however, neuroimaging data typically are not available. Hugdahl and Carolsson (1994) showed that in children with hemiplegic CP, ear advantage with dichotic listening could not be altered by forcing attention to the ear contralateral to the presumed lesion. Results indicate impairments in ability to direct attention that may reflect hemi-inattention caused by hypoarousal of the involved hemisphere or, alternatively, hyperarousal of the intact hemisphere. In a separate area of investigation, precise study of movement in children with hemiplegic CP has included recent support for a unique left-hemisphere role in forward movement planning (Steenbergen, Meulenbroek, & Rosenbaum, 2004).

NEURAL TUBE DEFECTS: SPINA BIFIDA

Spina bifida (SB) is one of two types of neural tube defects (NTDs), the other typically including defects involving cranial structures such as anencephaly and encephalocele. SB tends to be more common in girls than in boys at birth (Mitchell et al., 2004). Estimates of prevalence of NTDs at birth have varied geographically. For example, in London, prevalence at birth was 2.8 per 1,000, while in Northern Ireland, it was 7.1 per 1,000 (MacHenry, Nevin, & Merrett, 1979). Prevalence rates in the United Kingdom and North America have included peaks in rates, though the timing has differed. Groups with high risk who migrate from the British Isles do not keep their high risk for NTD. The prevalence of both types of NTDs has decreased dramatically, but statistics are based on prevalence at birth, often excluding spontaneous or elective termination data. The elective termination rate among identified cases of NTD doubled from 25% in 1986 to approximately 50% in 1999.

NTDs as a whole are described as complex genetic disorders with both genetic and environmental etiologies. Family history of NTD is one of the strongest risk factors (Mitchell et al., 2004). There are specific NTD syndromes that are clearly associated with genetic abnormalities (Frey & Hauser, 2000). There is strong evidence for a protective effect of folate supplementation, including randomized controlled trials; however, there also is evidence for a lack of folate efficacy for obese and Hispanic women (Frey & Hauser, 2003) and in the prevention of lipomyelomeningocele (McNeely & Howes, 2004). Other nutrients also have been associated with NTD risk, including low maternal vitamin B_{12} (Suarez, Hendricks, Felkner, & Gunter, 2003). Mitchell et al. (2004) note that SB is the only birth defect for which there has been significant success in both treatment and prevention.

The NTD risk associated with age is regarded as low, with some studies showing elevated rates in older or very young mothers. Lower socioeconomic status, across geographic regions, has been associated with increased risk. In the United States, risk for NTD is low among African Americans and high among Hispanics. Increased risk has consistently been associated with maternal obesity and high body mass index (Frey & Hauser, 2003). Increased risk has also been associated with illness, as well as hot tub use in the first trimester. Interestingly, a consistent finding is that smoking lowers NTD risk, and there is no evidence that alcohol or "recreational" drug use increases risk (Kallen, 1998; Shaw, Velie, & Schaffer, 1996). Antiseizure medication increases risk for NTDs (Samren, van Duijn, Lieve Christiaens, Hofman, & Lindhout, 1999).

Myelomeningocele entails substantial risk for paraplegia, bowel and bladder dysfunction, and orthopedic abnormalities including contractures and scoliosis. Chiari malformation and hydrocephalus are among the most prominent neuropathologies and complications associated with myelomeningocele. Among Chiari subtypes, Chiari type II is the most common, consisting of caudal shift of portions of the medulla oblongata and cerebellum into the foramen magnum (Sarnat, 1992). The most common preoperative symptoms associated with Chiari II are pain, weakness, sensory loss, and ataxia (Dyste, Menezes, & Van Gilder, 1989). Concomitant with Chiari II malformation, there can be elongation and compression of the cranial nerves and distortion of the fourth ventricle, probably contributing to hydrocephalus; more than 90% of children with Chiari II will develop hydrocephalus. Hydrocephalus, identified in approximately 80% of children with myelomeningocele, is associated with brain abnormalities that include thinning of the cortical mantle, dysplasia of the corpus callosum, and reduced cerebral blood flow in frontal regions (Del Bigio, 1993). There is some evidence that *in utero* SB repair is associated with lower incidence of significant hindbrain herniation and hydrocephalus (Tulipan et al., 1999).

Neuropsychology

Neuropsychological studies of SB have largely focused on the study of children with myelomeningocele (MM). In the subpopulation with nonhydrocephalic MM, higher level lesions have been associated with lower intellect (Shaffer, Friedrich, Shurtleff, & Wolf, 1985). The multiple brain anomalies associated with MM, including hydrocephalus, thinning of the corpus callosum, and Chiari malformations, entail cognitive risks. Hydrocephalus is a significant predictor of cognitive impairment in MM (Iddon, Morgan, Loveday, Sahakian, & Pickard, 2004), and the reader is referred to excellent reviews of the neuropsychology of hydrocephalus (e.g., Fletcher, Dennis, & Northrup, 2000). There is risk for lower Performance than Verbal IQs (Dennis et al., 1981; Donders, Canady, & Rourke, 1990) and an increasing verbal–nonverbal discrepancy with age (Wills, Holmbeck, Dillon, & McLone, 1990). That said, approximately two-thirds of children with mixed etiology shunted hydrocephalus do not exhibit a consistent significant Verbal–Performance IQ discrepancy over time (Brookshire et al., 1995). Fletcher et al. (1992) found that children with nonhydrocephalic MM had higher visuoperceptual skills than those with hydrocephalic MM. In the general population with shunted hydrocephalus, size of the corpus callosum is associated with Performance but not Verbal IQ (Fletcher et al., 1996), and frequency of shunt revisions has not been shown to affect intelligence, but similar to the findings in children with CP, presence of seizures is a significant negative predictor (Ralph, Moylan, Canady, & Simmons, 2000).

Recent studies of MM have focused on specific neuropsychological domains. Children with MM are at risk for impairments in multiple aspects of attention when compared with non-MM siblings (Loss, Yeates, & Enrile, 1998). Anatomical and medical variables including lesion level, oculomotor abnormalities, shunt revisions, and infections and dysgenesis of the corpus callosum are predictive of attentional risks. Hydrocephalic MM also is associated with memory and language deficits; however, at this point, there is not strong evidence that deficits in these domains differ between groups with hydrocephalic MM versus other types of hydrocephalus.

In an elegant study of specific aspects of visual perception in children with hydrocephalic SB, Dennis, Fletcher, Rogers, Hetherington, and Francis (2002) showed that there was specific risk of impairment in action-based versus object-based perception. Findings were consistent with the hypothesized greater compromise of the dorsal visual system in this population.

PSYCHOLOGICAL AND SOCIAL OUTCOMES

Children with neurodevelopmental disorders are at increased risk for psychological and social difficulties (Lavigne & Faier-Routman, 1992; McAndrew, 1979). McDermott and colleagues (1996), in a rare population-based study, showed that children with CP were five times more likely to have "behavior problems" (25.5 vs. 5.4%) than typically developing peers, although this represents a lower rate than previous estimates based on clinic sampling. Children with CP were more likely to exhibit both externalizing and internalizing behaviors and greater dependency. Those with CP and mental retardation had the greatest risk for anxiety, hyperactivity, and peer conflict. Interpretation of findings was limited by relatively global behavioral ratings.

Regarding depression and low self-esteem, Manuel, Balrishnan, Camacho, Smith, and Koman (2003) found that most of their adolescent sample with CP was reporting positive psychological status, but approximately 30% scored low, and greater concerns were associated with female gender, lower functional status, and higher perception of impact of disability. However, in a multivariate analysis, only perceived impact of disability was significantly associated with internalizing symptoms.

Older children and adolescents with SB are at risk for internalizing features (Ammerman et al., 1998; Appleton et al., 1997). Holmbeck et al. (2003) have recently found that preadolescents with SB appear to be at lower risk than older adolescents with SB. The preadolescents, however, did exhibit poorer social skills and greater isolation, and these social concerns may place the child with SB at specific risk for depression in adolescence. Typically, the associations between severity of physical condition and psychological adjustment have been weak or nonsignificant in children with disabilities; however, Hommeyer, Holmbeck, Wills, and Coers (1999) showed that severity of neurological condition can have indirect effects on psychosocial outcomes. For example, presence of a shunt in SB is associated with greater attentional difficulties, which in turn are associated with social problems. In parallel, studies of traumatic brain injury have begun to reveal similar indirect paths. The reader is referred to Chapter 13, this volume, for further description of social risks and interventions for children with neurodevelopmental conditions (NDCs).

Studies of family influences on child development in typically developing children have shown strong associations between positive family environments; specific parenting characteristics, including authoritative and permissive styles; higher socioeconomic status; and child outcomes (Baumrind & Black, 1967; Querido, Warner, & Eyberg, 2002). While there is evidence that family and socioeconomic factors are critical predictors of psychosocial outcomes for children with neurodevelopmental disorders, recent evidence suggests a complex set of moderating effects. A seminal set of studies with families of children with SB has shown both positive and negative family influences. McKernon et al. (2001) found that parental responsiveness was similarly associated with coping in typically developing children and children with SB. Stronger family cohesion was associated with increased use of problem-focused coping in both groups. Holmbeck, Coakley, Hommeyer, Shapera, and Westhoven (2002a) found that families of children with SB were less cohesive, particularly when of lower socioeconomic status. Children's verbal intellect mediated the greater passivity in family interactions noted in children with SB. In a related finding, Holmbeck et al. (2002b) showed that the child's verbal intellect partially mediated the greater parental overprotectiveness observed in families of children with SB. Overprotectiveness was associated with lower levels of preadolescent autonomous decision making. Subsequently, Coakley, Holmbeck, Friedman, Greenley, and Thill (2002), in a study of family transitions associated with onset of adolescence in SB, did not find the typical increased family conflict and decreased cohesion associated with perceived early puberty. At this point, it is not clear whether the Coakley et al. (2002) findings reflect a truncated or simply slower developmental process in these families.

This key issue of dependency and autonomy in children with NDCs also has been examined in the frequently overlooked nonverbal population. In addition to providing further support for a restricted and directed conversational pattern between mothers and their nonverbal children with CP, Pennington and McConachie (1999) showed that elicited conversational techniques were effective in increasing the children's communication. Findings highlight the importance of providing family members and other caregivers training to facilitate communication as one element in promoting optimal independence.

CLINICAL IMPLICATIONS AND FUTURE DIRECTIONS

Children with NDCs that include significant physical impairments often have unique assessment and intervention needs, particularly for those with a combination of motoric and communicative impairments. Standardized cognitive and psychological assessment instruments largely utilize verbal and/or motoric responses. The limitations to "universal assessment" practices have played out in schools, with continued psychological evaluation reports that essentially determine that "the child is not testable," leading to ongoing concerns that abilities and potential are underestimated and/or needs are underidentified. Recent alternative assessments offered in school settings at least partially address functional–adaptive skill levels but typically do not emphasize specific cognitive and academic skill needs. While there have been some attempts to develop accessible tests and evaluation strategies, there is a critical need for more standardized options in the presentation of stimuli and modality of response. For example, there are currently no standardized tests of phonological processing for nonverbal children with significant motoric impairments. To an extent, computerized assessments may have significant potential to address these needs, but this will involve careful psychometric study of these essentially new instruments.

Apart from accessibility concerns, the current review of neuropsychological studies highlights the importance of cognitive assessments that go beyond IQ. A significant portion of children with CP or SB have complex profiles that may include relative strength in some aspects of verbal functioning, impairments in others, impairments in some nonverbal functions, attentional difficulties, and types of executive dysfunction. Children with impairments in visuoperception and visuospatial skill may have unique needs in academic instruction, including early reading acquisition that may require additional strategies beyond the typical language-associated dyslexia interventions (Bakker, 1992; Rourke, 1995; Barnes, Faulkner, & Dennis, 2001).

At this point, it is not clear to what extent an NDC places the child at specific risk for attention-deficit/hyperactivity disorder (ADHD) or whether the underlying neuropsychological profiles of children with NDCs and ADHD are the same or different; for example, Are there ways in which motoric impairments and activity limitations mask the assessment of ADHD symptomatology on behavior rating scales? Yet there is recent evidence that for those who meet ADHD criteria, pharmacological intervention may be beneficial (Gross-Tsur, Shalev, Badihi, & Manor, 2002).

The clear evidence of risk for dependency in children with NDCs is met with a distinct paucity of assessment tools. The most common behavioral rating instruments completed by parents and teachers do not have subscales that assess dependency (Achenbach, 1991; Reynolds & Kamphaus, 1992). Interestingly, apart from specific social behavior rating instruments, these general screening instruments also do not assess assertiveness, a critical area of concern in children with disabilities. In addition to the need for new instruments that assess dependency and the associated family interaction patterns, NDC risks highlight the need to include a careful assessment of social integration in the school and community.

The combination of cognitive and/or communicative impairments, lack of assertiveness, and inflexible meeting structures usually preclude optimal participation of the adolescent with an NDC in school planning, and specifically in individualized education planning (IEP) meetings. However, technological advances present new opportunities for IEP participation, including the use of student-driven visual presentations using PowerPoint pictorial formats and video presentations of interests and capabilities. Clearly, some of the needs of children with NDCs will best be met by a willingness to "think outside the box."

The current review leads to a number of suggested directions for future research with the NDC population. In general, research with these populations has only recently begun to go beyond within-group descriptive analyses, and issues in choice of proper comparison groups have come to the fore. For example, little has been done to identify the separate contributions of physical and cognitive impairments and extrafamilial socioenvironmental factors on psychosocial development. Much of the work on cognitive predictors of psychosocial outcomes has utilized IQ, but clearly we are at the point where more refined neuropsychologically informed models can be tested. Studies of the neuropsychology of CP typically do not include neuroimaging data, limiting our understanding of brain–behavior relations in these conditions; however, there does appear to be an increasing literature utilizing a variety of imaging techniques.

There are other important differences within the NDC populations, such as those related to communicative impairments for which little is known about associated psychosocial risks and needs. Age at onset has important implications for psychosocial outcomes as well, and further study of acquired versus congenital group needs is recommended. Limited study of children with acquired conditions has suggested gender differences in outcomes and needs (Bohnert, Parker, & Warschausky, 1997; Donders & Woodward, 2003); there remains a paucity of study of gender-specific needs in the NDC population. Clearly, many of these research directions will be explored most effectively through collaborations between researchers who have traditionally functioned separately within the artificial boundaries of disciplines such as child development, pediatrics, and rehabilitation.

ACKNOWLEDGMENTS

Completion of this chapter was supported by U.S. Department of Education grants, including an Office of Special Education Programs model demonstration project (No. H324M020077) and field-initiated project (No. H324C0020026), and a National Institute on Disability and Rehabilitation field-initiated project award (No. H133G000038).

REFERENCES

Achenbach, T. M. (1991). *Manual for the Child Behavioral Checklist and 1991 Profile*. Burlington, VT: University of Vermont, Department of Psychiatry.

Allen, R. M. (1958). Suggestions for adaptive administration of intelligence tests for those with cerebral palsy: Part II. *Cerebral Palsy Review, 19*, 6–7.

Ammerman, R. T., Kane, V. R., Slomka, G. T., Reigel, D. H., Franzen, M. D., & Gadow, K. D. (1998). Psychiatric symptomatology and family functioning in children and adolescents with spina bifida. *Journal of Clinical Psychology in Medical Settings, 5*, 449–465.

Appleton, P. L., Ellis, N. C., Minchom, P. E., Lawson, V., Boll, V., & Jones, P. (1997). Depressive symptoms and concept in young people with spina bifida. *Journal of Pediatric Psychology, 22*, 707–722.

Bakker, D. J. (1992). Neuropsychological classification and treatment of dyslexia. *Journal of Learning Disabilities, 25*(2), 102–109.

Barnes, M. A., Faulkner, H. J., & Dennis, M. (2001). Poor reading comprehension despite fast word decoding in children with hydrocephalus. *Brain and Language, 76*, 35–44.

Baumrind, D., & Black, A. E. (1967). Socialization practices associated with dimensions of competence in preschool boys and girls. *Child Development, 38*, 291–327.

Bax, M. C. O. (1964). Terminology and classification of cerebral palsy. *Developmental Medicine and Child Neurology, 6*, 295–297.

Blair, E. (2001). Trends in cerebral palsy. *Indian Journal of Pediatrics, 68*, 433–437.

Bohnert, A., Parker, J., & Warschausky, S. (1997). Friendship and social adjustment of children following a traumatic brain injury; an exploratory investigation. *Developmental Neuropsychology, 13*, 477–486.

Brookshire, B. L., Fletcher, J. M., Bohan, T. P., Landry, S. H., Davidson, K. C., & Francis, D. J. (1995). Verbal and nonverbal skill discrepancies in children with hydrocephalus: A five year longitudinal follow-up. *Journal of Pediatric Psychology, 20*, 785–800.

Byrne, J. M., Dywan, C. A., & Connolly, J. F. (1995). An innovative method to assess the receptive vocabulary of children with cerebral palsy using event-related brain potentials. *Journal of Clinical and Experimental Neuropsychology, 17*, 9–19.

Carlsson, M., Hagberg, G., & Olsson, I. (2003). Clinical and etiological aspects of ep-

ilepsy in children with cerebral palsy. *Developmental Medicine and Child Neurology, 45*, 371–376.
Christ, S. E., White, D. A., Brunstrom, J. E., & Abrams, R. (2003). Inhibitory control following perinatal brain injury. *Neuropsychology, 17*, 171–178.
Coakley, R. M., Holmbeck, G. N., Friedman, D., Greenley, R. N., & Thill, A. W. (2002). A longitudinal study of pubertal timing, parent–child conflict, and cohesion in families of young adolescents with spina bifida. *Journal of Pediatric Psychology, 27*(5), 461–473.
Cowan, L. D., Bodensteiner, J. B., Leviton, A., & Doherty, L. (1989). Prevalence of the epilepsies in children and adolescents. *Epilepsia, 30*, 94–106.
Del Bigio, M. R. (1993). Neuropathological changes caused by hydrocephalus: A review. *Acta Neuropathologica, 85*, 573–585.
Dennis, M., Fitz, C., Netley, C., Sugar, J., Harwood-Nash, H., & Humphreys, R. (1981). The intelligence of hydrocephalic children. *Archives of Neurology, 38*, 607–615.
Dennis, M., Fletcher, J. M., Rogers, T., Hetherington, R., & Francis, D. J. (2002). Object-based and action-based visual perception in children with spina bifida and hydrocephalus. *Journal of the International Neuropsychological Society, 8*, 95–106.
Donders, J., Canady, A. J., & Rourke, B. P. (1990). Psychometric intelligence after infantile hydrocephalus: A critical review and reinterpretation. *Child's Nervous System, 6*, 148–154.
Donders, J., & Woodward, H. R. (2003). Gender as a moderator of memory after traumatic brain injury in children. *Journal of Head Trauma Rehabilitation, 18*(2), 106–115.
Dyste, G. N., Menezes, A. H., & Van Gilder, J. C. (1989). Symptomatic Chiari malformations: An analysis of presentation, management and long-term outcome. *Journal of Neurosurgery, 71*, 159–168.
Escobar, G. J., Littenberg, B., & Petitti, D. B. (1991). Outcome among surviving very low birth weight infants: A meta-analysis. *Archives of Disease in Childhood, 66*, 204–211.
Fedrizzi, E., Anderloni, A., Bono, R., Bova, S., Farinotti, M., Inverno, M., & Savoiardo, S. (1998). Eye-movement disorders and visual–perceptual impairment in diplegic children born preterm: A clinical evaluation. *Developmental Medicine and Child Neurology, 40*, 682–688.
Fletcher, J. M., Bohan, T. P., Brandt, M. E., Dramer, L. A., Brookshire, B. L., Thorstad, K., Davidson, K. C., Francis, D. J., McCauley, S. R., & Baumgartner, J. E. (1996). Morphometric evaluation of the hydrocephalic brain: Relationships with cognitive development. *Child's Nervous System, 12*, 192–199.
Fletcher, J. M., Dennis, M., & Northrup, H. (2000). Hydrocephalus. In K. O. Yeates, M. D. Ris, & H. G. Taylor (Eds.), *Pediatric neuropsychology: Research, theory, and practice* (pp. 25–46). New York: Guilford Press.
Fletcher, J. M., Francis, D., Thompson, N., Brookshire, B., Bohan, T., Landry, S., Davidson, K., & Milner, M. (1992). Verbal and nonverbal skill discrepancies in

hydrocephalic children. *Journal of Clinical and Experimental Neuropsychology, 14*, 593–609.

Frey, L., & Hauser, W. A. (2000). *Online Mendelian inheritance in man, OMIM.* McKusick–Nahans Institute for Genetic Medicine, Johns Hopkins University (Baltimore, MD) and National Center for Biotechnology Information, National Library of Medicine (Bethesda, MD). Retrieved from www.cnbi.nlm.nih.gov/omim.

Frey, L., & Hauser, W. A. (2003). Epidemiology of neural tube defects. *Epilepsia, 44*(Suppl. 3), 4–13.

Graham, E. M., Holcroft, C. J., Rai, K. K., Donahue, P. K., & Allen, M. C. (2004). Neonatal cerebral white matter injury in preterm infants is associated with culture positive infections and only rarely with metabolic acidosis. *American Journal of Obstetrics and Gynecology, 191*, 1305–1310.

Gross-Tsur, V., Shalev, R. S., Badihi, N., & Manor, O. (2002). Efficacy of methylphenidate in patients with cerebral palsy and attention-deficit hyperactivity disorder (ADHD). *Journal of Child Neurology, 17*(12), 893–866.

Hagberg, B., Hagberg, H., Beckung, E., & Uvebrant, P. (2001). Changing panorama of cerebral palsy in Sweden: VIII. Prevalence and origin in the birth year period 1991–1994. *Acta Paediatrica, 90*, 271–277.

Hagberg, B., Hagberg, G., & Olow, I. (1975). The changing panorama of cerebral palsy in Sweden (1954–1970): II. Analysis of the various syndromes. *Acta Paediatrica Scandanavica, 64*, 193–200.

Holmbeck, G. N., Coakley, R. M., Hommeyer, J. S., Shapera, W. E., & Westhoven, V. C. (2002a). Observed and perceived dyadic and systemic functioning in families of preadolescents with spina bifida. *Journal of Pediatric Psychology, 27*, 177–189.

Holmbeck, G. N., Johnson, S. Z., Wills, K. E., McKernon, W., Rose, B., Erklin, S., & Kemper, T. (2002b). Observed and perceived parental overprotection in relation to psychosocial adjustment in preadolesents with a physical disability: The mediational role of behavioral autonomy. *Journal of Consulting and Clinical Psychology, 70*, 96–110.

Holmbeck, G. N., Westhoven, V. C., Phillips, W. S., Bowers, R., Gruse, C., Nikolopoulos, T., Wienke, C. M., & Davison, K. (2003). A mulimethod, multi-informant, and multidimensional perspective on psychosocial adjustment in pre-adolescents with spina bifida. *Journal of Consulting and Clinical Psychology, 71*, 782–796.

Hommeyer, J. S., Holmbeck, G. N., Wills, K. E., & Coers, S. (1999). Condition severity and psychosocial functioning in pre-adolescents with spina bifida: Disentangling proximal functional status and distal adjustment outcomes. *Journal of Pediatric Psychology, 24*, 499–509.

Hugdahl, K. H., & Carlsson, G. (1994). Dichotic listening and focused attention in children with hemiplegic cerebral palsy. *Journal of Clinical and Experimental Neuropsychology, 16*, 84–92.

Hulme, C., Thomson, N., Muir, C., & Lawrence, A. (1984). Speech rate and the development of short-term memory span. *Journal of Experimental Child Psychology, 38*, 241–253.

Iddon, J. L., Morgan, D. J. R., Loveday, C., Sahakian, B. J., & Pickard, J. D. (2004). Neuropsychological profile of young adults with spina bifida with or without

hydrocephalus. *Journal of Neurology, Neurosurgery and Psychiatry, 75,* 1112–1118.
Ito, J.-I., Sayo, H., Araki, A., Tanaka, H., Tasaki, T., Cho, K., & Miyamoto, A. (1996). Assessment of visuoperceptual disturbance in children with spastic diplegia using measurements of the lateral ventricles on cerebral MRI. *Developmental Medicine and Child Neurology, 38,* 496–502.
Kallen, K. (1998). Maternal smoking, body mass index, and neural tube defects. *American Journal of Epidemiology, 147,* 1103–1111.
Krageloh-Mann, I., Hagberg, G., Meisner, C., Schelp, B., Haas, G., Eeg-Olofsson, K. E., Selbmann, H. K., Hagberg, B., & Michaelis, R. (1993). Bilateral spastic cerebral palsy—a comparative study between south-west Germany and eastern Sweden: I. Clinical patterns and disabilities. *Developmental Medicine and Child Neurology, 35,* 1037–1047.
Krageloh-Mann, I., Helber, A., Mader, I., Staudt, M., Wolff, M., Groenendaal, F., & DeVries, L. (2002). Bilateral lesions of thalamus and basal ganglia: Origin and outcome. *Developmental Medicine and Child Neurology, 44,* 477–484.
Kraus, F. T. (1997). Cerebral palsy and thrombi in placental vessels of the fetus: Insights from litigation. *Human Pathology, 28,* 246–248.
Lavigne, J. V., & Faier-Routman, J. (1992). Psychological adjustment to pediatric physical disorders: A meta-analytic review. *Journal of Pediatric Psychology, 17,* 133–157.
Loss, N., Yeates, K. O., & Enrile, B. G. (1998). Attention in children with myelomeningocele. *Child Neuropsychology, 4*(1), 7–20.
MacHenry, J. C. R. M., Nevin, N. C., & Merrett, J. D. (1979). Comparison of central nervous system malformations in spontaneous abortions in Northern Ireland and south-east England. *British Medical Journal, 1,* 1395–1397.
Manuel, J. C., Balkrishnan, R., Camacho, F., Smith, B. P., & Koman, L. A. (2003). Factors associated with self-esteem in pre-adolescents and adolescents with cerebral palsy. *Journal of Adolescent Health, 32,* 456–458.
McAndrew, I. (1979). Adolescents and young people with spina bifida. *Developmental Medicine and Child Neurology, 21,* 619–621.
McDermott, S., Coker, A. L., Mani, S., Krishnaswami, S., Nagle, R. J., Barnett-Queen, L. L., & Wuori, D. F. (1996). A population-based analysis of behavior problems in children with cerebral palsy. *Journal of Pediatric Psychology, 21,* 447–463.
McKernon, W. L., Holmbeck, G. N., Colder, C. R., Hommeyer, J. S., Shapera, W., & Westhoven, V. (2001). Longitudinal study of observed and perceived family influences on problem-focused coping behaviors of preadolescents with spina bifida. *Journal of Pediatric Psychology, 26,* 41–54.
McNeely, P. D., & Howes, W. J. (2004). Ineffectiveness of dietary folic acid supplementation on the incidence of lipomyelomeningocele: Pathogenetic implications. *Journal of Neurosurgery, 100,* 98–100.
Mitchell, L. E., Adzick, N. S., Melchionne, J., Pasquariello, P. S., Sutton, L. N., & Whitehead, A. S. (2004). Spina bifida. *Lancet, 364,* 1885–1895.
Mutch, L., Alberman, E., Hadberg, B., Kodama, K., & Perat, M. V. (1992). Cerebral palsy epidemiology: Where are we now and where are we going? *Developmental Medicine and Child Neurology, 34,* 547–551.

Nelson, K. B. (2002). The epidemiology of cerebral palsy in term infants. *Mental Retardation and Developmental Disabilities Research Reviews, 8*, 146–150.
Nelson, K. B., & Grether, J. K. (1997). Maternal infection and cerebral palsy in infants of normal birth weight. *Journal of the American Medical Association, 251*, 1843–1848.
Nelson, K. B., & Grether, J. K. (1998). Potentially asphyxiating conditions and spastic cerebral palsy in infants of normal birth weight. *American Journal of Obstetrics and Gynecology, 179*, 507–513
Palisano, R., Rosenbaum, P., Walter, S., Russell, D., Wood, E., & Galuppi, B. (1997). Gross Motor Function Classification System. *Developmental Medicine and Child Neurology, 39*, 214–223.
Paneth, N., Qui, H., Rosenbaum, P., Saigal, S., Bishia, S., Jetton, J., den Ouden, L., Broyles, S., Tyson, J., & Kugler, K. (2003). Reliability of classification of cerebral palsy in low-birth weight children in four countries. *Developmental Medicine and Child Neurology, 45*, 628–633.
Pennington, L., & McConachie, H. (1999). Mother–child interaction revisited: Communication with non-speaking physically disabled children. *International Journal of Language and Communication Disorders, 34*, 391–416.
Pharoah, P. O. (2001). Twins and cerebral palsy. *Acta Paediatrica Supplement, 90*, 6–10.
Pharoah, P. O. D., Price, T. S., & Plomin, R. (2002). Cerebral palsy in twins: A national study. *Archive of Diseases in Childhood: Fetal and Neonatal Edition, 87*, F122–F124.
Pueyo, R., Junque, C., & Ventrell, P. (2003). Neuropsychological differences between bilateral dyskinetic and spastic cerebral palsy. *Journal of Child Neurology, 18*, 845–850.
Querido, J. G., Warner, T. D., & Eyberg, S. M. (2002). Parenting styles and child behavior in African American families of preschool children. *Journal of Clinical Child Psychology, 31*, 272–277.
Ralph, K., Moylan, P., Canady, A., & Simmons, S. (2000). The effects of multiple shunt revisions on neuropsychological functioning and memory. *Neurological Research, 22*, 131–136.
Reynolds, C. R., & Kamphaus, R. W. (1992). *Behavioral Assessment System for Children manual.* Circle Pines, MN: American Guidance Service.
Rourke, B. P. (1995). Treatment program for the child with NLD. In B. P. Rourke (Ed.), *Syndrome of nonverbal learning disabilities* (pp. 497–508). New York: Guilford Press.
Sabbadini, M., Bonanni, R., Carolesimo, G. A., & Caltagirone, C. (2001). Neuropsychological assessment of patients with severe neuromotor and verbal disabilities. *Journal of Intellectual Disabilities Research, 45*, 169–179.
Samren, E. B., van Duijn, C. M., Lieve Christiaens, G. C. M., Hofman, A., & Lindhout, D. (1999). Antiepileptic drug regimens and major congenital abnormalities in the offspring. *Annals of Neurology, 46*, 739–746.
Sarnat, H. B. (1992). *Cerebral dysgenesis: Embryology and clinical expression.* New York: Oxford University Press.
Serdaroglu, G., Tekgul, H., Kitis, O., Serdaroglu, E., & Gokben, S. (2004). Correlative value of magnetic resonance imaging for neurodevelopmental outcome in

periventricular leukomalacia. *Developmental Medicine and Child Neurology, 46,* 733–739.

Shaffer, J., Friedrich, W. N., Shurtleff, D. B., & Wolf, L. Y. (1985). Cognitive achievement status of children with myelomeningocele. *Journal of Pediatric Psychology, 10,* 325–336.

Shaw, G. M., Velie, E. M., & Schaffer, D. (1996). Risk of neural tube defect-affected pregnancies among obsess women. *Journal of the American Medical Association, 275,* 1093–1096.

Steenbergen, B., Meulenbroek, R. G. J., & Rosenbaum, D. A. (2004). Constraints on grip selection in hemiparetic cerebral palsy: Effects of lesional side, end-point accuracy, and context. *Cognitive Brain Research, 19,* 145–159.

Suarez, L., Hendricks, K., Felkner, M., & Gunter, E. (2003). Maternal serum vitamin B12 levels and risk for neural tube defects in a Texas–Mexican border population. *Epidemiology, 13,* 81–88.

Surman, G., Newkick, H., & Johnson, A. (2003). Cerebral palsy rates among low-birth weight infants fell in the 1990s. *Developmental Medicine and Child Neurology, 45,* 456–462.

Tracht, V. S. (1948). Preliminary findings on testing cerebral palsied with Raven's Progressive Matrices. *Exceptional Child, 15,* 77–79

Tulipan, N., Bruner, J. P., Hernanz-Schulman, M., Lowe, L. H., Walsh, W. F., Nickolaus, D., & Oakes, W. J. (1999). The effect of intrauterine myelomeingocele repair on the central nervous system structure and neurologic function. *Pediatric Neurosurgery, 31,* 183–188.

Uvebrant, P. (1988). Hemiplegic cerebral palsy: Aetiology and outcome. *Acta Paediatrica Scandanavica, 345*(Suppl.), 1–100.

White, D. A., Craft, S., Hale, S., & Park, T. S. (1994). Working memory and articulation rate in children with spastic diplegic cerebral palsy. *Neuropsychology, 8,* 180–186.

Wills, K. E., Holmbeck, G. N., Dillon, K., & McLone, D. G. (1990). Intelligence and achievement in children with myelomeningocele. *Journal of Pediatric Psychology, 15,* 161–176.

6

Chronic Illness and Neurodevelopmental Disability

RONALD T. BROWN

Chronic disease and disability refer to disease states that have symptoms with a protracted course and involvement of one or more organ systems (e.g., brain, heart, lung, blood). A condition that persists for more than 3 months within 1 year and necessitates ongoing care from a health care provider is considered to be chronic (Wallander, Thompson, & Alriksson-Schmidt, 2003). Frequently, chronic conditions impact children's functioning for extended periods of time and sometimes for life (Wallander et al., 2003). While recent technologies in medical management sometimes have made possible control of symptoms and reductions in exacerbations of symptomatology and disease presentation, chronic disabilities and illnesses frequently cannot be cured (Wallander et al., 2003).

Each chronic physical condition has a distinct biological process and pathophysiology, and treatment is generally individually designed for a specific condition. The majority of research in pediatric psychology has focused on specific disease and diagnostic entities, although there is compelling support for several commonalities in psychosocial functioning across chronic conditions and disabilities. For this reason, many experts (Rolland, 1994) have recommended that the psychosocial study of children and adolescents with chronic disabilities and physical conditions follow a noncategorical approach. Wallander et al. (2003) have recommended that specific disease dimensions be the focus of investigation including psychosocial affects associated with the nature of onset and course of the disease, life threat potential, intrusiveness or plan of treatment, visibility and social stigma, stability versus crises, and secondary and functional cognitive disability. Thus, according to many experts (e.g., Rolland, 1994), it is the variance across each of these aforementioned dimensions that has implication for adjustment rather than the specific category of disease per se.

GENERAL EPIDEMIOLOGY AND PATHOPHYSIOLOGY

The percentage of children with severe long-term disease has more than doubled over the past two decades, in part due to technological advances in medical and surgical care. Specifically, several factors account for the increase, including advances in health care reflecting improved early diagnosis and treatment, the survival of infants of extreme prematurity or low birth weight, and new diseases, such as prenatal drug exposure and HIV/AIDS.

Approximately 10–20% of children and adolescents experience one or more chronic health conditions by the age of 17 years (Newacheck et al., 1998); about 2–4% of children have a disease of such severity that it regularly interferes with usual daily activities (Behrman & Vaughan, 1996). It has been estimated that approximately 1 million children in the United States have a chronic illness that may impair their daily functioning. Thus, the disease results in significant functional impairment or, for many children, neurodevelopmental impairments. An additional 10 million children have a less serious form of chronic conditions, including allergies that affect 10–15% of the total childhood population (Brown, 2004; Thompson & Gustafson, 1996).

Many chronic pediatric disorders are associated with marked neurological and psychological morbidity (i.e., disruption of normal developmental processes and adaptive competencies) and hence result in significant functional impairment (Brown, 1999; Roberts, 2003; Thompson & Gustafson, 1996). Behavioral factors (e.g., diet, treatment nonadherence, substance abuse, and neurological impairments) are important variables in predicting the onset, course, and prognosis of many disorders and injuries, and thus contribute to disease and injury onset as well as disease maintenance (Brannon & Feist, 1997). Table 6.1 presents a summary of disorders from major pediatric subspecialties, the incidence of the disorders, and examples of relevant psychological aspects for each of the disorders.

PSYCHOLOGICAL AND SOCIAL OUTCOMES ASSOCIATED WITH CHRONIC ILLNESS AND DISABILITY

Children and adolescents with chronic illness are predicted to have optimal adaptation to their disease state when protective or resistance factors out-

TABLE 6.1. Pediatric Disorders from Major Pediatric Subspecialty Populations with Examples of Relevant Psychological Aspects

Subspecialty	Condition	Representative psychological aspects
Trauma	Orthopedic trauma, burns	Coping with intense postinjury pain, adjustment to disfigurement, disability
Cardiology	Congenital heart defects	Impaired cognitive function secondary to hypoxia, parental guilt about responsibility for anomaly
	Acquired heart defects	Restriction of activity secondary to blood thinner used in valve replacement
	Hypertension	Cognitive/mood effects of antihypertensive medication
Endocrinology	Diabetes mellitus	Nonadherence with complex self-care regimen
	Short stature	Self-concept, peer relations
Gastroenterology	Encopresis	Coercive parent–child interactions around toileting, impaired child self-esteem
	Nonorganic recurrent abdominal pain	Reinforcement of child "sick" behavior, family dysfunction
	Ileitis (Crohn's disease)	Impaired self-esteem
Hematology	Sickle cell disease	Recurrent pain, cognitive changes
	Hemophilia	Chronic arthritic pain
Infectious disease	AIDS	Cognitive deterioration, depression
	Meningitis	Cognitive changes
Neonatology	Brochopulmonary dysplasia	Feeding disorders, developmental delays
	Apnea	Sleep regulation
Nephrology	Renal failure	Treatment nonadherence, cognitive symptoms
	Cushing syndrome	Muscle weakness, body composition changes
Neurology	Headaches	Stress
	Seizures	Medication-induced changes in cognitive functioning
Oncology	Leukemia	Coping with aversive medical diagnostic and treatment procedures
	Solid tumors	Pain, treatment-related cognitive changes, death and dying issues

weigh risk factors (Wallander et al., 2003). Protective or resistance factors include intrapersonal variables (e.g., temperament, problem-solving skills), social–ecological factors (e.g., stable family environment, adequate social support systems, and adequate financial resources), and stress processing (e.g., adaptive coping strategies). Risk factors include disease and disability parameters (e.g., disease type, severity of symptoms, and central nervous system involvement or neurological impairment), inadequate competencies, and a high frequency of psychosocial stressors.

A chronic illness that is comorbid with a neurological impairment is a risk factor that may predispose some children and adolescents to diminished self-concept and self-esteem (Nassau & Drotar, 1995). Social competencies and self-esteem are likely mediated by a number of biological and psychosocial variables, including the severity of the disease itself; functional limitations, including associated neurological impairments that are imposed by the disease; and the degree of social support available to the affected child from peers (Pendley, Dahlquist, & Dryer, 1997). The outcomes associated with chronic illness and disability include emotional and behavioral characteristics, school and academic outcomes that may be influenced by neurological impairments; familial factors; developmental changes over time; and, finally, child, family, and environmental factors.

Emotional, Behavioral, and Social Outcomes

Children with chronic illness as a group are at significant risk for difficulties in psychological adjustment, including behavioral and emotional problems; problems with self-esteem, social adjustment, and peer relationships; and difficulties with academic performance that may be secondary to neurological impairments (for review, see Wallander et al., 2003).

At the same time, only a minority of children with chronic illnesses evidence maladjustment (Wallander et al., 2003). Outcomes appear to be dependent on specific disease characteristics, including type of condition, severity of condition, comorbidities associated with the illness that may include neurological impairment, duration of disease, and the child's functional status. Other mediating and moderating variables have been posited: gender, age of the child or age of disease onset, the child's temperament, methods of coping with the disease, as well as cognitive processes including perceived stress and perceptions of physical appearance and stigma associated with a particular disease (Wallander et al., 2003).

Adequate assessment of children's adjustment and adaptation to chronic illness necessitates multiple methods of assessment and informants across settings and situations (Klinnert, McQuaid, McCormick, Adinoff, & Bryant, 2000). An important construct in this context is quality of life, but it can be difficult to discern what is and is not in fact disease-related (Wallander et al., 2003). Thus, neurological impairments, functional implications, and disease and treatment-related symptoms relevant to a specific disease, as well as how the disease impacts psychosocial adjustment, are important individual sources of information. These sources of information are critical for the purpose of understanding the whole child and not simply the child with a disease.

Academic and Cognitive Outcomes

For many chronic diseases and disabilities, either the illness itself or the treatment applied in its management exerts some type of influence on CNS functioning that in turn impacts cognition, learning, or emotional functioning that significantly affects classroom or academic performance. In this section, we review briefly those diseases in which a preponderance of research suggests that the disease or its associated treatment impacts cognition, learning, and hence school performance. We also review those diseases for which associated neurological impairments also may influence disease management. One chronic illness that is increasing in prevalence in school-age children is asthma, and there are several excellent reviews available on the topic (e.g., Annett, 2004; McQuaid & Walders, 2003). In general, the research suggests that poor asthma management, the use of steroid therapy, and a history of respiratory arrests are generally associated with poor cognitive outcome among these children and adolescents (Annett, 2004). Insulin-dependent diabetes mellitus (IDDM) is another chronic illness in which cognitive impairments have resulted from early disease onset and a history of poor disease management (for review, see Wysocki, Greco, & Buckloh, 2003; Young-Hyman, 2004). In another chronic illness that affects many children and adolescents, particularly in inner-city regions of the country, Smith, Martin, and Wolters (2004) have reviewed recent and innovative advances in the prognosis for children and adolescents with HIV/AIDS. For these children, specific issues related to school functioning include frequent absences and anxiety about social relationships that may be associated with disclosure of the illness. In addition, for children and adolescents with HIV/AIDS who have prolonged absences, facilitation of school reentry also is important. Finally, for all schoolchildren, the prevention of HIV/AIDS through safe health practices is a high priority and of relevance to pediatric psychologists.

Williams (2004) has provided a critical review of the literature in the area of seizure disorders, a frequently occurring neurological condition in childhood. Conclusions are that the disease, as well as its pharmacological management, significantly impacts the learning and school environment. In general, the influence of seizure disorders on cognitive and behavioral outcomes includes medication effects, ongoing seizures, and the stigma associated with the disease (Williams, 2004). Similarly, for children and adolescents with sickle cell disease and hemophilia, it has been demonstrated that a small, albeit significant, subgroup of children experiences marked difficulties in cognitive and psychosocial functioning due to significant neurological involvement (Brown, Mulhern, & Simonian, 2003; Casey & Brown, 2003). More recently, a program of research has delineated specific risk factors (e.g., severity of disease) and screening tools that assist in the identification of children and adolescents with sickle cell disease who are especially at risk for cognitive impairment (Casey & Brown, 2003; Kral et al., 2003). This screening and identification of central nervous system involvement are important, since such impairments are often indicative of further disease progression.

As has been noted previously, many pediatric diseases, such as childhood cancer, were fatal prior to current medical advances, but now a significant number of children can expect to live beyond these diseases. Armstrong and Briery (2004) have reviewed the literature on long-term survivors of childhood cancer. Generally, they conclude that the challenges previously faced by these children and adolescents only in hospitals must now be recognized in classrooms. Specifically, the long-term consequences of chemotherapy and radiation therapy on learning outcome are well documented (for review, see Brown, Mulhern, & Simonian, 2000), and as of recent, the emerging literature is beginning to address appropriate management of these learning problems (Butler & Copeland, in press; Mulhern et al., 2004). Clearly, those professionals working in school settings need to collaborate with physicians and other health care providers. This expanded treatment team can provide services for long-term survivors of cancer, and the collaboration represents the next step in the designation of cancer as a chronic illness rather than a fatal disease.

One prevalent, albeit under-researched disease in the area of pediatric chronic illness is congenital heart disease, which frequently affects neurocognitive functioning and classroom learning (DeMaso, 2004). DeMaso has concluded that children with congenital heart problems may manifest a number of vulnerabilities in cognition and emotional and social functioning, all of which affect adjustment and adaptation at school.

Familial Outcomes

Children do not seek health care in isolation from the environment in which they reside (Kazak et al., 2003). The family environment appears to be an important predictor of adaptation to the disease or disability by the children who are ill and their caregivers (Kazak et al., 2003). Alderfer and Kazak (in press) have asserted that disability or chronic illness occurs within a complex network of social systems, including the family. The family environment refers to family members' adaptation, social support systems, and family utilitarian resources (e.g., intact, divorced, presence of siblings, family income and health care financing, parental responsibilities and leisure time, and parental education level). There also has been compelling support for the interrelation of family structure, child adjustment, and disease management (for review, see Kazak et al., 2003). Specifically, greater levels of cohesive and adaptive family functioning have been demonstrated to buffer the potential detrimental effects of caring for hard-to-manage, chronically ill children (Ievers, Brown, Lambert, Hsu, & Eckman, 1998). Furthermore, adaptive family relationships and parental psychological adjustment have been found to be positively associated with better psychological adaptation for children with chronic disease (Kazak et al., 2003).

Rolland (1993) has emphasized that the complex mutual interaction between illness, the family member diagnosed with illness, and the family's conceptualization and adaptation to illness is a developmental process that unfolds across time. Health care beliefs provide coherence to family life and facilitate the continuity between the past, present, and future, and, most importantly, provide a means of negotiating the serious illness or disability (Alderfer & Kazak, in press).

Other important variables in understanding the influence of chronic illness on the family system include marital distress, sibling relationships, and parent–child relationships. For example, approximately 40% of couples report marital distress around the time of their child's diagnosis with cancer (Patistea, Makrodimitri, & Panteli, 2000), while siblings frequently experience feelings of marginalization throughout their brother's or sister's cancer experience (for review, see Alderfer & Kazak, in press). Finally, parenting and parent–child relationships often are influenced by a chronic illness whereby significant problems with parenting distress, overprotectiveness, problems with discipline, and confusion in communication between parent and child have been reported (see Alderfer & Kazak, in press). Family relations and family knowledge about disease also have been demonstrated to be key ingredients for adherence to disease or disability treatment regimens. However, few investigators have tested the family system as a means of enhancing adherence (La Greca & Schuman, 1995).

Developmental Changes over Time

Unlike their adult counterparts, children and adolescents with chronic physical and neurological conditions are developing organisms. The systems in which they interact, such as the family, also experience significant developmental milestones and critical periods (Wallander et al., 2003). Unfortunately, much of the research in the disability and chronic illness literature has not reflected developmental models and concepts within this research. As Wallander et al. have recommended, general developmental processes should become more salient features of the conceptualizations of adjustment for children and adolescents with chronic disease and disabilities. Greater research efforts need to focus on longitudinal designs, the course of the physical disorder or disability and its management, and, finally, the interaction of the disease, possible neurological involvement, the child's developmental course, and the family (Wallander et al., 2003). Finally, some investigators have conceptualized chronic illness or disability as a specific stressor or trauma that exerts particular influences on the developing child, the family, or specific subsystems within the family, such as siblings (Kazak et al., 2004).

With regard to children's development and changes of adjustment over the course of time, longitudinal studies are most important in addressing the cognitive and psychosocial prognosis of children with chronic illnesses. Longitudinal designs also may address an important issue in health and rehabilitation psychology, so as to determine specifically how psychosocial adjustment influences physical health (Wallander et al., 2003). For example, one study has provided important data to suggest that adjustment problems among adolescents with diabetes predict poor metabolic control during early adulthood (Bryden et al., 2001). Similarly, in a longitudinal investigation, Holmes, Overstreet, and Greer (1997) have demonstrated specific cognitive predictors of self-care behaviors among youth with diabetes. Such findings are particularly valuable in predicting later disease adaptation and specific risk factors for poor disease management.

Interestingly, while few longitudinal studies are available in the pediatric chronic disease and disability literatures, the majority of available studies in the extant literature have generally reported good adjustment and adaptation of children and adolescents at follow-up assessment (for review, see Wallander et al., 2003). One exception to this body of literature is the program of research conducted by Thompson and associates (Thompson et al., 1994a, 1994b), who found that adjustment problems in children with cystic fibrosis and sickle cell disease were fairly constant over the course of a 1-year follow-up period.

Clearly the longitudinal research in the chronic illness and disability literatures, still actually in its infancy, is characterized by heterogeneity in samples, chronic conditions, developmental functioning of the samples, as well as the length of follow-up period evaluated (Wallander et al., 2003). Greater research efforts are sorely needed that will test the association of chronic illness and psychosocial adjustment by examining critical developmental periods and transitions through longitudinal research designs. This is clearly a research agenda that awaits development over the next decade.

INDIVIDUAL FACTORS AFFECTING PSYCHOSOCIAL OUTCOME

Over the past several years, the chronic illness literature has been characterized by an examination of the variability in the psychosocial adjustment and adaptation of children with chronic illnesses. In part, the purpose of this program of research has been to understand better the psychological correlates of disease and disability, as well as to accumulate data for the purpose of developing and implementing intervention efforts for these children and their families. Some investigators have conceptualized three broad dimensions in our understanding of those mediators and moderators associated with a chronic condition or disability (Wallander et al., 2003). These dimensions include disease condition, specific child parameters, and social–ecological parameters. We now turn our attention to specific conditions or disease parameters that include disease severity, functional status, and duration of disease.

Condition Parameters

Findings have revealed few differences in adjustment or adaptation among specific disease categories (Perrin, Ayoub, & Willett, 1993; Wallander et al., 2003). A notable exception, however, is children with chronic illnesses or disabilities that involve the central nervous system. Specifically, children with central nervous system involvement have been found to evidence a greater frequency of behavioral problems and social difficulties than those children without neurological disorders (Nassau & Drotar, 1997). Moreover, cognitive impairment also has been demonstrated to impact disease management (for review, see Rovet & Fernandes, 1999; Young-Hyman, 2004). With regard to severity of condition, in general, the data have been mixed, with some investigations demonstrating compelling support for a significant association between adjustment and severity of disease for children, including those with seizure disorders and asthma, while other research has yielded inconsistent findings for children and adolescents with sickle cell disease, diabetes, and spina bifida (for review, see Thompson & Gustafson, 1996).

One variable that consistently appears to be associated with children's psychological adjustment is their functional status, including neurological status, severity of physical disabilities, and motor skills. For example, for children with hydrocephaly, Fletcher et al. (1995) provided important data to suggest that motor skills are associated with behavioral problems. Wallander et al. (2003) have advocated for the use of functional status as a means of operationalizing disease severity across chronic disability and illness conditions. They have cautioned, however, about the importance of basing such functional measures on objective biomedical parameters, including degree of ambulation, pulmonary functioning, or metabolic control, so as to maintain functional status as independent from psychological adjustment and perceived disease severity. Academic performance is one critical functional outcome that also is associated with disease management, particularly for children and adolescents with IDDM (for review, see Rovet & Fernandes, 1999)

Finally, with regard to duration of disease or disability, the dearth of research in this area is primarily due to the few longitudinal studies with pediatric populations. The majority of these investigations have been correlational in design. In general, findings have suggested a significant association between psychological adjustment and duration of disease. Findings from these samples have generally revealed an increase in adjustment difficulties and depressive symptoms with longevity of disease (for review, see Wallander et al., 2003). Furthermore, for some diseases, including cancer and sickle cell disease, cognitive functioning has been found to be associated with duration of disease; greater disease duration has been associated with more impaired cognitive functioning (Brown, 1999). Again, the important question with regard to the relationship of psychological adjustment, cognitive functioning, and duration of illness begs longitudinal research that specifically addresses the direct influence of various disease condition parameters on psychological adaptation (Hommeyer, Holmbeck, Wills, & Coers, 1999).

Child Parameters

Gender

The majority of studies in the extant literature generally reveal no significant differences in reports of behavioral problems or adjustment difficulties as a function of gender (for review, see Wallander et al., 2003). Child reports, however, have influenced gender outcome, with girls generally reporting a higher frequency of distress symptoms than their male counterparts (for review, see Brown, Mulhern, & Simonian, 2000; Casey & Brown, 2003). For example, females with sickle cell disease have reported greater concerns about sexual development than their male counterparts, which in turn may be associated with findings of dissatisfaction with body image (for review, see Brown et al., 2006; Casey & Brown, 2003). Finally, female survivors of cancer have been found to suffer from greater cognitive impairments than their male counterparts, particularly females diagnosed and treated during the preschool years (Brown et al., 1998). In part, these findings have been attributed to hormonal influences on adolescent females.

Age

While the corpus of literature for children with chronic illness and disabilities has generally failed to provide support for an age effect on variables of psychological adjustment, including externalizing behavioral problems and self-esteem, there have been some mixed findings with regard to age of disease onset and psychological adjustment (for review, see Wallander et al., 2003). The majority of research in this area has examined children with IDDM, with some studies demonstrating support for greater externalizing behavioral difficulties among boys with disease onset after the age of 4 years, while other studies have failed to provide empirical support for such a relationship between chronological age and adjustment difficulties. Children with type 1 IDDM diagnosed during preschool have been found to evidence greater cognitive impairments than their peers identified during later childhood and adolescence (Rovet & Fernandes, 1999). In part, this is attributed to the development of the central nervous system during the preschool years. All of these aforementioned studies employed correlational designs. Clearly, longitudinal designs are necessary, particularly those studies that examine specific developmental tasks during critical developmental periods, including school entry, transition from middle school to high school, and transition to college (Wallander et al., 2003).

Coping and Cognitive Appraisals

Coping has been studied extensively in the pediatric literature, particularly as it affects management, as well as adaptation to the stressors and the demands, of a disease (Harbeck-Weber, Fisher, & Dittner, 2003). The association between styles of coping and children's adjustment in negotiating the stressors of a chronic illness or disability has been the topic of numerous investigations in the field of pediatric psychology (for review, see Harbeck-Weber et al., 2003), and research has clearly affirmed the importance of coping in the prediction of psychological and social adjustment in children with chronic illness and disability. For example, a positive relationship has been demonstrated between the use of avoidance coping and psychosocial problems (Frank, Blount, & Brown, 1997; Lewis & Kliewer, 1996), with coping also moderating the negative association between hope and anxiety in children and adolescents with sickle cell disease (Lewis & Kliewer, 1996). The assessment and measurement of coping is a major methodological issue in this literature, and a greater understanding is needed with regard to what specifically constitutes coping and the developmental changes of coping patterns (Wallander et al., 2003).

It also has been demonstrated that children and adolescents who feel control over their illness evidence better adjustment and adaptation than those who do not experience such control (Weithorn & McCabe, 1998). A self-perceived lack of a predictable association between one's behavior and the outcome of events may lead to feelings of helplessness in the child and may also pose a viable risk factor for depression or other psychopathology (for review, see Wallander et al., 2003). Thus, perceived stress of negative life events or daily hassles has been associated with poor psychological adjustment for various chronic diseases and disabilities (for review, see Wallander et al., 2003).

Social-Ecological Parameters

In this chapter, we conceptualize social factors as basic demographic variables that may predict either psychological adjustment or critical adaptations to disease, including health outcome. These social factors include social class or socioeconomic status; rural versus urban settings; access to health care; interaction of the health system, the child, and the family; family functioning; and peer support.

Socioeconomic Factors

Socioeconomic status represents a cluster of variables including education, occupation, and income that serve as an indicator of an individual's position within a social system (House & Williams, 2000). Socioeconomic and cultural factors have been demonstrated to be salient determinants of health outcome and adaptation to illness, with health outcome being positively associated with socioeconomic standing (Wingood & Keltner, 1999). Specifically, low socioeconomic status affects health care outcomes, because it limits access to preventive health care due to factors such as poor or no insurance coverage, exposure to less optimal environmental conditions (e.g., lead exposure, pollutants, and toxic wastes), and greater occupational hazards (e.g., disadvantaged individuals are more likely to perform manual labor in which there is greater risk of injury). Furthermore, children with disabilities and chronic illness from less affluent families have decreased access to quality health care, mental health care, and evidence-based diagnostic and treatment procedures (Wingood & Keltner, 1999). Finally, evidence also exists that children from more rural areas have less access to medical care, placing them at greater risk for poor health and adjustment difficulties that are associated with chronic disease and disability (Brown, Ojeda, Wynn, & Levan, 2000; Burns, Costello, Angold, Tweed, & Stangl, 1995).

Health Access in Underserved Rural Areas

A number of explanations have been offered for the persisting and increasing racial and ethnic disparities in health and mental health care. For instance, lower socioeconomic status, and living in rural areas in which there are a shortage of specialty care providers, including mental health providers and the lack of access to quality health care, are considered to be primary contributing factors to racial and ethnic disparities (Giachello & Arrom, 1997). Access to services for many children in rural and disadvantaged communities is sometimes exceedingly difficult because of a shortage of health care providers in these areas (American Academy of Pediatrics, 2000). Poor education and insufficient economic resources limit access to health insurance, connection to health care systems, and quality medical care, which further limit mental health promotion, disease prevention, and psychological adaptation to chronic disease and disability. Moreover, for ethnic and racial minorities and vulnerable populations, such as children with chronic disease and disabilities, environmental risks (e.g., crowded living conditions and substandard housing) also may pose risk factors for poor health, chronic stress, and poor coping. Notwithstanding these aforementioned risk factors, it is equally likely that the broader social, cultural, and political climate may influence racial and ethnic disparities in health care delivery. Societal racism, discrimination, and a dearth of culturally competent care within most of our health care system also contribute to this state of affairs (Giachello & Arrom, 1997).

Health Care Systems and Utilization Patterns

Relative to their Caucasian counterparts, children and their families from racial and ethnic minority groups are generally reported to have fewer visits to health care providers for ambulatory care, fewer well-child screenings, fewer immunizations, and a higher frequency of hospitalizations (Health Care Financing Administration, 1995). Of interest are the findings that these children and their families also wait longer to seek necessary medical care, present to medical providers with a greater frequency of acute medical health problems, and also tend to use more "home remedies" as a first response to illness. Furthermore, underreporting and denial of discomfort are frequent means of coping behavior for some minority and ethnic groups (Wilson, Rodrigue, & Taylor, 1997).

Racial and ethnic minority disparities have only recently been addressed among pediatric populations. Unfortunately, limited epidemiological data are available on the health status and access to care of minority populations (Giachello & Arron, 1997). In fact, children and adolescents have been underrepresented in clinical, biomedical, and health services research (Lohr, Dougherty, & Simpson, 2001). It is anticipated that recognition of these disparities will provide direction for future practice, policy, and research within the field of pediatric and rehabilitation psychology.

Parental Adjustment

Much of the developmental, psychopathology, and clinical literature has supported an association between children's adjustment and parental distress/stress. Such findings have been reported for children and adolescents with sickle cell disease (for review, see Brown, Mulhern, & Simonian, 2000; Casey & Brown, 2003) and cystic fibrosis (Thompson et al., 1994b), and children with congenital heart disease (Davis, Brown, Bakeman, & Campbell, 1998). It is likely that the association between child adjustment and parental adjustment changes over time in response to both parental and child stressors. Chaney et al. (1997), who examined both maternal and paternal adjustment longitudinally, have found that for children with diabetes, child adjustment was associated with paternal adjustment and not maternal adjustment. In conducting research on the association between parent and child adjustment, again, it is critical to incorporate both child and maternal reports, and to examine self-reports across multiple informants.

Peer Relationships

A review of the recent literature has indicated that peers may serve as protective factors for providing support for ongoing disease management for children and adolescents. Recent research, for example, has focused on peer support among adolescents with diabetes (Bearman & La Greca, 2002; Schuman & La Greca, 1999), indicating that adolescents perceive their friends as providing greater support than their families for "feeling good about diabetes" (for review, see Schuman & La Greca, 1999). In fact, findings with ethnic minority youth (Thompson, La Greca, & Shaw, 1997) have provided compelling support to indicate that African American adolescents with diabetes who reported higher levels of peer support for dietary adherence, insulin administration, and exercise regimens evidenced significantly better levels of metabolic control than their counterparts without such peer support. Bearman and La Greca (2002) also have found friendship support to be associated with adherence for blood glucose testing.

Given the important influences of the peer group on disease adaptation and management, greater research efforts are needed. In addition, peers also may serve as risk factors for poor disease management, particularly for those youth with strong conformity needs, who may resist the daily tasks associated with disease management. As Schuman and La Greca (1999) have noted, research is especially needed that goes beyond correlational designs to examine specifically the bidirectional influence of disease on peer relationships and the influence of peers on children's and adolescents' adaptation to disease. Both experimental intervention studies and longitudinal designs will be necessary to address this next stage of research.

CLINICAL IMPLICATIONS

Studies of children and adolescents with chronic illness recently have entered a tertiary stage of evolution, with the development of empirically validated treatment research. It has been recommended that this type of research be conducted for the purpose of testing theoretical models that previously were correlational or descriptive in design (Thompson & Gustafson, 1996). There have been various programs of intervention research for children and adolescents with chronic illness and disabilities. While a complete discussion of these studies is not possible within the scope of this particular chapter, the reader is referred to Part III (this volume). Intervention studies have been conceptualized within the domains of school performance and peer relations, parenting and family systems research, adherence research, and pain management (Brown & Macias, 2000; Thompson & Gustafson, 1996).

Brown, Boeving, La Rosa, and Carpenter (2006) conceptualize intervention studies in pediatric chronic illness as primary, secondary, and tertiary prevention efforts. The goal of primary prevention efforts is to alter risk factors prior to the onset of disease, thereby preventing disease onset or decreasing severity of disease. Examples of primary prevention include injury and accident prevention, substance abuse, risky sexual behavior, and reducing cardiovascular risk (for review, see Brown et al., 2006).

Secondary prevention efforts focus on the identification and treatment of health problems prior to the progression of disease (see Brown et al., 2006). Examples of secondary prevention efforts include addressing alcohol use in college students and the initiation of intensive problem-solving strategies for the management of newly diagnosed children with diabetes and their families (for review, see Brown et al., 2006).

Finally, tertiary prevention efforts focus on diseases or conditions that may cause long-term or irreversible damage (e.g., serious injuries, substance dependence, chronic diseases) (Brown et al., 2006). Examples of tertiary intervention programs include intervention programs for school performance and peer relations, parenting stressors for children with disabilities and chronic disease, and adherence to medical procedures and pain management (for review, see Brown & Macias, 2000). A frequent challenge in the development and implementation of empirically supported intervention efforts is integration and adaptation of interventions to real-world or ecologically valid settings (i.e., maintaining external validity), while adhering to the rigors of controlled clinical trials (internal validity).

CONCLUSIONS AND FUTURE RESEARCH DIRECTIONS

In this chapter, we have reviewed the epidemiology and pathophysiology literatures related to chronic diseases and disabilities, and conclude that approximately 10–20% of youth experience one or more chronic health conditions. Fewer children and adolescents have diseases of such severity that result in functional impairments. There exist several approaches from which to predict adaptation, although a noncategorical approach to classification will likely prove useful in predicting psychosocial adjustment. As a group, children and adolescents with chronic physical conditions are at significant risk for adjustment difficulties. Fortunately, however, only a minority of this group evidences maladjustment difficulties. Much of the research over the past 10 years has focused on those variables that predict both good adaptation to disease and disability, as well as poor adaptation. A major issue with regard to adjustment is the adequate assessment of children's adjustment and quality of life.

For many chronic diseases, there are academic and cognitive morbidities, some of which result from the disease itself, while others are associated with iatrogenic effects of treatment. Because children now survive diseases that previously had a much more guarded prognosis, school re-entry and later academic concerns are likely to be a major research forefront for investigators. Thus, the impact of diseases on classroom learning and socialization will be an important research agenda over the next several years.

An important issue is that various chronic illnesses occur within the context of various systems, including schools and families. Family relations and adaptation frequently predict children's coping and adjustment to an illness. Clearly, correlational studies have provided very compelling data to suggest significant associations between the capacity of the family system to cope and adapt to illness, and the overall adjustment in the child. Recent research has incorporated longitudinal designs, as well as clinical trials, so that the correlational data that have guided this program of research might later be demonstrated to be causal.

Other important issues within the field of chronic illness include developmental course and adjustment over time, as well as the interaction of specific developmental markers and milestones, and adaptation to illness. In addition to developmental factors are those variables that incorporate specific disease parameters. These include children's functional status, duration and severity of disease, as well as specific child parameters that have been demonstrated to be important mediators and moderators of disease adaptation, including children's gender, age, temperament, and coping style. Finally, social class, health access and utilization patterns, parental adjustment, and peer relationships also influence adjustment to children's illness.

The field of pediatric chronic illness is in an exciting tertiary stage of development in which longitudinal studies and experimental investigations have become the "gold standard" of innovative research protocols. In particular, studies that include the examination of children with chronic illness longitudinally within systems and demonstrate the reciprocal interactions of children and adolescents within these systems represent an important next direction of research efforts with this population. Moreover, empirically validated treatments at the primary, secondary, and tertiary levels that provide support for practice also are an important next research direction across the majority of chronic diseases and disabilities. This type of intervention research will be necessary not only to provide support for prevention, clinical practice, and setting a standard of care for the delivery of psychological services, but also I hope, provide verification of the theoretical models in pediatric psychology and developmental disabilities that have been developed over the past two decades.

REFERENCES

Alderfer, M. A., & Kazak, A. E. (in press). Family issues when a child is on treatment for cancer. In R. T. Brown (Ed.), *Pediatric hematology/oncology: A biopsychosocial approach*. New York: Oxford University Press.

American Academy of Pediatrics. (2000). Insurance coverage of mental health and substance abuse services for children and adolescents: A consensus statement (RE0090). *Pediatrics, 106,* 860–862.

Annett, R. D. (2004). Asthma. In R. T. Brown (Ed.), *Handbook of pediatric psychology in school settings* (pp. 149–167). Mahwah, NJ: Erlbaum.

Armstrong, F. D., & Briery, B. G. (2004). Childhood cancer and the school. In R. T. Brown (Ed.), *Handbook of pediatric psychology in school settings* (pp. 149–167). Mahwah, NJ: Erlbaum.

Bearman, K., & La Greca, A. (2002). Assessing friend support of adolescents' diabetes care: The Diabetes Social Support Questionnaire—Friend's Version. *Journal of Pediatric Psychology, 27,* 417–428.

Behrman, R. F., & Vaughan, V. C. (1996). *Nelson textbook of pediatrics*. Philadelphia: Saunders.

Brannon, L., & Feist, J. (1997). *Health psychology* (3rd ed.). Pacific Grove, CA: Brooks/Cole.

Brown, E. R., Ojeda, V. D., Wynn, R., & Levan, R. (2000). *Racial and ethic disparities in access to health insurance and health care.* Retrieved December 23,

2001, from University of California, Los Angeles, Center for Health Policy, www.healthpolicy.ucla.edu.
Brown, R. T. (1999). *Cognitive aspects of chronic illness in children.* New York: Guilford Press.
Brown, R. T. (2004). *Handbook of pediatric psychology in school settings.* Mahwah, NJ: Erlbaum.
Brown, R. T., Boeving, A., LaRosa, A., & Carpenter, A. (2006). Adolescent health and chronic illness. In D. A. Wolfe & E. J. Mash (Eds.), *Behavioral and emotional disorders in children and adolescents: Nature, assessment, and treatment* (pp. 505–531). New York: Guilford Press.
Brown, R. T., & Macias, M. (2001). Chronically ill children and adolescents. In J. N. Hughes, A. M. La Greca, & J. C. Conoley (Eds.), *Handbook of psychological services for children and adolescents* (pp. 353–372). New York: Oxford University Press.
Brown, R. T., Madan-Swain, A., Walco, G. A., Cherrick, I., Ievers, C. E., Conte, P. M., et al. (1998). Cognitive and academic late effects among children previously treated for acute lymphocytic leukemia receiving chemotherapy as CNS prophylaxis. *Journal of Pediatric Psychology, 23,* 330–340.
Brown, R. T., Mulhern, R. K., & Simonian, S. (2000). Diseases of the blood and blood-forming organs. In T. J. Boll (Ed.), *Handbook of clinical healthy psychology: Vol. 1. Medical disorders and behavioral applications* (pp. 101–141). Washington, DC: American Psychological Association.
Bryden, K. S., Preveler, R. C., Stein, A., Neil, A., Mayou, R. A., & Dunger, D. B. (2001). Clinical and psychological course of diabetes from adolescence to young adulthood: A longitudinal cohort study. *Diabetes Care, 24,* 1536–1540.
Burns, B. J., Costello, E. J., Angold, A., Tweed, D., & Stangl, D. (1995). Children's mental health service use across service sectors. *Health Affairs, 14,* 147–159.
Butler, R. W., & Copeland, D. R. (in press). Interventions for cancer late effects and survivorship. In R. T. Brown (Ed.), *Pediatric hematology/oncology: A biopsychosocial approach.* New York: Oxford University Press.
Casey, R., & Brown, R. T. (2003). Psychological aspects of hematological diseases. *Psychiatric Clinics of North America, 12,* 567–584.
Chaney, J. M., Mullins, L. L., Frank, R. G., Peterson, L., Mace, L. D., Kashani, S. H., et al. (1997). Transactional patterns of child, mother, and father adjustment in insulin-dependent diabetes mellitus: A prospective study. *Journal of Pediatric Psychology, 22,* 229–244.
Davis, C. C., Brown, R. T., Bakeman, R., & Campbell, R. (1998). Psychological adaptation and adjustment of mothers of children with congenital heart disease: Stress, coping, and family functioning. *Journal of Pediatric Psychology, 23,* 219–228.
DeMaso, D. R. (2004). Pediatric heart disease. In R. T. Brown (Ed.), *Handbook of pediatric psychology in school settings* (pp. 283–297). Mahwah, NJ: Erlbaum.
Fletcher, J. M., Brookshire, B. L., Landry, S. H., Bohan, T. P., Davidson, K. C., Francis, D. J., et al. (1995). Behavioral adjustment of children with hydrocephalus: Relationships with etiology, neurological and family status. *Journal of Pediatric Psychology, 20,* 109–125.

Frank, N. C., Blount, R. L., & Brown, R. T. (1997). Attributions, coping, and adjustment of children with cancer. *Journal of Pediatric Psychology, 22,* 563–576.

Giachello, A. L., & Arrom, J. O. (1997). Health service access and utilization among adolescent minorities. In D. K. Wilson, J. R. Rodrigue, & W. C. Taylor (Eds.), *Health promoting and health compromising behaviors among minority adolescents* (pp. 303–320). Washington, DC: American Psychological Association.

Harbeck-Weber, C., Fisher, J. L., & Dittner, C. A. (2003). Promoting coping and enhancing adaptation to illness. In M. C. Roberts (Ed.), *Handbook of pediatric psychology* (3rd ed., pp. 99–118). New York: Guilford Press.

Health Care Financing Administration. (1995). *Summary Report to Congress: Monitoring the impact of medicare physician payment reform on utilization and access.* Baltimore: Author.

Holmes, C. S., Overstreet, S., & Greer, T. (1997). Cognitive predictors of self-care behaviors 3 years later in youth with IDDM. *Diabetes, 46,* 263A.

Hommeyer, J. S., Holmbeck, G. N., Wills, K. E., & Coers, S. (1999). Condition severity and psychosocial functioning in preadolescents with spina bifida: Disentangling proximal functional status and distal adjustment outcomes. *Journal of Pediatric Psychology, 24,* 499–509.

House, J. S., & Williams, D. R. (2000). Understanding and reducing socioeconomic and racial/ethnic disparities in health. In B. D. Smedley & S. L. Syme (Eds.), *Promoting health: Intervention strategies from social and behavioral research* (pp. 81–124). Washington, DC: National Academy Press.

Ievers, C. E., Brown, R. T., Lambert, R. G., Hsu, L., & Eckman, J. R. (1998). Family functioning and social support in the adaptation of caregivers of children with sickle cell syndromes. *Journal of Pediatric Psychology, 23,* 378–381.

Kazak, A., Alderfer, M., Streisand, R., Simms, S., Rourke, M., Barakat, L., et al. (2004). Treatment of posttraumatic stress symptoms in adolescent survivors of childhood cancer and their families: A randomized clinical trial. *Journal of Family Psychology,* 493–504.

Kazak, A. E., Rourke, M. T., & Crump, T. (2003). Families and other systems in pediatric psychology. In M. Roberts (Ed.), Handbook of pediatric psychology (3rd ed., pp. 159–175). New York: Guilford Press.

Klinnert, M. D., McQuaid, E. L., McCormick, D., Adinoff, A. D., & Bryant, N. E. (2000). A multimethod assessment of behavioral and emotional adjustment in children with asthma. *Journal of Pediatric Psychology, 25,* 35–46.

Kral, M. C., Brown, R. T., Nietart, P. J., Abboud, M. R., Jackson, S. M., & Hynd, G. W. (2003). Transcranial Doppler ultrasonography and neurocognitive functioning in children with sickle cell disease. *Pediatrics, 112,* 324–331.

La Greca, A. M., & Schuman, W. B. (1995). Adherence to prescribed medical regimens. In M. C. Roberts (Ed.), *Handbook of pediatric psychology* (2nd ed., pp. 55–83). New York: Guilford Press.

Lewis, H. A., & Kliewer, W. (1996). Hope, coping, and adjustment among children with sickle cell disease: Tests of mediator and moderator variables. *Journal of Pediatric Psychology, 21,* 25–41.

Lohr, K. N., Dougherty, D., & Simpson, L. (2001). Methodologic challenges in health services research in the pediatric populations. *Ambulatory Pediatrics, 1,* 36–38.

McQuaid, E. L., & Walders, N. (2003). Pediatric asthma. In M. Roberts (Ed.), *Handbook of pediatric psychology* (3rd ed., pp. 269–285). New York: Guilford Press.

Mulhern, R. K., Khan, R. B., Kaplan, S., Helton, S., Christensen, R., Bonner, M., et al. (2004). Short-term efficacy of methylphenidate: A randomized double-blind, placebo-controlled trial among survivors of childhood cancer. *Journal of Clinical Oncology, 22,* 4743–4751.

Nassau, J. H., & Drotar, D. (1995). Social competence in children with IDDM and asthma: Child, teacher, and parent reports of children's social adjustment, social performance, and social skills. *Journal of Pediatric Psychology, 20,* 187–204.

Newacheck, P. W., Strickland, B., Shonkoff, J. P., Perrin, J. M., McPherson, M., McManus, M., et al. (1998). An epidemiologic profile of children with special health care needs. *Pediatrics, 102,* 117–123.

Patistea, E., Makrodimitri, P., & Panteli, V. (2000). Greek parents' reactions, difficulties and resources in childhood leukaemia at the time of diagnosis. *European Journal of Cancer Care, 9,* 86–96.

Pendley, J. S., Dahlquist, L. M., & Dryer, Z. (1997). Body image and psychosocial adjustment in adolescent cancer survivors. *Journal of Pediatric Psychology, 22,* 29–43.

Perrin, E. C., Ayoub, C. C., & Willett, J. B. (1993). In the eyes of the beholder: Family and maternal influences on perceptions of adjustment of children with a chronic illness. *Journal of Developmental and Behavioral Pediatrics, 14,* 94–105.

Roberts, M. C. (Ed.). (2003). *Handbook of pediatric psychology* (3rd ed.). New York: Guilford Press.

Rolland, J. S. (1993). Mastering family challenges in serious illness and disability. In F. Walsh (Ed.), *Normal family processes* (2nd ed., pp. 444–473). New York: Guilford Press.

Rolland, J. S. (1994). *Families, illness, and disability: An integrative treatment model.* New York: Basic Books.

Rovet, J., & Fernandes, C. (1999). Insulin-dependent diabetes mellitus. In R. T. Brown (Ed.), *Cognitive aspects of chronic illness in children* (pp. 142–171). New York: Guilford Press.

Schuman, W., & La Greca, A. M. (1999). Social correlates of chronic illness. In R. T. Brown (Ed.), *Cognitive aspects of chronic illness in children* (pp. 289–311). New York: Guilford Press.

Smith, R. A., Martin, S. C., & Wolters, P. L. (2004). Pediatric and adolescent HIV/AIDS. In R. T. Brown (Ed.), *Handbook of pediatric psychology in school settings* (pp. 195–221). Mahwah, NJ: Erlbaum.

Thompson, A. M., La Greca, A. M., & Shaw, K. H. (1997). *Ethnic differences in family and friend support of adolescents with diabetes.* Unpublished manuscript, Department of Psychology, University of Miami, Coral Gables, FL.

Thompson, R. J., Jr., Gil, K. M., Keith, B. R., Gustafson, K., George, L. K., & Kinney, T. R. (1994a). Psychological adjustment of children with sickle cell disease: Stability and change over a 10-year period. *Journal of Consulting and Clinical Psychology, 62,* 856–860.

Thompson, R. J., Jr., & Gustafson, K. (1996). *Adaptation to chronic childhood illness.* Washington, DC: American Psychological Association.

Thompson, R. J., Jr., Gustafson, K., George, L. K., & Spock, A. (1994b). Changes over a 12–month period in the psychological adjustment of children and adolescents with cystic fibrosis. *Journal of Pediatric Psychology, 19,* 189–203.

Wallander, J. L., Thompson, R. J., Jr., & Alriksson-Schmidt, A. (2003). Psychosocial adjustment of children with chronic physical conditions. In M. Roberts (Ed.), *Handbook of pediatric psychology* (3rd ed., pp. 141–158). New York: Guilford Press.

Weithorn, L. A., & McCabe, M. A. (1998). Emerging ethical and legal issues in pediatric psychology. In D. K. Routh (Ed.), *Handbook of pediatric psychology* (pp. 567–606). New York: Guilford Press.

Williams, J. (2004). Seizure disorders. In R. T. Brown (Ed.), *Handbook of pediatric psychology in school settings* (pp. 221–239). Mahwah, NJ: Erlbaum.

Wilson, D. K., Rodrigue, J. R., & Taylor, W. C. (1997). *Health promotion and health compromising behaviors among minority adolescents.* Washington, DC: American Psychological Association.

Wingood, G. M., & Keltner, B. (1999). Sociocultural factors and prevention programs affecting the health of ethnic minorities. In J. M. Raczynski & R. J. DiClemente (Eds.), *Handbook of health promotion and disease prevention* (pp. 561–577). New York: Kluwer Academic/Plenum Press.

Wysocki, T., Greco, P., & Buckloh, L. M. (2003). Childhood diabetes in psychological context. In M. C. Roberts (Ed.), *Handbook of pediatric psychology* (3rd ed., pp. 304–320). New York: Guilford Press.

Young-Hyman, D. (2004). Diabetes and the school-age child and adolescent: Facilitating good glycemic control and quality of life. In R. T. Brown (Ed.), *Handbook of pediatric psychology in school settings* (pp. 169–193). Mahwah, NJ: Erlbaum.

7

Hard-of-Hearing, Deafness, and Being Deaf

PETER C. HAUSER
KAREN E. WILLS
PETER K. ISQUITH

Hearing loss, particularly early in childhood, can have some of the most far-reaching and complex consequences of any sensory deficit. Hearing loss alone implies a developmental difference in awareness of sound, including speech and environmental noise. Hearing loss does not directly or necessarily result in developmental, behavioral, cognitive, or psychiatric problems. A number of potential comorbid conditions that may accompany hearing loss and multiple environmental conditions, including linguistic, social, cultural, familial, and academic, can substantially modify the child's developmental trajectory.

"Deaf" and "hard-of-hearing" are difficult to define, because they are not used simply to refer to degrees of hearing loss. These terms carry specific linguistic and cultural meanings. For many individuals with hearing loss, the terms "Deaf" and "hard-of-hearing" do not connote levels of hearing loss but are associated with cultural values or identity. Individuals with hearing loss who value the norms of the general "hearing" culture (i.e., speech intelligibility and spoken English-related behaviors) often identify themselves as "hard-of-hearing" even if they have profound hearing loss. On the other end of the spectrum, some individuals with mild hearing loss whose first language was American Sign Language (ASL) might call themselves "Deaf," referring to their cultural identity rather than to their degree of hearing loss.

In this chapter, hearing "loss" refers to a reduction in the functional aspects of audition, "deaf" refers to hearing loss sufficient to prevent access to and/or reliance upon auditory channels for understanding speech, "hard-of-hearing" refers to a more modest hearing loss that allows for auditory input, and "Deaf" refers to a cultural identification of oneself with the Deaf Community, a recognized linguistic minority that shares a culture. Deaf culture, like all cultures, is neither monolithic nor static. It is a rich, vibrant culture with traditions of gathering; sharing jokes and poetry and stories, extending support and affiliation to members of the in-group and acceptance to some extent of out-group members (i.e., hearing signers and deaf nonsigners) who appreciate and participate in some aspects of Deaf culture (Lane, Hoffmeister, & Bahan, 1996; Padden & Humphries, 1988). The term "hearing impaired" will not be used, since this has long been considered offensive by many deaf and hard-of-hearing individuals because of its emphasis on "impairment."

COMMON DEVELOPMENTAL, COGNITIVE, AND SOCIAL OUTCOMES

The incidence of hearing loss and hearing loss etiologies has historically been difficult to determine and estimates vary widely. Approximately one in 1,000 children is born with severe or profound deafness (Kitson & Fry, 1990), and as many as one in 300 children is born with at least some degree of hearing loss (Thiringer, Kankhunen, Liden, & Niklasson, 1984). Another one in 1,000 children become deaf before adulthood (Petit & Weil, 2001). Less than 5% of all children with hearing loss have a deaf or hard-of-hearing parent (Mitchell & Karchmer, 2002).

Substantial strides have been made in the past decade in the identification of genetic causes of hearing loss. Over 350 different genetic conditions associated with hearing loss are described in the literature (Martini, Mazzoli, & Kimberling, 1997). At least 50% of children born deaf have genetic bases for their hearing loss (Morton, 1991; Steel & Bussoli, 1999). There are also many nonhereditary causes of hearing loss: (1) congenital infections such as cytomegalovirus and rubella; (2) postnatal infections such as bacterial meningitis; (3) pre-, peri- or postnatal anoxia; (4) the use of ototoxic drugs pre- or postnatally; or (5) premature birth (for discussion, see King, Hauser, & Isquith, in press; Wills & Wills, 2005). Nonhereditary forms of hearing loss are often associated with other, sometimes severe, neurological sequelae that affect behavioral, cognitive, and psychiatric functioning.

Hearing loss has an impact on cognitive organization but not on intellectual functioning (Braden, 1994; Maller, 1999). The reorganization of some cognitive functions has been evident in functional magnetic resonance imaging (fMRI), event-related potential (ERP), and cognitive-behavioral studies (e.g., Bavelier et al., 2000; Neville & Lawson, 1987a, 1987b, 1987c; Proksch & Bavelier, 2002). Subtle effects of hearing loss and sign language have been found with some visual skills such as enhancement of peripheral visual attention (Bosworth & Dobkins, 1999; Neville & Lawson, 1987a, 1987b, 1987c; Bavelier et al., 2000, 2001), mental rotation (Chamberlain & Mayberry, 1994; McKee, 1988), image generation (Emmorey, Kosslyn, & Bellugi, 1993; Emmorey & Kosslyn, 1996), and face processing (Bellugi et al., 1990; Parasnis, Samar, Bettger, & Sathe, 1996).

There are often indirect behavioral and developmental consequences of growing up with hearing loss in a world that relies heavily on audition. Compared with the general population, children with hearing loss, particularly those from hearing families, are more apt to be exposed to risk factors that can lead to adjustment disorders in adolescence. These risk factors include academic failure, low self-esteem, inconsistent discipline, delay of age-appropriate development, and sexual and physical abuse. Most of these are secondary to negative attitudes toward deafness and failure to develop age-appropriate language fluency (du Feu & Fergusson, 2003; Goldberg, Lobb, & Kroll, 1975; Powers, Elliott, Patterson, & Shaw, 1995). The psychosocial impact of growing up with hearing loss is described in the following sections.

First 3 Years

Most parents cannot distinguish infants who are deaf or hard-of-hearing from those who are hearing, because their production of early cooing and babbling sounds much the same to individuals not familiar with infants with hearing loss (Kimbrough & Eilers, 1988). Family members and pediatricians typically become concerned when the development of word imitation, first words, and first sentences are delayed. In recent years, the average age at diagnosis of hearing loss has been about 18 months (Mertens, Sass-Lehrer, & Scott-Olson, 2000). With the advent of universal hearing screening for newborns in many states, hearing loss is being detected earlier. In some instances, hearing loss can be detected even during the neonatal period.

Parents often go through a process of mourning for the idyllic hearing child whom they have lost (Harvey, 2003; Mertens et al., 2000; Schirmer, 2001). For a typical hearing parent, at least initially, having a deaf child can seem like a tragedy. Feelings of grief, anger, and betrayal, as well as feelings of love and acceptance, are likely to alternate in "waves" rather than follow a set, predictable sequence with a clear timetable for resolution. Feelings of loss can recur at intervals throughout the child's lifespan, particularly at times of normal developmental transition (starting kindergarten, going to high school, graduating, getting married, etc.), or when parents perceive the hearing loss as obstructing or complicating the child's ability to accomplish these expected developmental transitions.

The processes parents go through are different when one or both parents are deaf or hard-of-hearing. Some deaf parents may hope for a child who is deaf like themselves, whereas others hope for a child who is hearing. Regardless of their wishes, deaf parents tend to be at least conscious of, and prepared for, the possibility that their child may be deaf. Deaf toddlers develop secure attachments and independence from their deaf parents similar to hearing children of hearing parents (Meadow, Greenberg, & Erting, 1984). In contrast, the diagnosis of hearing loss often has a negative impact on hearing parents' attachment with their deaf or hard-of-hearing child (Azar, 1995; Meadow-Orlans, 1990). Hearing parents who have more accepting attitudes about deafness in general, and those who communicate more successfully with their deaf or hard-of-hearing child, tend to show more positive and mutually responsive parent–child interactions (Samuel, 1996).

Preschool and Elementary School Years

During the preschool years, dramatic, interactive play with siblings and peers becomes increasingly important for the development of social skills, preacademic learning, phonological awareness, vocabulary, syntax, pragmatic skills, and general knowledge. Children with hearing loss who have not developed adequate language skills, regardless of modality, will have difficulties in self-regulation and social communication (Rhine-Kahlback, 2004). This is the age at which deaf children typically come to the attention of psychologists.

One of the first decisions that many parents of a child with hearing loss will make is whether and how to augment the child's hearing. With newer digital amplifiers, hearing aids can provide substantial benefit for some children, while others will benefit little. In the 1990s, cochlear implants were approved for use in children; within 10 years, the average age at which children received cochlear implant prostheses decreased from about 6 years old to about 1 year old. While not qualitatively replicating acoustic hearing, cochlear implants can be an effective means of enabling sound awareness and fostering auditory skills for some children. They are not, however, a panacea for all children.

Another decision that hearing parents in the United States make is whether or not they want their child to be bilingual (English and ASL) or monolingual (English only). The other decision is how to provide access to spoken English. Parents in urban areas typically are faced with an array of options for helping children develop interpersonal communication skills. These options typically include oral–aural communication methods, visible English communication systems (signed English and cued English), and ASL. Often parents are not fully educated about all of these choices but tend to be limited by the choices preferred by the professionals working with their child.

Since the passing of the Rehabilitation Act of 1973 and the Individuals with Disabilities Education Act of 1975, children with hearing loss have been educated more frequently within neighborhood schools. Some attend self-contained classrooms for children with hearing loss within a public school, and many are mainstreamed into nondeaf classes, often with an oral, sign language, or cued English interpreter or transliterator to ensure access to all of the content information and instructions spoken by the teacher. It has been argued that this is not necessarily the "least restrictive environment," as defined by Public Law 94-142. Children and adolescents who have a significant amount of hearing loss do not have full access to communication (social and educational) within a mainstream setting even with an interpreter/transliterator.

Residential schools might be considered the appropriate placement for full inclusion of some deaf children, because the children are within an accessible language environment at almost all times. In the mainstream, children with hearing loss are left out of much conversational exchange, experience frequent communication barriers, and miss most information that is not explicitly directed to them; therefore, they may be inadvertently "excluded" rather than "included" in academic groups, social interaction, group decision making, and other aspects of daily life. On the other hand, children in residential schools often have to travel a long distance to get to the school and be separated from their family. It is difficult to advocate for a specific educational placement, because the "pros and cons" vary widely across different residential or mainstreamed settings; however, these examples illustrate the complexity of decision making and some of the issues regarding educational options for children with hearing loss.

Middle and High School Years

Adolescent friendships increasingly depend upon shared interests, extracurricular activities, and values. Within this period of development, communication among peers becomes critical. Social comparison with peers increasingly forms a basis for self-perception and self-esteem. If an adolescent with hearing loss has poor language skills, he or she may encounter peer neglect, rejection, or ridicule, and might experience loneliness, academic failure, and diminished self-worth (e.g., Bat-Chava, 1993). Three factors have been found to be associated with better and healthier self-esteem among deaf children and adolescents: (1) parents who have a positive attitude toward deafness; (2) availability of clear and accessible communication within the home; and (3) whether the deaf child or adolescent identifies with others within the Deaf Community and has a rich sense of language and heritage as a part of a vital cultural group (see Bat-Chava, 1993, for review).

The impact of Deaf cultural pride is not surprising given that minority individuals who identify with their minority group have higher self-esteem than those who do not (Crocker & Major, 1989). The experiences of hard-of-hearing individuals with moderate to severe hearing loss are different from those of deaf individuals with profound hearing loss. Many hard-of-hearing individuals feel that they are stuck between two worlds, the auditorily oriented "hearing world" and the visually oriented "Deaf world" (Laszlo, 1995). Hard-of-hearing identity is distinct from the Deaf identity that is rooted in signed languages and Deaf culture. Hearing parents of deaf children who are aware of and concerned about these cultural issues may make a point of exposing their children to Deaf role models, involving the child from infancy onward in gatherings and celebrations of the Deaf Community.

The explosion of computer technology in the past 20 years, coupled with social policies such as the Americans with Disabilities Act of 1990, has broadened educational and vocational options and opportunities for many deaf and hard-of-hearing adolescents and young adults. At the same time, these changes have increased the importance of literacy and English-language communication skills for successful employment. Deaf and hard-of-hearing high school graduates' average reading levels have remained around the fourth-grade level for the past 100 years (Holt, Traxler, & Allen, 1997; Pintner & Patterson, 1916) but Deaf undergraduate college students from Deaf families read on average at an 11th grade level (Hauser, 2001). Postsecondary educational and vocational choices reflect the deaf or hard-of-hearing adolescent's mastery of language and literacy. Many deaf and hard-of-hearing individuals from various backgrounds experience a satisfactory quality of life. Today there are even deaf and hard-of-hearing clinical neuropsychologists and physicians, some of whom use sign language interpreters on a regular basis to communicate with their hearing patients, staff, and colleagues.

CLINICAL IMPLICATIONS

Historically, many deaf people with poor written, spoken or sign language skills were found in psychiatric institutional care (Denmark, 1985, 1994; Vernon & Diagle-King, 1999). The most recent study of the prevalence of psychiatric disorders among deaf people was conducted in the United Kingdom. Based on a sample of 62 children ages 11–16 years, the study found the prevalence to be as high as 50.3%, with higher prevalence among children in mainstreamed educational settings than among those at schools for the deaf (Hindley, Hill, McGuigan, & Kitson, 1994). The deaf and hard-of-hearing groups with higher prevalence of psychiatric disturbances tended to come from dysfunctional families involved in substance abuse, physical abuse, verbal abuse, parental psychiatric difficulties, and parental refusal to learn the child's language or communication (Goldberg et al., 1975; Powers et al., 1995). Given the limited availability of professionals versed in working with deaf and hard-of-hearing children, many such children are evaluated or treated by professionals who do not specialize in individuals with hearing loss. In the following sections, we attempt to illustrate some of the dangers of evaluating or treating a deaf or hard-of-hearing child or adolescent if one is not familiar with this population.

Psychological Assessment

Hearing loss is an important historical factor in the clinical evaluation of deaf and hard-of-hearing children. Certain etiologies are more likely than others to carry additional neurological complications such as visual, motor, or cognitive deficits. In some cases, hearing loss is just one manifestation of a complex medical condition or syndrome. The deaf and hard-of-hearing community is widely heterogeneous in terms of (1) degree, onset, and cause of hearing loss; (2) amplification; (3) communication mode; and (4) language fluency. All of these factors need to be taken into consideration when selecting, administering, and interpreting tests.

The psychological assessment of deaf and hard-of-hearing children and adolescents requires specialized training. The psychologist needs to have in-depth knowledge regarding the complex interaction between deafness, language accessibility, and family dynamics that impact both cognitive and psychosocial development. Assessment of these areas is imperative to make appropriate clinical judgments, decisions, and interpretations. Misdiagnoses of mental retardation and learning disabilities in deaf children are frequent when psychologists unfamiliar with the issues of intelligence testing with this population attempt to make the diagnosis (Vernon & Andrews, 1990).

The existence of hearing loss threatens the validity of many psychological instruments. For example, the most widely used test for children with hearing loss, the Wechsler Intelligence Scale for Children, third edition (WISC-III; Wechsler, 1991; Braden & Hannah, 1998; Gibbins, 1989), has been reported to measure the construct of intelligence differently at the item and factor structure levels with deaf children (Maller, 1999; Maller & Ferron, 1997). Other intelligence batteries also have similar validity issues when used with this population (for reviews, see Maller, 2003; Simeonsson, Wax, & White, 2001). The use of psychological tests with verbal content has long been strongly discouraged when evaluating a client from this population. Nonverbal psychological tests have been considered the most appropriate tool to use with children and adolescents with hearing loss (Blennerhassett, 1990; Maller, 2003; Vernon & Brown, 1964).

The psychologist who works with deaf and hard-of-hearing children and adolescents must attempt to put together an appropriate set of assessment procedures, customized to the individual client, to provide a comprehensive evaluation (see Miller, Thomas-Presswood, Hauser, & Hardy-Braz, in press, for an in-depth discussion of the evaluation of deaf and hard-of-hearing children and adolescents). A greater reliance must be placed upon qualitative data obtained through observations, knowledge, and discernment to support clinical hypotheses, diagnoses, and recommendations. Those who are less familiar with the far-ranging and multifaceted aspects of hearing loss should refer patients or seek consultation.

Psychotherapy

When children and adolescents with hearing loss are referred for psychotherapy, hearing loss might appear to be the necessary focus of therapy for a professional who is not familiar with this population. These children and adolescents have the same variety of treatment issues as their hearing peers, and hearing loss should not necessarily be the focus of the therapy. Most psychotherapeutic approaches can be used to treat deaf or hard-of-hearing children and adolescents successfully (Anderson & Watson, 1985; Gough, 1990; Levin, 1981; Sussman, 1988). The child or adolescent's communication skills need to be taken into consideration when selecting the appropriate therapeutic approach.

Professionals who require interpreting (sign) or transliterating (oral or cue) services need to be aware that the use of these services does not simply solve communication barriers. The use of interpreters has a direct impact on the individual therapeutic process by diluting and distorting the patient–therapist relationship (Leigh, Corbett, Gutman, & Morere, 1996; Wohl, 1995). Deaf or hard-of-hearing individuals need to look at the interpreter instead of the therapist, impacting the ease and development of rapport between the therapist and the child or adolescent (Sussman & Brauer, 1999). In family therapy, it is often necessary to use interpreting or transliterating services if the familial unit lacks adequate skills to communicate with the family member with hearing loss (Harvey, 2003).

The use of interpreters or manual communication skills alone does not qualify a professional to provide appropriate treatment. If the professional is not familiar with this population, then it is likely that the treatment progress will be slow and possibly misleading, or even cause harm. It is necessary to seek a professional who specializes in working with this unique population (see Glickman, 1996, for discussion on culturally affirmative psychotherapy; Harvey, 2003; Leigh et al., 1996; Sussman & Brauer, 1999).

FUTURE DIRECTIONS

Early diagnosis of hearing loss makes it possible to provide early linguistic intervention and support to parents. Growing numbers of parent–infant/early childhood education programs provide instruction to parents with deaf or hard-of-hearing infants/toddlers at school and in their home. These programs typically teach parents how to communicate and relate with their child, provide the support they need to adjust to the fact that they have a child with hearing loss, and provide adult deaf or hard-of-hearing role models and contacts with the deaf community. This is important because, as this chapter has illustrated, hearing loss itself is often not the most disabling factor. Rather, various combinations of related biopsychosocial factors may impede or facilitate development of children who are deaf or hard-of-hearing, including coexisting neurodevelopmental problems; family acceptance, knowledge, communication, and parenting skills; and medical, educational, and social policies. Assessment and diagnosis of cognitive, social, emotional, or behavioral disorders in a child who is deaf or hard-of-hearing requires acute awareness of the special characteristics, resources, and obstacles of this complex "ecology" within which they develop.

After the initial diagnosis of hearing loss, professionals should create an active intervention plan that is implemented immediately, with regular follow-up. It is critical to identify ways to create parental involvement in classes related to learning how to communicate with children with hearing loss. Families might also benefit from support groups and meeting other families with deaf or hard-of-hearing children. Local schools for the deaf, mainstream educational programs, and deaf and hard-of-hearing clubs and organizations often have information on where families and friends can receive communication education and/or support.

The community of individuals with hearing loss needs to be recognized as an underserved population. Professionals need to advocate for more programs and social policies to provide parents with the much needed information and emotional support vital to raising a child with hearing loss. More funding is needed for research, training, and community programs that provide specialization in the assessment and psychotherapeutic treatment of deaf and hard-of-hearing individuals. There is a great need for more studies on how to evaluate deaf and hard-of-hearing individuals appropriately, such as experiments on the validity of various psychological instruments when used with this population.

REFERENCES

Anderson, G. B., & Watson, D. (1985). *Counseling deaf people: Research and practice.* Little Rock: Arkansas Rehabilitation Research and Training Center on Deafness and Hearing Impairment, University of Arkansas.

Azar, H. (1995). Attitudes toward deafness and security of attachment relationships among deaf children and their parents. *Early Education and Development, 2,* 181–191.

Bat-Chava, Y. (1993). Antecedents of self-esteem in deaf people: A meta-analytic review. *Rehabilitation Psychology, 38,* 221–234.

Bavelier, D., Brozinsky, C., Tomann, A., Mitchell, T., Neville, H., & Liu, G. (2001). Impact of early deafness and early exposure to sign language on the cerebral organization for motion processing. *Journal of Neuroscience, 21,* 8931–8942.

Bavelier, D., Tomann, A., Hutton, C., Mitchell, T. V., Corina, D. P., Liu, G., & Neville, H. J. (2000). Visual attention to the periphery is enhanced in congenitally deaf individuals. *Journal of Neuroscience, 20,* 1–6.

Bellugi, U., O'Grady, L., Lillo-Martin, D., O'Grady, M., van Hoek, K., & Corina, D. (1990). Enhancement of spatial cognition in deaf children. In V. Volterra & C. Erting (Eds.), *From gesture to language in hearing and deaf children* (pp. 278–298). New York: Springer-Verlag.

Blennerhassett, L. (1990). Intellectual assessment. In D. Moores & K. Meadow-Orlans (Eds.), *Educational and developmental aspects of deafness* (pp. 255–280). Washington, DC: Gallaudet University Press.

Bosworth, R., & Dobkins, K. (1999). Left hemisphere dominance for motion processing in deaf signers. *Psychological Science, 10,* 256–262.

Braden, J. P. (1994). *Deafness, deprivation, and IQ.* New York: Plenum Press.

Braden, J. P., & Hannah, J. M. (1998). Assessment of hearing-impaired and deaf children with the WISC-III. In A. Prifitera & D. Saklofske (Eds.), *WISC-III clinical use and interpretation* (pp. 175–201). San Diego: Academic Press.

Chamberlain, C., & Mayberry, R. I. (1994, May). *Do the deaf "see" better?: Effects of deafness on visuospatial skills.* Poster presented at TENNET V, Montreal, Quebec.

Crocker, J., & Major, B. (1989). Self-blame, self-efficacy, and adjustment to abortion. *Journal of Personality and Social Psychology, 57,* 1059–1068.

Denmark, J. C. (1985). A study of 250 patients referred to a department of psychiatry for the deaf. *British Journal of Psychiatry, 146,* 282–286.

Denmark, J. C. (1994). *Deafness and mental health.* London: Jessica Kingsley.

du Feu, M., & Fergusson, K. (2003). Sensory impairment and mental health. *Advances in Psychiatric Treatment, 9,* 95–103.

Emmorey, K., & Kosslyn, S. M. (1996). Enhanced image generation abilities in deaf signers: A right hemisphere effect. *Brain and Cognition, 32,* 28–44.

Emmorey, K., Kosslyn, S. M., & Bellugi, U. (1993). Visual imagery and visual–spatial

language: Enhanced imagery abilities in deaf and hearing ASL signers. *Cognition, 46,* 139–181.
Gibbins, S. (1989). The provision of school psychological assessment services for the hearing impaired: A national survey. *Volta Review, 91,* 95–103.
Glickman, N. S. (1996). What is culturally affirmative psychotherapy? In N. S. Glickman & M. A. Harvey (Eds.), *Culturally affirmative psychotherapy with deaf persons* (pp. 1–55). Mahwah, NJ: Erlbaum.
Goldberg, B., Lobb, H., & Kroll, H. (1975). Psychiatric problems of the deaf child. *Canadian Psychiatric Association Journal, 20,* 75–83.
Gough, D. L. (1990). Rational–emotive therapy: A cognitive-behavioral approach to working with hearing impaired clients. *Journal of Rehabilitation of the Deaf, 23,* 96–104.
Harvey, M. (2003). *Psychotherapy and deaf and hard-of-hearing persons: A systemic model* (2nd ed.). Mahwah, NJ: Erlbaum.
Hauser, P. C. (2001). Deaf readers' phonological encoding: An electromyogram study of covert reading behavior. *Dissertation Abstracts International, 62,* 4B. (UMI No. AAI3012772)
Hindley, P., Hill, P. D., McGuigan, S., & Kitson, N. (1994). Psychiatric disorder in deaf and hearing impaired children and young people: A prevalence study. *Journal of Psychiatry and Psychology, 35,* 917–934.
Holt, J. A., Traxler, C. B., & Allen, T. E. (1997). *Interpreting the scores: A user's guide to the 9th Edition Stanford Achievement Test for educators of deaf and hard-of-hearing students* (Gallaudet Research Institute Technical Report 97-1). Washington, DC: Gallaudet University Press.
Kimbrough, O. D., & Eilers, R. E. (1988). The role of audition in infant babbling. *Child Development, 59,* 441–449.
King, B. H., Hauser, P. C., & Isquith, P. K. (in press). Deaf and hard of hearing. In C. E. Coffey & R. A. Brumback (Eds.), *Textbook of pediatric neuropsychiatry.* Washington, DC: American Psychiatric Association.
Kitson, N., & Fry, R. (1990). Prelingual deafness and psychiatry. *British Journal of Hospital Medicine, 44,* 353–356.
Lane, H. L., Hoffmeister, R., & Bahan, B. J. (1996). *A journey into the deaf-world.* San Diego: Dawn Sign Press.
Laszlo, C. (1995). Is there a hard-of-hearing identity? *Journal of Speech–Language Pathology and Audiology, 18,* 248–252.
Leigh, I. W., Corbett, C. A., Gutman, V., & Morere, D. A. (1996). Providing psychological services to deaf individuals: A response to new perceptions of diversity. *Professional Psychology: Research and Practice, 27,* 364–371.
Levin, F. M. (1981). Insight-oriented psychotherapy with the deaf. In L. K. Stein, E. G. Mindel, & T. Jabaley (Eds.), *Deafness and mental health* (pp. 113–132). New York: Grune & Stratton.
Maller, S. J. (1999, April). *The validity of WISC-III subtest analysis for deaf children.* Paper presented at the annual meeting of the American Educational Research Association, Montreal, Canada.
Maller, S. J. (2003). Intellectual assessment of deaf people: A critical review of core concepts and issues. In M. Marshark & P. E. Spencer (Eds.), *Oxford handbook of deaf studies, language, and education* (pp. 451–463). New York: Oxford University Press.

Maller, S. J., & Ferron, J. (1997). WISC-III factor invariance across deaf and standardization samples. *Educational and Psychological Measurement, 7*, 987–994.

Martini, A., Mazzoli, M., & Kimberling, W. (1997). An introduction to the genetics of normal and defective hearing. *Annals of the New York Academy of Sciences, 830*, 361–374.

McKee, D. E. (1988). An analysis of specialized cognitive functions in deaf and hearing signers. *Dissertation Abstracts International, 49*, 768.

Meadow, K. P., Greenberg, M. T., & Erting, C. (1984). Attachment behavior of deaf children of deaf parents. *Journal of the American Academy of Child Psychiatry, 22*, 23–28.

Meadow-Orlans, K. P. (1990). Research on developmental aspects of deafness. In D. F. Moores & K. P. Meadow-Orlans (Eds.), *Education and developmental aspects of deafness* (pp. 283–298). Washington, DC: Gallaudet University Press.

Mertens, D. M., Sass-Lehrer, S., & Scott-Olson, K. (2000). Sensitivity in family-professional relationships: Potential experiences of families with young deaf and hard of hearing children. In P. T. Spencer, C. J. Erting, & M. Marschark (Eds.), *The deaf child in the family at school* (pp. 133–150). Mahwah, NJ: Erlbaum.

Miller, M., Thomas-Presswood, T., Hauser, P. C., & Hardy-Braz, S. (in press). *Assessment of deaf and hard of hearing children and adolescents: Psychological and educational evaluation practices*. Washington, DC: Gallaudet University Press.

Mitchell, R. E., & Karchmer, M. A. (2002). Chasing the mythical ten percent: Parental hearing status of deaf and hard of hearing students in United States. *Sign Language Studies, 4*, 138–163.

Morton, N.E. (1991). Genetic epidemiology of hearing impairment. *Annals of the New York Academy of Sciences, 630*, 16–31.

Neville, H. J., & Lawson, D. S. (1987a). Attention to central and peripheral visual space in a movement detection task: An event-related potential and behavioral study: I. Normal hearing adults. *Brain Research, 405*, 253–267.

Neville, H. J., & Lawson, D. S. (1987b). Attention to central and peripheral visual space in a movement detection task: An event related potential and behavioral study: II. Congenitally deaf adults. *Brain Research, 405*, 268–283.

Neville, H. J., & Lawson, D. S. (1987c). Attention to central and peripheral visual space in a movement decision task: III. Separate effects of auditory deprivation and acquisition of a visual language. *Brain Research, 405*, 284–294.

Padden, C. A., & Humphries, T. (1988). *Deaf in America: Voices from a culture*. Cambridge, MA: Harvard University Press.

Parasnis, I., Samar, V. J., Bettger, J. G., & Sathe, K. (1996). Does deafness lead to enhancement of visual spatial cognition in children?: Negative evidence from deaf nonsigners. *Journal of Deaf Studies and Deaf Education, 1*, 145–152.

Petit, C., & Weil, D. (2001). Deafness. In *Encyclopedia of life sciences*. New York: Nature Publishing Group. Retrieved August 22, 2004, from www.els.net.

Pintner, R., & Patterson, D. (1916). A measure of the language ability of deaf children. *Psychological Review, 23*, 413–436.

Powers, A. R., Elliott, R. N., Patterson, D., & Shaw, S. (1995). Family environment and deaf and hard-of-hearing students with mild additional disabilities. *Journal of Childhood Communication Disorders, 17*, 15–19.

Proksch, J., & Bavelier, D. (2002). Changes in the spatial distribution of visual attention after early deafness. *Journal of Cognitive Neuroscience, 14*, 687–701.
Rhine-Kahlback, S. (2004). *The assessment of developmental language differences, executive functioning, and social skills in deaf children.* Unpublished doctoral dissertation, Gallaudet University, Washington, DC.
Samuel, K. A. (1996). The relationship between attachment in deaf adolescents, parental sign communication and attitudes, and psychosocial adjustment. *Dissertation Abstracts International, 57*, 2182B. (UMI No. 9623718)
Schirmer, B. R. (2001). *Psychological, social, and educational dimensions of deafness.* Needham, MA: Allyn & Bacon.
Simeonsson, R. J., Wax, T. M., & White, K. (2001). Assessment of children who are deaf or hard of hearing. In R. J. Simeonsson & S. L. Rosenthal (Eds.), *Psychological and developmental assessment: Children with disabilities and chronic conditions* (pp. 248–266). New York: Guilford Press.
Steel, K. P., & Bussoli, T. J. (1999). Deafness genes: Expressions of surprise. *Trends in Genetics, 15*, 207–211.
Sussman, A. E. (1988). Approaches in counseling and psychotherapy revisited. In D. Watson, G. Long, M. Taff-Watson, & M. Harvey (Eds.), *Two decades of excellence 1967–1987: A foundation for the future* (pp. 2–15). Little Rock, AR: American Deafness and Rehabilitation Association.
Sussman, A. E., & Brauer, B. A. (1999). On being a psychotherapist with deaf clients. In I. W. Leigh (Ed.), *Psychotherapy with deaf clients from diverse groups* (pp. 3–22). Washington, DC: Gallaudet University Press.
Thiringer, K., Kankhunen, A., Liden, G., & Niklasson, A. (1984). Perinatal risk factors in the etiology of hearing loss in preschool children. *Developmental Medical Child Neurology, 26*, 799–807.
Vernon, M., & Andrews, J. F. (1990). *The psychology of deafness: Understanding deaf and hard of hearing people.* New York: Longman.
Vernon, M., & Brown, D. W. (1964). A guide to psychological tests and testing procedures in the evaluation of deaf and hard-of-hearing children. *Journal of Speech and Hearing Disorders, 29*, 414–423.
Vernon, M., & Diagle-King, B. (1999). Historical overview of inpatient care of mental patients who are deaf. *American Annals of the Deaf, 144*, 51–61.
Wechsler, D. (1991). *WISC-III: Manual for Wechsler Intelligence Scale for Children* (3rd ed.). San Antonio, TX: Psychological Corporation.
Wills, L., & Wills, K. (2005). Hearing impairment. In S. Parker, B. Zuckerman, & M. Augustyn (Eds.), *Developmental and behavioral pediatrics: A handbook for primary care* (pp. 215–221). Philadelphia: Lippincott Williams & Wilkins.
Wohl, J. (1995). Traditional individual psychotherapy with ethnic minorities. In J. F. Aponte, R. Y. Rivers, & J. Wohl (Eds.), *Psychological interventions and cultural diversity* (pp. 74–91). Boston: Allyn & Bacon.

8

Visual Impairments

SCOTT J. HUNTER
NORA GRIFFIN-SHIRLEY
LISA NOLL

With increased success at promoting survival in youngsters born prematurely, the rate of neurodevelopmental disabilities affecting the sensory systems has increased in the last 20 years (Simeonsson & Rosenthal, 2001); in particular, rates of visual impairment, secondary to causes such as retinopathy of prematurity (ROP) and periventricular white matter damage, have been identified as much more common than previously observed (Msall & Tremont, 2000; Silberman, 2000). As a result, greater numbers of children with partial or complete vision loss are attending mainstream or inclusive academic environments. Throughout this chapter, it is our intent to assist the reader in better understanding the etiology of commonly experienced forms of visual impairment, their epidemiology, and their impact on the neuropsychological and psychosocial aspects of childhood development. However, in line with the emphasis of this volume on the neurodevelopmental disorders, we focus solely on visual impairments that occur early in life.

BACKGROUND INFORMATION

The infant's developmental progress is marked by changes across all neural systems, with the visual system dominating in terms of importance (Sonksen, 1997). Disruption of the visual system is most often associated with a principal disruption in early neurodevelopment (Dale & Sonksen, 2002); however, this is not always the case. As a result, there are differences in the degree to which sight is fully impaired, and when impairment takes place, that can strongly influence the pace and challenge of child development. Also, the presence of additional disability conditions plays a very strong role in the development of skill and competence across time.

Visual impairment impacts the range and variety of experiences a child may have, including the ability to move freely and interact with the environment (Lowenfeld, 1975), as well as affecting attachment, social engagement, and language acquisition. A child with a visual impairment is "forced" to use other sensory modalities to learn form and function, in order to effectively develop an understanding of his or her environment and its requirements. Similarly, a child with visual impairment processes changes in the environment at a less successful level than the child with intact vision. This leads to a limited range of exploration and experience with the environment. Socialization is another concern for the child with visual impairment; he or she is unable to rely upon the subtle, often physical cues accompanying vocalizations and intents, and as a result, the ability to maneuver social interactions may be significantly impacted. While children with visual impairments (including children classified as partially sighted) have been identified as being "at risk" for a developmentally delayed classification across assessments (Reynell, 1978), alternative developmental pathways may arise, thereby compensating for sensory and experiential deficits secondary to visual impairment. Such pathways allow for functional behaviors to present differently; as such, traditional means of assessment may not be sensitive to these alternative skills (Perez-Pereira & Conti-Ramsden, 1999).

Definitions

"Visual acuity" refers to the level of visual detail a person sees; it is calculated as a ratio between what is actually seen by the person being tested, and what an individual with normal vision would see at the same distance. It is typically described as an equation, with 20 designated as the first number, reflecting the distance (in feet) at which a visual acuity measurement is taken. The second number designates the distance in feet at which a normal sighted person can see the specific detail being identified by the person being assessed (e.g., identification of letters commonly seen at 35 feet by a sighted person). Using the Snellen chart, the most typical acuity measurement, visual acuity is measured ranging from 20/15 to 20/200. The United States has defined legal blindness as visual acuity falling at or below 20/200 in the better eye, with best correction made (Tielsch, 2000).

The notion of visual impairment in childhood has changed over the past 30 years (Rahi & Dezateux, 1998), with fewer children displaying an isolated visual problem, and a greater number of children presenting with both a visual impairment and a coexisting neurological disability (Rogers, 1996). What constitutes visual impairment in children is often determined by the laws where the child lives or where the research protocols are conducted (Flanagan, Jackson, & Hill, 2003). West and Sommer (2001) identify four terms conveying blindness, including "registrable blindness," "educational blindness," "total functional blindness," and "economic blindness." Each refers to the pattern of cognitive, social, and environmental factors underlying the loss of vision. In line with these classifications, the assessment and means by which visual impairments are quantified may be achieved through formal assessment by a pediatric ophthalmologist to assess visual acuity and visual fields, or by pediatricians and educators, looking at more functional descriptions of the impact of the visual impairment (Flanagan et al., 2003).

Given the comorbidity of visual impairment with neurological compromise, the task of classifying visual impairment and quantifying visual function in children is further complicated. Measuring visual acuity is complicated in infants with sensory and motor difficulties. Additionally, definitions of deficit across levels of vision vary internationally. A desire to establish criteria that could be utilized across national boundaries for purposes of epidemiology, as well as research and support, led the World Heath Organization (WHO), in 1966, to look at the definitions of "blindness." The result was the uniform classification of visual impairment, which is now internationally accepted, illustrated in Table 8.1.

Epidemiology

According to the WHO (1992), nearly 1.5 million children in the world are blind, with a majority of them in the poorest countries of Africa and Asia. While medical and ophthalmic care has reduced the prevalence and effect of visual impairment in children with congenital and acquired ocular problems, the number of children with visual impairment secondary to neurological impairments continues to place demands on rehabilitative and educational systems (Flanagan et al., 2003; Rogers, 1996). Community surveys have found higher prevalence rates of children with visual impairments than are actually registered, with higher rates of children with cortical visual impairments typically not accounted for (Flanagan et al., 2003; Rahi & Dezateux, 1998).

According to the *Twenty-fourth Annual Report to Congress* (U.S. Department of Education, 2004) concerning disability conditions, only 0.5% of children requiring individualized education plans under the Individuals with Disabilities Education Act (IDEA) are classified as visually impaired.

TABLE 8.1. World Health Organization Classification of Vision

Category	Grade	Criteria
Normal vision	0	20/25 or better
Near-normal vision	0	20/30 to 20/60
Low vision		
Moderate visual impairment	1	20/70 to 20/160
Severe visual impairment (legal blindness in the United States)	2	20/200 to 20/400
Blindness		
Profound visual impairment	3	20/500 to 20/1,000 or a visual field less than 10 degrees
Near-total visual impairment	4	Worse than 20/1,000 or a visual field less than 5 degrees
Total visual impairment	5	No light perception (NLP)

Note. Data from World Health Organization (1977).

Thus, children with visual impairments represent a low incidence population. In 2003, more than 53,000 children in the United States were eligible for federal support for educational materials.

Of children with visual impairments, 50–75% also have additional disabilities (Silberman, 2000). Ferrell (1998) conducted a longitudinal study of 202 children with visual impairments from birth to age 5. Of these children, 59% had at least one additional medical condition or disability diagnosed, in addition to their visual impairment, ranging from cerebral palsy to diabetes mellitus to traumatic brain injury. Children are affected by these conditions in different ways, with sight being one sensory system seen to be at risk. Children with visual impairment are often observed to display a number of comorbid difficulties, such as motor deficits, autistic-like behaviors, emotional disorders, behavioral disturbances, and learning disabilities.

Racial and ethnic diversity are major issues when educating, habilitating, and rehabilitating children and adults with visual impairments. For example, Kirchner and Schmeidler (1999) reported in the data from the National Center for Health Statistics for 1994–1995 that the occurrence of visual impairments was higher among Hispanics and African Americans than among Caucasians. They also found that as the population aged beyond 22 years, the frequency of visual impairments became higher among minority groups.

In Ferrell's (1998) longitudinal study, Project PRISM, 61% of the children were White; 15.9% were Hispanic; 4.9% were African American; 1.1% were Native American; and 17% were of mixed races. Slightly over 5% of the children came from Spanish-speaking homes; 2.6% were from

English- and Spanish-speaking homes; and 3.6 were from homes where other languages were spoken. The most common eye disease found among African Americans was coloboma; for Hispanics, ROP, and for mixed races, optic nerve hypoplasia.

Hence, it appears that one very important criterion for developing an appropriate intervention plan is to understand the cultural demands placed on the child and his or her family, and how disability is addressed within the culture itself.

COMMON PSYCHOLOGICAL AND SOCIAL OUTCOMES

Children with visual impairments are children first. They have the same need to be loved, to learn, and to be independent, both physically and socially, as other children. However, children with visual impairment acquire skills at a rate that often differs from that of their sighted peers, and they require supports for meeting goals and expectations of maturity. Children with normal vision perceive their world primarily through their vision and the resulting incidental learning that vision supports; children with visual impairments do not have the same set of cognitive experiences. They instead explore their world using their other senses and, as a result, come to acquire a very different "conceptual understanding" of the environment and its expectations. For example, children who are totally blind use their hearing, touch, smell, and taste to explore their environments to a much greater degree than do their sighted peers (Sacks & Silberman, 1998). As a result, the gestalt of an object or a situation is not fully gained, because children with visual impairments receive information that is inconsistent and fragmented.

Specific areas affected by a vision loss are the acquisition of some expressive language skills, due to an inability to learn through observation and subsequent imitation; concept development; sensory–motor integration, particularly in terms of visual–motor sequencing and awareness of spatial orientation; socialization; locomotion; and career or vocational preparation (Corn, Hatlen, Huebner, Ryan, & Siller, 1995). Griffin-Shirley, Trusty, and Rickard (2000) indicated through their research that a consequence of visual impairment is the restriction in one's ability to maneuver through physical and social environments, and to participate and exercise control over dangerous experiences and situations. This hampers opportunities to learn through experience and engagement, and limits options in terms of behavior and skill development.

To foster independent mobility and to encourage more effective cognitive development, children with vision impairments need to be taught the compensatory skills and the techniques needed to adapt to their vision loss

(Corn et al., 1995). For example, children with visual impairments tend to engage more frequently in solitary play and stereotypical behaviors than children with normal vision. As a consequence, early intervention is often a key strategy for supporting engagement with the environment and peers. Another difficulty has to do with parenting supports; the naturally overprotective parent of a child with visual impairment may be unsure how to encourage his or her child to move about within the home, or how to demonstrate and support efforts at imitation and skills learning. Often, an orientation and mobility specialist can be consulted to instruct the parents in activities that will motivate their children to reach out and explore their environments more actively. The parents can then better teach their children how to engage in purposeful movement, leading to manipulative play rather than only solitary play.

Traditionally, research has compared the growth and development of children with visual impairments to children with normal vision. This approach has been questioned by researchers such as Warren (1984) and Ferrell (1998) in the area of vision education. These researchers have suggested that the development of children with visual impairment should not just be compared to the development of children with normal vision, due to the range of experiential differences each group presents. In a longitudinal study of children ages 1 day to 5 years, Ferrell (1998) found that while many of these children had some delays in the acquisition of developmental milestones, these differences disappeared over time. Most children with visual impairment acquired typical levels of cognitive and adaptive functioning. When difficulties persisted, it appeared that additional disabilities played a significant role.

Early education for children with visual impairment and their parents is crucial to facilitate continual growth toward independence. Opportunities for exploration of the environment, modeling and guidance of language usage, engagement and interaction, and instruction in how to take in information more effectively using the sensory channels that remain unimpaired are crucial for promoting independence and learning. Supportive educational programming that includes instruction in braille and makes use of appropriate adaptive technologies, while also instilling opportunities for successful mastery, serves to minimize the deficiencies children with visual impairment experience.

Over time, vision loss can have a negative impact on the ability of children to complete independent living skills. For example, Lewis and Iselin (2002) found that children with visual impairments performed only 44% of the skills assessed independently, whereas, 84% of the children with normal vision performed these skills independently. This highlights a substantial need for guidance and support around acquiring daily living skills, including bathing, toileting, and food preparation. Limitations in the acquisition of such skills frequently contribute to difficulties in meeting learning and vocational goals.

As children with visual impairments age, they go through the same changes as children with normal vision; however, some special challenges may arise, such as the inability to obtain a driver's license, lack of acceptance by peers due to a physical flaw (deformed eyes), or socially unacceptable stereotypical mannerisms such as rocking (Rosenblum, 2000). Additional concerns include the need to use adaptive equipment (i.e., a magnifier, a long cane) to accomplish everyday tasks such as reading, writing, and walking. Social concerns include a lack of a number of friends their own age and an inability to observe nonverbal behavior, facial expressions, or "body language" due to vision loss. This may interfere with dating. Last, the need for children with low vision to want to "pass" as children with normal vision often isolates them from peers, due to the difficulty they have in doing so.

To facilitate the development of children with visual impairments, Sacks and Wolffe (1988) have suggested that parents and other mentors–caregivers need to provide support in mobility and transportation; instruction in social skills; and to offer feedback about objects, people, and events in the environment that these youngsters may not perceive. Encouraging children to be risk takers, to problem-solve on their own, and to strive for independence were additional suggestions made by these authors.

A paucity of research concerning the social and emotional development of children with vision loss exists. Longitudinal studies to date have shown that younger children with visual impairment who do not present with additional disabilities do not differ greatly from their sighted peers with regard to behavioral or social development (Freeman, Goetz, Richards, & Groenveld, 1991; Sacks & Wolffe, 1988). This suggests that for children who have only visual impairment, there is less of an impact of their disability condition on their range of social and affectional outcomes; however, the findings to date are sparse and quite variable, leading to uncertainty as to whether this assumption truly holds. It is also possible that developmental level plays an important role given the changes in socialization and emotional maturity that accompany the onset of adolescence. Research examining differences between adolescents with visual impairment and their sighted peers has identified a greater level of impact, and a greater degree of difference in the development of friendships, opportunities for socialization, and affectional relationships (Ferrell, 1998; Griffin-Shirley, Nes, & Siew, 2004).

Research completed to date addressing adolescents with visual impairment has found that adolescents with low vision have more difficulty with social and personal aspects of adjustment than do totally blind children (Griffin-Shirley et al., 2004). These adolescents, who have some level of sight, tend to engage in more passive activities and spend less time in social situations than do fully blind adolescents. In terms of social experiences, adolescents with vision loss rely more on the telephone than on engaging in one-to-one or social group experiences, are more sedentary, and are more homebound than their sighted peers.

Some developmental tasks are learned more slowly and at a later age by children with visual impairments (Tuttle & Tuttle, 1996). The direct effects of a vision loss with respect to the practical impact on day-to-day activities such as mobility and money management are first related to the family in the context of helping to develop self-concept and self-esteem in children and adults with visual impairments. Tuttle and Tuttle (1996) and Warren (1984) suggest that children with visual impairments are often more socially immature and remain more egocentric. Often, these children have difficulty observing and imitating peers; therefore, they may experience more problems with the development of a positive self-esteem than children with sight. Families, friends, and professionals play a key role in the affective responses of a person who is visually impaired.

Since the majority of children with visual impairments have additional disabilities, it is important to understand how these disabilities affect their learning and opportunities for social and emotional growth. Characteristics of children with visual impairments and additional disabilities often include difficulty with the generalization of skills. Children with visual impairment tend to rely on concrete, direct interpretations of requests and statements made, rather than being able to make use of abstract learning drawn from observation; when multiple sensory or physical handicaps accompany visual impairment, the degree to which other input can be used is strongly limited. Some youngsters with visual impairment show a negative response to sensory stimulation; this may lead to difficulties such as distractibility, tactile defensiveness, or oppositionality.

Some children have difficulty understanding the cause and effect of behaviors and objects. As well, many youngsters with visual impairments exhibit learned helplessness over time. These further limitations serve to isolate more clearly the child in question and add hardship to the task of educating and engaging the child with multiple disabilities, beyond just the impact of the visual impairment itself.

CLINICAL IMPLICATIONS

In line with academic and social difficulties frequently seen in youngsters with complex visual impairments, there is often a need for educators and clinicians to be particularly sensitive to adaptive and functional concerns with these children. While advances in perinatal and neonatal management have resulted in a greater number of "fragile infants" surviving, with accompanying sensory and motor concerns, these youngsters often require multiple levels of support and accommodation in order to meet daily living demands. As a result, school districts and pediatric practices have had to work collaboratively in order to ensure that appropriate remediation is available. Most public school districts now have available the use of a visual itinerant consultant, who is trained in the rehabilitation needs of the youngster with visual impairment. Additionally, special education programs make use of available consulting resources, such as the Lighthouse, to provide necessary training in support for teachers and aides. Nonetheless, there remain a number of areas where children with visual impairments are less successfully served, including counseling support and sensitivity to emotional distress and mood concerns.

In terms of addressing cognitive needs, it is important to keep in mind that many youngsters with visual impairments such as blindness present with delays in the emergence of self-help skills and adaptive functions, due to not only their lack of vision but also their dependency on others (Davidson & Dolins, 1993). While early intellectual skills development is less likely to be impacted solely because of a loss of visual acuity, age of visual impairment and the degree of loss experienced interact to determine how likely it is that a child will miss developmental goals. Additionally, the co-occurrence of visual impairment with other sensory disabilities serves as a significant mediator in terms of cognitive developmental status (Msall, Bier, LaGasse, Tremont, & Lester, 1998). Because early intervention programs are the norm in the United States for children born with disability conditions, it is also more common that potential sources of deficiency are more effectively addressed, and from an earlier point in time (Vohr & Msall, 1997). This has led to a need for re-examining the outcome data in terms of visual impairment and academic success; because children with neurodevelopmental disabilities are often more aggressively supported and accommodated given the provisions of federal guidelines, long-term outcomes are more effectively optimized for these children (Msall et al., 1998).

The extant literature concerning academic success of children with complex visual disabilities is quite diverse in terms of its findings. Research examining children born with very low birth weight (VLBW) and developed visual impairments due to ROP were observed to do reasonably well with regard to reaching kindergarten readiness when factors such as a supportive family and social resources, and the lack of environmental barriers (i.e., improved family economic status, availability of educational programs, low social stress) were considered. In contrast, children with visual disabilities secondary to VLBW, and its consequent sequelae, who also experience impoverishment economically and socially, fare much worse in terms of learning readiness (Vohr & Msall, 1997; Msall & Tremont, 2000).

Similarly, children born with visual impairment and co-occurring motor impairment, such as cerebral palsy, experience the least successful outcomes in terms of meeting adaptive and educational goals when family and environmental supports are weak (Chaudry & Davidson, 2001).

It has been noted in the assessment-related literature that children with complex disabilities are often quite difficult to evaluate using standardized measures (Chaudry & Davidson, 2001); this is particularly the case with youngsters who have visual impairments, due to the fact that many measures used by psychologists and diagnosticians are dependent on visual processing. When children present with multiple disabilities, such as blindness and an inability to use language, the use of many standardized measures is typically precluded. Similarly, significant motor impairment accompanied by visual impairment often means that more commonly used measures of intellectual development are, at best, inappropriate. Instead, clinicians must rely on more qualitative means of understanding the affected child's needs; observation and modifications in the administration of measures used are often the only means available for effectively tapping into children's skills and describing their ability level and potential. Additionally, despite the fact that many psychologists receive some academic training pertinent to working with children with disabilities, few have any real hands-on experience in working with children with multiple disabilities; this often restricts what can be done by such clinicians and hampers their effectiveness when asked to evaluate a child with multiple disabilities.

Despite these concerns, which have been previously discussed in the literature (Simeonsson & Rosenthal, 2001), there is a reasonably extensive clinical literature available that discusses how best to approach assessment in children with visual impairments and combined sensory and motor disabilities. Given this need, a series of published review chapters and dissertations have discussed how best to examine cognitive and neuropsychological functioning, in addition to adaptive and academic skills development in children with visual impairments (Chaudry & Davidson, 2001; Moore, 1999). As a result, clinicians and school personnel, in particular, have been provided with rough guidelines for approaching such assessment protocols. Unfortunately, few studies have been done to assess the efficacy of these recommendations.

When considering how best to understand the neuropsychological status of a youngster with visual impairments, it is necessary to be specific about what is affected in terms of the child's particular disability, in order to address effectively what is impacted, and what is more typically developing and thus in need of less support. For a child with blindness but no other clear sensory or processing concerns, the social and academic expectations are similar to what would be seen with a sighted child. In contrast, more severely impacted children, such as ones who, following a premature birth, have experienced ROP, often experience a greater impact on their development of cognitive and social milestones (Davidson & Dolins, 1993; Msall & Tremont, 2000). Typically, these children develop blindness, but at least 50% also show multisensory impact (Msall & Tremont, 2000), further hampering their success developmentally. As a result, the most important first step is to gather extensive information about medical and developmental background before attempting to determine what measures will be helpful in assessment. For a more detailed discussion of appropriate measures for assessment of intellectual and academic skills development in children with visual impairments, the reader is referred to Sacks and Silberman's (1998) excellent review of educational programming for children with visual impairments.

Federal legislation has provided a system for young adults with visual impairments to transition from the educational system to independent adulthood. At the age of 14, visually impaired children receiving special education services must have transition services identified within their individualized education plans (IEPs). These transition services usually include rehabilitation services from a state vocational rehabilitation agency that serves people with disabilities, including those persons who are blind or visually impaired. To receive these rehabilitation services, young adults must meet the eligibility criteria established by the state vocational rehabilitation agency where they reside. The eligibility criteria usually include the fact that a young adult's blindness interferes with his or her ability to obtain employment; this person would benefit from, and requires, these services to prepare for and to seek employment. Rehabilitation counselors, upon completion of an ecological evaluation of adults with visual impairments, develop an individual written rehabilitation program, stating a vocational goal and objectives, services, and technology needed to obtain this goal. Adults with visual impairments must sign these contracts to receive rehabilitation services. To assist persons with visual impairments to become gainfully employed, rehabilitation services may include training, payment for technology to improve an adult's functioning level, counseling, services from a job coach, and supported employment. Once adults meet their vocational goal and objectives, their rehabilitation services are terminated (Miller, 2001; Moore & Wolfe, 1996).

Young adults with visual impairments face many barriers when seeking and retaining employment. Negative attitudes of the general public and prospective employers toward people with visual impairments, low wages, lack of accessible technology, and unwillingness of employers to make reasonable accommodations within the workplace are some of the challenges people with visual impairments face (Moore & Wolfe, 1996). Adults with visual impairments who possess a high level of self-efficacy and self-confidence, independent living skills, job skills, and self-advocacy skills are better prepared to overcome these barriers. Yet according to the National Longitudinal Transition Study, the employment rates for young adults with visual impairments 3–5 years after high school graduation is 29% (Heward, 2003).

When individuals with visual impairment transition to adulthood, professionals look at living arrangements, supportive employment, coordination between school and adult service agencies, parental involvement, and guardianship issues, and select age-appropriate recreational and leisure activities and procure disability entitlements. Supported living, coupled with working in a sheltered workshop setting, is a realistic goal. The supportive living arrangement provides a natural support, while the sheltered workshop offers employment, training in functional skills, and opportunities for engaging in recreational and leisure-time activities.

DIRECTIONS FOR FUTURE RESEARCH

Research to improve the quality of life for children and young adults with visual impairments is being conducted in various fields by many different types of professionals. For example, medical researchers are trying to find cures for conditions that cause blindness (i.e., retinitis pigmentosa, glaucoma, macular degeneration, diabetes) by investigating the use of stem cells in retinal transplantation. Additionally, improving medications to control eye conditions, such as glaucoma, is another area of focus. Outcome-based research to validate current instructional methods, and the development and adaptation of assessment instruments for children with visual impairments, are just a few areas educators are investigating. Looking at the accessibility of computer software to enable children with visual impairments to use a computer easily is another area that educators are currently exploring. Bioengineers and rehabilitation engineers are interested in improving prostheses and redesigning wheelchairs and scooters to assist with mobility. Low vision therapists focus on the improvement of low vision aids (i.e., monoculars, magnifiers, closed circuit televisions) to help children with low vision read more efficiently.

The training of qualified personnel to work with children and young adults with visual impairments is a major issue. Specifically, the recruitment of potential students for university training programs, the funding of these programs, the use of distance education to deliver the training programs, and increasing the numbers of these university programs are primary concerns for researchers and policymakers (Kelley, Ward, & Griffin-Shirley, 2000). The best service delivery model for educating children with visual impairments is also under consideration.

Socialization and effective supports for meeting the developmental needs of adolescence and adulthood are areas that require substantial emphasis, particularly given that most youngsters with visual impairment present with multiple disabilities. Because it is still far from certain whether visual impairment hampers the youngsters' opportunities for successful social development, particularly in the early years of childhood, further research is strongly needed. Additionally, research concerning the role that inclusion experiences play in supporting better socialization and interpersonal skills development is strongly needed. Transition issues and employment are primary concerns for rehabilitation teachers and counselors of young adults with visual impairments. Universal design advocates suggest that a more pedestrian, friendly environment not only meets the needs of people with disabilities but is also helpful for all people, especially our aging population (Bentzen, 1997).

In summary, many professionals representing various disciplines are interested in improving the quality of life of children and young adults with visual impairments. Through their collaboration and sharing of research, the future direction of research in the field of blindness and visual impairment is dynamic and hopeful.

REFERENCES

Bentzen, B. L. (1997). Environmental accessibility. In B. B. Blasch, W. R. Wiener, & R. L. Welsh (Eds.), *Foundations of orientation and mobility* (pp. 317–358). New York: American Foundation for the Blind Press.

Chaudry, N. M., & Davidson, P. W. (2001). Assessment of children with visual impairment or blindness. In R. J. Simeonsson & S. L. Rosenthal (Eds.), *Psychological and developmental assessment: Children with disabilities and chronic conditions* (pp. 225–247). New York: Guilford Press.

Corn, A. L., Hatlen, P., Huebner, K. M., Ryan, F., & Siller, M. A. (1995). *The national agenda for the education of children and youths with visual impairments, including those with multiple disabilities.* New York: American Foundation for the Blind Press.

Dale, N., & Sonksen, P. (2002). Developmental outcome, including setback, in young children with severe visual impairment. *Developmental Medicine and Child Neurology, 44,* 613–622.

Davidson, P. W., & Dolins, M. (1993). Assessment of the young child with visual impairment and multiple disabilities. In J. Culbertson & D. Willis (Eds.), *Testing young children: A reference guide for developmental, psychoeducational, and psychosocial assessments* (pp. 237–261). New York: Guilford Press.

Ferrell, K. (1998). *Project PRISM: A longitudinal study of developmental patterns of children who are visually impaired.* Greeley: University of Northern Colorado Press.

Flanagan, N. M., Jackson, A. J., & Hill, A. E. (2003). Visual impairment in childhood:

Insights from a community-based survey. *Child: Care, Health, and Development, 29,* 493–499.
Freeman, R. D., Goetz, E., Richards, D. P., & Groenveld, M. (1991). Defiers of negative prediction: A 14–year follow-up of legally blind children. *Journal of Visual Impairment and Blindness, 85,* 365–370.
Griffin-Shirley, N., Nes, S., & Siew, L. K. (2004). *Exploring self-esteem and empathy: Preadolescents with and without vision loss.* (Unpublished manuscript).
Griffin-Shirley, N., Trusty, S., & Rickard, R. (2000). Orientation and mobility. In A. J. Koenig & M. C. Holbrook (Eds.), *Foundations of education: Vol. II. Instructional strategies for teaching children and youths with visual impairments* (pp. 529–560). New York: American Foundation for the Blind Press.
Heward, W. L. (2003). *Exceptional child.* Upper Saddle River, NJ: Pearson Education.
Kelley, P., Ward, M., & Griffin-Shirley, N. (2000). Personnel preparation and the national agenda. *Review, 32,* 102–114.
Kirchner, C., & Schmeidler, E. (1999). Life chances and ways of life: Statistics on race, ethnicity, and visual impairment. *Journal of Visual Impairment and Blindness, 93,* 319–324.
Lewis, S., & Iselin, S. A. (2002). A comparison of the independent living skills of primary students with visual impairments and their sighted peers: A pilot study. *Journal of Visual Impairment and Blindness, 96,* 335–344.
Lowenfeld, B. (1975). *The changing status of the blind.* Springfield, IL: Thomas.
Miller, J. (2001). The use of self-reports and parent observations in assessing performance outcomes for teenagers who received vision rehabilitation services. *Journal of Visual Impairment and Blindness, 95,* 229–234.
Moore, J. E., & Wolfe, K. E. (1996). Employment considerations for adults with low vision. In A. L. Corn & A. J. Koenig (Eds.), *Foundations of low vision: Clinical and functional perspectives* (pp. 340–362). New York: American Foundation for the Blind Press.
Moore, M. C. (1999). Assessing the preschool child with visual impairment. In E. V. Nuttal, I. Romero, et al. (Eds.), *Assessing and screening preschoolers: Psychological and educational dimensions* (2nd ed., pp. 360–380). Needham Heights, MA: Allyn & Bacon.
Msall, M. E., Bier, J. A., LaGasse, L., Tremont, M., & Lester, B. (1998). The vulnerable preschool child: The impact of biomedical and social risks on neurodevelopmental function. *Seminars in Pediatric Neurology, 5,* 52–61.
Msall, M. E., & Tremont, M. R. (2000). Functional outcomes in self-care, mobility, communication, and learning in extremely low-birth weight infants. *Clinics in Perinatology, 27,* 381–401.
Perez-Pereira, M., & Conti-Ramsden, G. (1999). *Language development and social interaction in blind children.* Hove, UK: Psychology Press.
Rahi, J. S., & Dezateux, C. (1998). Epidemiology of visual impairment in Britain. *Archives of Disease in Childhood, 78,* 381–386.
Reynell, J. (1978). Developmental patterns of visually handicapped children. *Child: Care, Health and Development, 4,* 291–303.
Rogers, M. (1996). Vision impairment in Liverpool: Prevalence and morbidity. *Archives of Disease in Childhood, 74,* 299–303.

Rosenblum, L. P. (2000). Perceptions of the impact of visual impairment on the lives of adolescents. *Journal of Visual Impairment and Blindness, 94*, 434–445.

Sacks, S. Z., & Silberman, R. K. (1998). *Educating students who have visual impairments with other disabilities*. Baltimore: Brookes.

Sacks, S. Z., & Wolffe, K. E. (1988). Lifestyle of adolescents with visual impairments: An ethnographic analysis. *Journal of Visual Impairment and Blindness, 92*, 7–17.

Silberman, R. K. (2000). Children and youths with visual impairments and other exceptionalities. In M. C. Holbrook & A. J. Koenig (Eds.), *Foundations of education: History and theory of teaching children and youths with visual impairments* (pp. 173–196). New York: American Foundation for the Blind Press.

Simeonsson, R. J., & Rosenthal, S. L. (2001). *Psychological and developmental assessment: Children with disabilities and chronic conditions*. New York: Guilford Press.

Sonksen, P. M. (1997). Developmental aspects of visual disorders. *Current Pediatrics, 7*, 18–22.

Tielsch, J. M. (2000). The epidemiology of vision impairment. In B. Silverstone, M. A. Lang, B. P. Rosenthal, & E. E. Faye (Eds.), *The lighthouse handbook on vision impairment and vision rehabilitation* (Vol. 1, pp. 5–17). New York: Oxford University Press.

Tuttle, D. W., & Tuttle, N. R. (1996). *Self-esteem and adjusting with blindness: The process of responding to life's demands* (2nd ed.). Springfield, IL: Thomas.

U.S. Department of Education. (2004). *Twenty-fourth annual report to Congress on the Implementation of the Individuals with Disabilities Education Act*. Washington, DC: Author.

Vohr, B. R., & Msall, M. E. (1997). Neuropsychological and functional outcomes of very low birth weight infants. *Seminars in Perinatology, 21*, 202–220.

Warren, D. H. (1984). *Blindness and children: An individual differences approach*. New York: Cambridge University Press.

West, S., & Sommer, A. (2001). Prevention of blindness and priorities for the future. *Bulletin of the World Health Organization, 79*, 244–248.

World Health Organization. (1977). *Manual of the international classification of diseases, injuries, and causes of death*. Geneva: Author.

World Health Organization. (1992). *International statistical classification of diseases and health related problems*. Geneva: Author.

Part III

Innovative Treatment Strategies

9

Pediatric Family-Centered Rehabilitation

SYLVIE NAAR-KING
JACOBUS DONDERS

Pediatric family-centered rehabilitation is an approach to the provision of services to children and adolescents that started developing in the mid-1980s in response to increasing dissatisfaction on the part of families with traditional health care delivery. Common complaints were lack of involvement in decision-making processes, insufficient information, and fragmentation of care (Thomas, 1987; Turnbull & Turnbull, 1985). This chapter describes the core elements of pediatric family-centered rehabilitation that were developed to address these concerns. We also provide suggestions for evaluation, review research on outcomes, and discuss barriers to successful implementation. We describe these rehabilitation efforts as they may apply to both hospital organizations and outpatient community settings.

CORE ELEMENTS

The Association for the Care of Children's Health outlined the basic philosophy of family-centered care in 1987 (Shelton, Jeppson, & Johnson, 1987). Subsequently, the Commission for the Accreditation of Rehabilitation Facilities (CARF) started accrediting organizations in 1997 for the provision of family-centered services in pediatric rehabilitation. These programs serve children and adolescents with significant functional limitations as the result of congenital or acquired impairments, and aim to prevent further impairment, reduce activity limitations, and minimize participation restrictions, while maximizing growth and development (CARF, 2003).

Several authors have provided a description of the key principles of -pediatric family-centered rehabilitation (PF-CR; Hostler, 1999) and family-centered care (FCC) in general (Bruce et al., 2002; Patterson & Hovey, 2000; Rosenbaum, King, Law, King, & Evans, 1998; Shelton, 1999). There are also websites that offer similar information, such as CanChild (www.fhs.mcmaster.ca/canchild/) and the Institute for Family-Centered Care (www.familycenteredcare.org). Table 9.1 presents a brief summary of those guiding fundamental principles.

PF-CR represents a fundamental departure from the traditional way of providing rehabilitation services to children and adolescents. Instead of being passive recipients of care, families are involved in all phases of planning and decision-making processes. As such, they are considered integral members of the rehabilitation team, regardless of the diagnosis of the child or the nature of the family unit. This requires that families not only have access to appropriate and necessary information in a timely manner but also that organizations and staff are genuinely committed to share control and responsibility with families. The underlying motivation is that when families are directly involved in decisions and plans about the care of their children, physical and psychosocial health outcomes are expected to improve,

TABLE 9.1. Principles of Pediatric Family-Centered Rehabilitation

1. The family is recognized as the main constant in a child's life, whereas rehabilitation systems and the personnel within those systems are transient and fluctuate.
2. Collaboration between families and health care professionals is facilitated throughout the rehabilitation process.
3. Complete and unbiased information about the child is shared with families on an ongoing basis in an appropriate and supportive manner.
4. Comprehensive policies and programs are implemented that provide emotional and financial support to meet the needs of families.
5. Families' unique strengths and individuality are recognized, and their different coping mechanisms, as well as cultural values and customs, are respected.
6. The developmental needs of infants, children, and adolescents and their families are understood and incorporated into rehabilitation systems.
7. Parent-to-parent support is encouraged and facilitated.
8. Rehabilitation systems are designed such that they are flexible, accessible, and responsive to families.

while remaining cost-effective (Shelton, 1999). From a rehabilitation perspective, this makes intuitive sense, because the purpose is to enhance families' ability to provide care and support for their children in the home and in the community.

A few practical examples may be helpful to illustrate how these principles can be implemented in the rehabilitation setting. In context of rehabilitation, team conferences are typically held on a regular basis to discuss the current status and recent progress of the child, to identify barriers to further improvement, and to establish short- and long-term goals. In the traditional rehabilitation model, such team conferences usually involve the physician, nursing and therapy staff, and possibly a case manager, whereas family members are excluded and are supposed to wait until after the team conference to learn what decisions have been made about their child. In a PF-CR model, families may be encouraged or even expected to be present during, and participate actively in, the entire team conference. With advancing age and development, it may also be appropriate to include the child. Rather than handing down decisions about interventions, the team may ask families about the desirability or feasibility of certain treatment options, giving them an opportunity to be actively involved in the decision-making process. As another example, rather than encouraging families simply to trust the expertise an experience of the medical and clinical staff, a PF-CR program may make active attempts at providing educational materials to parents about their child's specific condition, local and state special education process guidelines, and parent support groups. The program may also develop requirements of specific competencies for the entire staff, including both developmental training and formal continuing education in family-centered practice.

EVALUATING FCC

There are various ways in which PF-CR programs can evaluate themselves. Program evaluation is made through the application of methods of systematic inquiry into program processes and program outcomes. A process evaluation describes the degree to which the program is being implemented as intended and helps developers understand how programs are successfully implemented in the real world (Scheirer, 1994). Outcome evaluation focuses on the impact of the program, including consumer satisfaction, clinical outcomes, and cost-effectiveness.

Rosenbluth and colleagues (1991) described the process components considered essential in the evaluation of medical programs, including productivity, utilization, accountability, continuity of care, and coordination.

Each component can be readily adapted for the evaluation of multidisciplinary health care programs including PF-CR. The "coordination component" is most relevant to PF-CR and is defined as the degree to which team members, including staff and family members, communicate with each other. The least time-intensive way to evaluate coordination may be to determine the percentage of clinic charts with documented contact with the family or referring physician (e.g., team meeting notes, a "cc:" on a letter). In addition to assessing these process variables using systematic record reviews and available hospital statistics, a qualitative component can yield rich data about potential barriers to successful implementation of the program. However, the most accurate estimate of coordination with the family and other health care providers is to ask directly.

King, Rosenbaum, and King (1996) developed the Measure of Processes of Care (MPOC), a self-administered questionnaire for families to quantify their experience with the FCC they received. While the original scale included 56 items, a revised version includes 20 items with similar psychometric properties (King, King, & Rosenbaum, 2004). Subscales include enabling and partnership, providing general information, providing specific information about the child, coordinated and comprehensive care for child and family, and respectful and supportive care. This instrument has also been adapted to a 27-item version that can be used to measure the perceptions of pediatric health care providers in this regard (Woodside, Rosenbaum, King, & King, 2001). The Family-Centered Care Questionnaire—Revised (FCCQ-R; Bruce et al., 2002) was also designed to assess provider perceptions. The FCCQ-R includes 45 items over 9 subscales with good psychometric properties. There are two formats: one for provider perceptions, and the other for provider practices. Finally, the Family-Centered Program Rating Scale (Murphy, Lee, Turnbull, & Turbiville, 1995), a 59-item measure that can be administered to parents and providers, includes 11 subscales; the authors report good reliability and construct validity. However, the measure was designed only for programs serving children ages 0–5.

Outcome evaluation of PF-CR may rely on nonexperimental, quasi-experimental, or experimental designs. The most relevant nonexperimental design is outcome monitoring, the routine measurement of important indicators of the impact of the program (Affholter, 1994). Outcome monitoring allows evaluators to determine whether the program is meeting outcome goals, and, along with a process evaluation, is a critical component of quality improvement. Examples of outcome monitoring include reports on the number of clients served, revenue generated, number of emergency room or hospitalization visits, percentage of children with certain competencies, school absences, and percentage of parents–staff satisfied.

Clinical outcome comparisons help determine whether the program has been able to induce change. Experimental and quasi-experimental designs, in which the evaluator randomizes participants to different conditions, are often not possible in evaluations of existing programs. Evaluators must rely on naturally occurring comparison groups, such as patients at two different hospital sites or students whose teachers chose to participate in a program versus those who did not. Potential confounding variables and unexpected differences on pretest scores (if available) should be measured and controlled statistically to improve the odds that differences in outcomes are due to the program.

Consumer satisfaction is a critical part of an outcome evaluation, and parents, children, and providers are all considered consumers of the program. Ware, Snyder, Wright, and Davies (1983) outline three reasons for measuring consumer satisfaction with health care services. First, it is often argued that the satisfaction of program recipients, along with health status, is an ultimate outcome of service delivery. Second, there may be a number of behavioral consequences of patient dissatisfaction, such as poor adherence. Third, satisfaction ratings from consumers contain useful information about the structure, process, and outcomes of care.

Several measures of patient satisfaction with good psychometric properties are appropriate for parents, including the Client Satisfaction Questionnaire and the Services Satisfaction Scale (Attkisson & Greenfield, 1994), and the Patient Satisfaction Questionnaire (Ware et al., 1983). Relatively few measures of child satisfaction with medical care and even fewer measures of staff satisfaction have good psychometric properties. A set of three psychometrically sound measures was developed to assess parent, child, and staff perceptions of medical specialty care (Naar-King, Siegel, Smyth, & Simpson, 2000). The Parent Perceptions of Specialty Care (PPSC) includes 18 items loading on three factors: General Satisfaction, Worth of the Time Involved, and Access. The General Satisfaction scale includes items specific to PF-CR, such as communication with the treatment team and the teams' attention to parents' concerns. The Child Perceptions of Specialty Care (CPSC), a single scale of nine items, addresses communication with the team, perceived helpfulness of staff, and understanding of condition. The Staff Perceptions of Specialty Care (SPSC) includes nine items reflecting General Satisfaction and four items reflecting satisfaction with the multidisciplinary team. The General Satisfaction scale asks about issues relevant to PF-CR, such as how services meet patients' needs and how families are informed of recommendations, while the Team scale asks about how team members work collaboratively. Table 9.2 summarizes the measures available for evaluating PF-CR. In the next section, we will review the research on the effectiveness of FCC on satisfaction and patient outcomes.

TABLE 9.2. Summary of Measures for Evaluating PF-CR

Measure	Items/informant	Content	Subscales
Measures of Processes of Care (MPOC)	56 items/parent	Parents' experience with the family-centered care they received.	5 subscales for both MPOC and MPOC—short form: Enabling and Partnership; Providing General Information; Providing Specific Information about the Child; Coordinated and Comprehensive Care for Child and Family; and Respectful and Supportive Care.
MPOC—Short Form	20 items/parent	Parents' perceptions of the extent to which specific provider behaviors occur.	4 scales: Showing Interpersonal Sensitivity; Providing General Information; Communicating Specific Information about the Child; and Treating People Respectfully.
MPOC for Service Providers (MPOC-SP)	27 items/provider	Pediatric providers' reported implementation of family-centered service.	
Family-Centered Care Questionnaire—Revised (FCCQ-R)	45 items/provider	Providers' perceptions and practices of family-centered care.	9 subscales: Family Is the Constant; Parent–Professional Collaboration; Family Individuality; Sharing Info w/ Parents; Parent-to-Parent Support; Developmental Needs; Emotional and Financial Support for Families; Design of Health Care Delivery System; Emotional Support for Staff.
Family-Centered Program Rating Scale	59 items/parent and provider	Rating programs serving children ages 0–5.	11 subscales: Flexibility and Innovation in Programming; Providing and Coordinating Responsive Services; Individualizing Services and Ways of Handling Complaints; Providing Appropriate and Practical Information; Communication Timing and Style; Developing and Maintaining Comfortable Relationships; Building Family–Staff Collaboration; Respecting the Family as Decision Maker; Respecting the Family's Expertise and Strengths; Recognizing the Family's Need for Autonomy; Building Positive Experiences.

Client Satisfaction Questionnaire (CSQ)	8, 18, or 31 items/patients, parents	Client satisfaction across a wide range of services.	9 domains: Physical Surroundings; Procedures; Support Staff; Kind or Type of Service; Treatment Staff; Quality of Service; Amount, Length, or Quantity of Service; Outcome of Service; General Satisfaction.
Services Satisfaction Scale (SSS-30)	30 items/patients, parents	Patients/parents rate characteristics of services on a 5-point scale ("Delighted" to "Terrible").	2 subscales: Practitioner Manner and Skill; Perceived Outcome.
Patient Satisfaction Questionnaire (PSQ)	55 items/older patient or parent	Attitudes toward the more salient characteristics of doctors and medical care services as well as general satisfaction with care.	7 subscales: Access to Care (nonfinancial); Financial Aspects; Availability of Resources; Continuity of Care; Technical Quality; Interpersonal Manner; Overall Satisfaction.
Parent Perceptions of Specialty Care (PPSC)	18 items/parent	Parents' perceptions of medical specialty care.	3 subscales: General Satisfaction; Worth of Time Involved; Access.
Child Perceptions of Specialty Care (CPSC)	9 items/child	Child's perceptions of medical specialty care including relationships and communication with the treatment team.	None.
Staff Perceptions of Specialty Care (SPSC)	13 items/staff	Assess staff perceptions of medical specialty care, including how services meet family needs and relationships between team members.	2 subscales: General Satisfaction; Satisfaction with the Multidisciplinary Team.

OUTCOMES OF PF-CR

Studies have documented the effects of FCC on satisfaction with services, parent outcomes, and child outcomes (see King, Teplicky, King, & Rosenbaum, 2004, for a review). Naar-King, Siegel, and Smyth (2000) documented parent, child, and provider satisfaction with a multidisciplinary, FCC program for children receiving specialty care for a wide range of chronic and disabling conditions. Responses were compared to an a priori, defined minimum standard of 80% satisfaction. More than 80% of parents were satisfied with care. Even though FCC may take more time in clinic than traditional services, families felt that the time involved was worthwhile. However, child satisfaction approached but did not meet the criterion, suggesting that FCC programs must not only focus on parents but also help children to feel included in decision making. Staff satisfaction met the 80% criterion for quality of care and for components of the multidisciplinary team approach, but staff members were less satisfied with training, a potential barrier to implementing PF-CR.

Williams and colleagues (1995) found that the best predictors of parent satisfaction with epilepsy clinic services were parents' experience of staff attitudes as positive and the amount of information they received about the condition. Other studies have confirmed that components of FCC, particularly parent perceptions of supportive and collaborative communication with providers, are associated with increased satisfaction with services (Carrigan, Rodger, & Copley, 2001; DeChillo, Koren, & Schultze, 1994). Studies using the MPOC, described earlier, have consistently found that parents who perceived care to be family-centered were more likely to report satisfaction with services (King et al., 1996; King, King, Rosenbaum, & Goffin, 1999).

Using more advanced statistical techniques, Law and colleagues (2003) analyzed the effects of FCC of children with disabilities on parent satisfaction. They assessed parents' perceptions of PF-CR based on the MPOC. They also assessed the family-centered culture of the organization based on provider questionnaires about beliefs about FCC and services provided, and questionnaires from CEOs/managers about the consistency of their organizational structure with FCC. Structural equation modeling suggested that these two variables were the key determinants of parent satisfaction with services.

Studies suggest that parents of children with a wide range of chronic or disabling conditions who receive interventions grounded in FCC principles show better adjustment. Using structural equation modeling, King et al. (1999) found that parents' perceptions of FCC were associated with improved parent well-being. Similarly, Van Riper (1999) found that mothers who perceived their relationships with providers as positive were more likely to report higher levels of parent well-being and family adjustment. Even the amount of information received about the child's condition could be associated with improved parent well-being (Miller, Gordon, Daniele, & Diller, 1992). Finally, a key outcome of FCC is the parents' ability to take care of their child at home. Two studies have documented that FCC is associated with increased self-efficacy in parents (Dunst, Trivette, Davis, & Cornwall, 1988; Washington & Schwartz, 1996).

There are a few controlled studies of the effect of family-centered care on child outcomes. Parker, Zahr, Cole, and Brecht (1992) tested the effects of a home-based program for prematurely born infants from families of low socioeconomic status that included education, skills building based on parents' strengths, and individualizing services. Infants in the developmental intervention showed greater gains in mental and motor development compared to children in a home-based attention control and no intervention groups. Assessing a wider age range, Pless and colleagues (1994) found that children with chronic physical conditions receiving a family-centered nursing intervention demonstrated lower levels of internalizing symptoms, greater academic competence, and greater self-worth than children in the control condition.

Stein and Jessop (1984) compared children with chronic conditions who received a home-based, interdisciplinary, family-centered program to children receiving standard hospital care. The intervention group not only showed higher satisfaction with care but also higher levels of child and parent psychological adjustment. Even stronger support for the program was demonstrated by a dose–response effect and long-term follow-up. Families in the program for the longest period of time had the best outcomes. Data from a 4- to 5-year follow-up showed even greater differences between the intervention and the control condition (Stein & Jessop, 1991).

Finally, Naar-King, Siegel, Smyth, and Simpson (2003) compared families who attended family-centered clinics with families attending clinics that followed a traditional model in the same hospital setting. Children had a wide range of chronic or disabling conditions. There were no differences between groups on demographic variables or health status. Children in the FCC clinics had significantly fewer behavioral symptoms than children attending traditional clinics. Significantly fewer children from the FCC clinics were in the clinical range for poor school functioning compared to children in nonintegrated clinics.

There have not been published studies of the impact of family-centered services on frequency of hospitalizations and emergency room visits or length of hospital stays. However, one study demonstrated the effect of family-centered service on utilization in residential psychiatric treatment program using a quasi-experimental design (Landsman, Groza, Tyler, & Malone, 2001). Children assigned to the family-centered service program based on county of origin had shorter lengths of stay in residential treatment than families assigned to standard care. Table 9.3 summarizes the research available on the outcomes of PF-CR.

BARRIERS TO IMPLEMENTATION

Implementation of PF-CR is no panacea. Enablement and empowerment are easily endorsed buzzwords, but genuine commitment to PF-CR is a demanding requirement for the program and participating health care professionals, involving significant changes in terms of philosophy of care and day-to-day service delivery (Hostler, 1999). Thus, it is not surprising that there may emerge discrepancies between what is preached and what is practiced (Bruce et al., 2002; Lawlor & Mattingly, 1997; O'Neil & Palisano, 2000). Clinical rehabilitation staff may be more inclined to expect compliance from, as opposed to collaboration with families, and program administrators often provide limited education regarding the underlying principles of PF-CR and especially how to apply them (Bruder, 2000). Rather than changing themselves, many health care professionals expect families to change, or they may feel that they have more pressing priorities, such as getting paperwork done (Campbell & Halbert, 2002). Researchers have also determined that practitioners are at risk for making blanket, unfounded assumptions about a family's cultural or ethnic background, and do not always ask families specifically about their health beliefs and practices (Garwick, Jennings, & Theisen, 2002). Ethnic or cultural groups also differ considerably in the extent to which extended family members are typically involved in the child's care, and rehabilitation professionals are not always sufficiently sensitive or open to this (Ochieng, 2003).

PF-CR requires a team of professionals who are able to work together, as well as with the family. It is difficult to include families as team members when the pediatric rehabilitation team is not integrated across disciplines in the first place. Some rehabilitation professionals tend to be "turf-protective," which does not facilitate a collaborative team process (Richards, Elliott, Cotliar, & Stevenson, 1995). Physicians in particular may be reluctant to relinquish the traditional hierarchy, but allied health professionals may also value their own expertise more than coordination of services with other providers (Letourneau & Elliott, 1996; Marvel & Morphew, 1993). Various models of collaborative team models have been described, ranging from multidisciplinary to interdisciplinary to transdisciplinary, and although there is little empirical support for the superiority of one over the

TABLE 9.3. Summary of Key Findings on PF-CR

Study	Sample	Setting	Key outcome variables	Results
Law et al. (2003)	Parents of children with disabilities (N = 494); service providers (N = 324); CEOs (N = 15).	16 family-centered services (FCS) centers; urban and rural centers in Ontario, Canada.	Parents: • Measure of beliefs about participation in FCS (parent perceptions of FCS). • Client Satisfaction Questionnaire. • Measure of Processes of Care (MPOC). Service providers and CEOs: • Measure of beliefs about FCS • CEOs' beliefs about FCS • Information about physical, procedural, and strategic characteristics of organization. • MPOC—service providers.	• Parent satisfaction with services was strongly influenced by the perception that services were family centered. • They had more positive perceptions of family centeredness when there were fewer places where services were received (fewer sources) and fewer health and development problems for their child. • Key determinants of parent satisfaction with services: family-centered culture of the organization (providers' beliefs about FCS and services provided), and consistency of their organizational structure with FCS (CEOs).
Stein & Jessop (1984)	Families of children with chronic conditions (N = 219; at 6 months and 1-year, 80% completed all three interviews).	University-affiliated hospital- and home-based program; longitudinal clinical trial comparing home-based interdisciplinary family-centered program or standard hospital care.	• Satisfaction with care. • Personal Adjustment and Role Skills Scale II (child's psychological adjustment). • Psychiatric Symptom Index of mother. • The Impact on Family Scale. • Functional status measure.	• Families in the family-centered program showed higher satisfaction with care, and higher levels of child and parent psychological adjustment. • Families in program for the longest period of time had the best outcomes.

(continued)

TABLE 9.3. (continued)

Study	Sample	Setting	Key outcome variables	Results
Stein & Jessop (1991)	Follow-up study of Stein & Jessop (1984) ($N = 81$, 68% of original sample).	Same as above; follow-up study (4.5–5 years after original enrollment).	• Personal Adjustment and Role Skills Scale II (child's psychological adjustment).	• Results from the 4.5- to 5-year follow-up showed even greater differences between the family-centered program and the control condition.
Williams et al. (1995)	Parents of children with epilepsy ($N = 136$).	Urban multidisciplinary clinic.	• Epilepsy Clinic Satisfaction Questionnaire.	• Best predictor of satisfaction was the amount of information they had on their child's condition given by providers. • Staff attitude was also significantly related to parental satisfaction.
Van Riper (1999)	Families of children with Down syndrome ($N = 94$).	Families were recruited from Down syndrome support groups, through family study referrals and the Association for the Care of Children's Health Parent Resource Directory.	• Family–Provider Relationships Instrument. • Psychological well-being (parent). • Center for Epidemiologic Studies Depression Scale (parent). • General Scale of the Family Assessment Measurement.	• Positive relationships with providers were related to family satisfaction, parent well-being, and family adjustment.

Miller et al. (1992)	Mothers of children with physical disabilities ($N = 69$).	Rehabilitation hospital and outpatient occupational therapy treatment center; part of larger study comparing parents of children with disabilities and those without.	• Single 6-point Likert scale item about information parent received regarding the child's medical condition. • Brief Symptom Inventory.	• Parents who reported receiving more information about their child's medical condition reported lower psychological distress.
Dunst et al. (1988)	Two families of children with special health care needs (autosomal recessive disorder, multiple severe neurological disorders).	Families involved with multi-disciplinary FCS.	Family interview: • Prehelping attitudes and beliefs. • Helping behaviors. • Posthelping resources and consequences.	• Parents felt more able to care for their child at home because of PF-CR.
Pless et al. (1994)	Families of children (ages 4–16) with chronic physical disorders ($N = 332$).	Outpatients in 9 clinics at Montreal Children's Hospital with families randomized to specialized family-centered nursing for 1 year versus routine nursing services.	Psychosocial functioning: Parents: • Achenbach Child Behavior Checklist. • Personal adjustment. • Role skills. Children: • Self-Perception Profile (Harter), ages 4–7 and ages 8–16	• Families receiving family-centered nursing had parents with lower levels of internalizing symptoms and children with greater academic competence and greater self-worth.

(*continued*)

TABLE 9.3. (continued)

Study	Sample	Setting	Key outcome variables	Results
Landsman et al. (2001)	REPARE group (experimental group): family-based residential treatment (N = 82); Northside program (comparison group) (N = 57).	Four Oaks Residential Treatment Center quasi-experminental design.	• Length of stay. • Family visits on the unit.	• Children in the REPARE group had shorter lengths of stay in residential treatment than families assigned to standard care. They also had more family visits on the unit.
Naar-King et al. (2002)	Parents of children with special health care needs (N = 345); children with special health care needs over age 8 (N = 63); staff working in specialty clinics (N = 67).	16 family-centered specialty clinics in an urban pediatric university hospital.	Satisfaction with family-centered specialty care (FCC): • Parent perceptions of specialty care. • Child perceptions of specialty care. • Staff perceptions of specialty care.	• More than 80% of parents were satisfied. • Parents felt that the time involved with FCC was worthwhile. • Child satisfaction approached but did not meet criterion, suggesting that FCC programs must also help children to feel included in decision making. • Staff satisfaction met 80% criterion for quality of care and for components of the multidisciplinary team approach. • Staff were less satisfied with training.
Naar-King et al. (2003)	Families in family-centered specialty clinics (FCCs) (N = 80); families in clinics that followed a traditional model (N = 36)	Specialty clinics at an urban, university-affiliated, midwestern tertiary care center.	Parents and child completed: • Behavior Assessment Scale for Children. • Coping Strategies Inventory. Parents completed: • Child Vulnerability Scale—parents' perceptions of child vulnerability. • Parent Well-Being Scale. • Functional Status II—Revised.	• Children in the FCC clinics had significantly fewer behavioral symptoms than children attending traditional clinics. • Significantly fewer children from the FCC clinics were in the clinical range for poor school functioning compared to children in traditional clinics.

King et al. (1996)	Pilot test: Parents of children who attended 13 ambulatory rehabilitation centers ($N = 749$).	Ambulatory rehabilitation centers (plus one residential facility) across Ontario, Canada.	• Measure of Processes of Care (MPOC): assess parents' experiences and perceptions of specific behaviors of health care professionals, particularly those judged by parents to be most important.	• Parents who perceived care to be family-centered were more likely to report satisfaction with services.
King et al. (1999)	Parents of children with nonprogressive neurodevelopmental disorders ($N = 164$).	Six publicly funded children's family-centered (FCC) rehabilitation centers in Ontario, Canada.	• Caregiving process (MPOC). • General Functioning scale of the Family Assessment Device and satisfaction with social support. • Psychosocial life stressors. • Coping strategies. • Satisfaction with care. • Parent emotional well-being.	• Parents' perceptions of FCC were associated with improved parent well-being.
Parker et al. (1992)	Mothers of preterm infants with low socioeconomic status ($N = 41$).	Neonatal intensive care unit, randomized controlled study (home-based, family-centered care-FCC vs. control group with no intervention).	• Bayley Scales of Infant Development (measures infant cognitive and motor development).	• Infants in FCC intervention showed greater gains in mental and motor development compared to children in the no-intervention group.

(*continued*)

TABLE 9.3. (continued)

Study	Sample	Setting	Key outcome variables	Results
Carrigan et al. (2001)	Parents of children ($N = 11$) who had received at least one school term of occupational therapy.	A family-centered occupational therapy children's life skills clinic (OTCLSC) focus group and interviews.	Focus group sessions, telephone interviews, and face-to-face interviews: • Overall level of satisfaction of services.	• Parents' perceptions of the positive change in their child and the personal qualities of the therapists and students (communication skills, competence, rapport, and friendliness) were associated with increased satisfaction with services.
DeChillo et al. (1994)	Caregivers of children with severe emotional disorders ($N = 455$).	Organizations that provide services to families whose children have emotional, behavioral, or mental disorders in three states (Research and Training Center on Family Support and Children's Mental Health—RTC).	Families assessed the services of two professionals (one person that they found to be easiest to work with, and the other the most difficult to work with): • Family empowerment was measured. • Assessed the two professionals they worked with. • Assessed the service delivery process. • Satisfaction with services. • Availability of resources.	• Components of FCC, particularly parent perceptions of supportive and collaborative communication with providers, were associated with increased satisfaction with services.
Washington & Schwartz (1996)	Two adoptive mother–therapist dyads.	Two facilities providing family-centered services (FCC) to families with young children (home- or center-based physical and occupational therapy, as well as other multidisciplinary services).	Interviews were conducted with the mothers and therapists: • Describe ways in which physical or occupational therapy services addressed their caregiving concerns, and how their perceptions of caregiving competency may have changed since being involved in FCC program.	• FCC was associated with increased self-efficacy in parents.

others, it is generally agreed that administrative and physician leadership, as well as specific staff training in team processes, are often key to facilitating a team environment that is integrated and collaborative, as opposed to fragmented and discipline-centered (Allen, Wilczynski, & Evans, 1997). Ideally, however, training in the principles and practicalities of PF-CR should start during the graduate training of those pursuing a career in rehabilitation, with the understanding that ongoing continuing education will be required for all practicing clinicians.

The gap between superficial endorsement of the importance of family involvement and actual incorporation of the values of PF-CR is often due to a large extent to insufficient staff preparation and training. Bruce et al. (2002) found that one of the elements of PF-CR least agreed upon and least practiced by professionals was parent–professional collaboration. Several authors have suggested that lack of preparation of health care professionals about the need to assume more flexible roles and to relinquish some control can typically be traced to insufficient preparation of, and support for, staff before and during attempts at implementing a family-centered model of care (Bruder, 2000; Caty, Larocque, & Koren, 2001; Lawlor & Mattingly, 1997; Patterson & Hovey, 2000). Thus, it is essential that all members of the rehabilitation team, from therapy assistants to medical directors, receive specific training and continuing education in areas such as family dynamics, cultural competency, interpersonal communication, and other aspects of PF-CR. Developmental issues also need to be addressed in this context, because it may become increasingly appropriate and desirable to actively include children into the decision-making process with advancing age. Periodic reminders of the rehabilitation team that children typically go home with their families, and that it is therefore essential to give families the tools to manage after they leave the clinic or the hospital, are probably a useful adjunct intervention as well.

One of the most challenging aspects of PF-CR is the need to work truly collaboratively with families, regardless of their constellation, cultural background, or degree of cohesiveness. It is easy to dismiss family members' involvement on the grounds that they are not experts and, especially, that they tend to be "dysfunctional." Implementation of PF-CR requires an emphasis on families' strengths rather than their deficits (Dunst, 1997). Rather than blaming or excluding family members, health care professionals need to explore all factors that reduce the efficacy and efficiency of the rehabilitation process, and address barriers that prevent family members from being active team members. For example, many families of children with special health care needs experience considerable burden and lack of control, which may make them appear angry, naive, and unreasonable in their demands, and this may make some professionals reluctant to ask or consider their input or participation (Patterson & Hovey, 2000). Meeting with families on the day of admission, not only to explain the roles of various professionals but also to inquire about families' concerns and priorities, and to encourage their active participation in the rehabilitative planning and decision process, is one feasible way of dealing with such issues in a proactive and constructive manner. This allows for expectancies, contingencies, and boundaries to be clarified up front, and it sets a framework for communication that can address troublesome issues as, or even before, they emerge.

CONCLUSIONS AND FUTURE DIRECTIONS

FCC is emerging as the "best practices" model for pediatric rehabilitation services. PF-CR represents a fundamental diversion from traditional rehabilitation service delivery that requires considerable staff training and genuine commitment to fully involved families in all phases of decision-making processes regarding their children. Barriers to implementation include internal prejudices affecting behavior toward families and other disciplines, ability of staff and family members to work as a team, and staff training and resources. Evaluation of programs is critical to determining whether services are provided as intended, as well as documenting outcomes. Existing evidence suggests that PF-CR results in enhanced child and family functioning and increased parent satisfaction.

There are a number of avenues for future research. Child perspectives in particular warrant further study, because most of the outcome studies have focused on the perspectives of parents and health care providers. Since an understanding of the developmental needs of children, and incorporation of those needs into the rehabilitation process, is considered a key element of PF-CR, it is crucial that instruments be developed that can obtain reliable and valid input from children at different age levels about their perceptions of the services that they received. Future research could assess the degree to which PF-CR programs include children and whether this variable is associated with outcomes. Also, there have been no studies of programs that involve extended family members, a component that may be especially relevant for families of ethnic minority groups. This would address another key principle of PF-CR, namely, the need to respect cultural diversities of families. Outcome studies should include a process evaluation component, so that the link between process and outcome may be assessed, as in King et al. (1999). Finally, studies must also focus on the impact of PF-CR on health care utilization (including length of hospital stay and/or outpatient therapy expenditures) to demonstrate the potential cost-effectiveness of this service model.

REFERENCES

Affholter, D. P. (1994). Outcome monitoring. In J. S. Wholey, H. P. Hatry, & K. E. Newcomer (Eds.), *Handbook of practical program evaluation* (pp. 96–118). San Francisco: Jossey-Bass.

Allen, K. D., Wilczynski, S. M., & Evans, J. H. (1997). Pediatric rehabilitation: Defining a field, a focus, and a future. *International Journal of Rehabilitation and Health, 3,* 25–40.

Attkisson, C. C., & Greenfield, T. K. (1994). The Client Satisfaction Questionnaire–8 and the Service Satisfaction Questionnaire–30. In M. E. Maruish (Ed.), *The use of psychological testing for treatment planning and outcome assessment* (pp. 120–128). Hillsdale, NJ: Erlbaum.

Bruce, B. B., Letourneau, N., Ritchie, J., Larocque, S., Dennis, C., & Elliott, M. R. (2002). A multisite study of health care professionals' perception and practices of family-centered care. *Journal of Family Nursing, 8,* 408–429.

Bruder, M. B. (2000). Family-centered early intervention: Clarifying our values for the new millennium. *Topics in Early Childhood Special Education, 20,* 105–122.

Campbell, P. H., & Halbert, J. (2002). Between research and practice: Provider perspectives on early intervention. *Topics in Early Childhood Special Education, 22,* 213–226.

Carrigan, N., Rodger, S., & Copley, J. (2001). Parent satisfaction with a paediatric occupational therapy service: A pilot investigation. *Physical and Occupational Therapy in Pediatrics, 21,* 51–76.

Caty, S., Larocque, S., & Koren, I. (2001). Family-centered care in Ontario general hospitals: The views of pediatric nurses. *Canadian Journal of Leadership, 14,* 10–18.

Commission for the Accreditation of Rehabilitation Facilities. (2003). *Medical rehabilitation standards manual.* Tucson, AZ: Rehabilitation Accreditation Commission.

DeChillo, N., Koren, P. E., & Schultze, K. H. (1994). From paternalism to partnership: Family and professional collaboration in children's mental health. *American Journal of Orthopsychiatry, 64,* 564–576.

Dunst, C. J. (1997). Conceptual and empirical foundations of family-centered practice. In R. Illback, C. Cobb, & J. H. Joseph (Eds.), *Integrated services for children and families: Opportunities for psychological practice* (pp. 75–91). Washington, DC: American Psychological Association.

Dunst, C. J., Trivette, C. M., Davis, M., & Cornwall, J. (1988). Enabling and empowering families of children with health impairments. *Children's Health Care, 17,* 71–81.

Garwick, A., Jennings, J. M., & Theisen, D. (2002). Urban American Indian family caregivers' perceptions of the quality of family-centered care. *Children's Health Care, 31,* 209–222.

Hostler, S. L. (1999). Pediatric family-centered rehabilitation. *Journal of Head Trauma Rehabilitation, 14,* 384–393.

King, G., King, S., Rosenbaum, P., & Goffin, R. (1999). Family-centered caregiving and well-being of parents of children with disabilities: Linking process with outcome. *Journal of Pediatric Psychology, 24,* 41–53.

King, S., King, G., & Rosenbaum, P. (2004). Evaluating health service delivery to children with chronic conditions and their families: Development of a refined Measure of Processes of Care (MPOC-20). *Children's Health Care, 33,* 35–57.

King, S., Rosenbaum, P., & King, G. (1996). Parents' perceptions of caregiving: Development and validation of a measure of processes. *Developmental Medicine and Child Neurology, 38,* 757–772.

King, S., Teplicky, R., King, G., & Rosenbaum, P. (2004). Family-centered service for children with cerebral palsy and their families: A review of the literature. *Seminars in Pediatric Neurology, 11,* 78–86.

Landsman, M. H., Groza, V., Tyler, M., & Malone, K. (2001). Outcomes of family-centered residential treatment. *Child Welfare, 80,* 351–379.

Law, M., Hanna, S., King, G., Hurley, P., King, S., Kertoy, M., & Rosenbaum, P. (2003). Factors affecting family-centered service delivery for children with disabilities. *Child: Care, Health and Development, 29,* 357–366.

Lawlor, M. C., & Mattingly, C. F. (1997). The complexities embedded in family-centered care. *American Journal of Occupational Therapy, 52,* 259–267.

Letourneau, N., & Elliott, M. (1996). Pediatric health care professionals' perceptions and practices of family-centered care. *Children's Health Care, 25,* 157–174.

Marvel, M., & Morphew, P. (1993). Levels of family involvement by resident and attending physicians. *Family Medicine, 25,* 26–30.

Miller, A. C., Gordon, R. M., Daniele, R. J., & Diller, L. (1992). Stress, appraisal, and coping in mothers of disabled and nondisabled children. *Journal of Pediatric Psychology, 17,* 587–605.

Murphy, D. L., Lee, I. M., Turnbull, A. P., & Turbiville, V. (1995). The Family-Centered Program Rating Scale: An instrument for program evaluation and change. *Journal of Early Intervention, 19,* 24–42.

Naar-King, S., Siegel, P. T., & Smyth, M. (2002). Consumer satisfaction with a collaborative, interdisciplinary health care program for children with special needs. *Children's Services: Social Policy, Research, and Practice, 5,* 189–200.

Naar-King, S., Siegel, P. T., Smyth, M., & Simpson, P. (2000). Evaluating collaborative health care programs for children with special needs. *Children's Services: Social Policy, Research, and Practice, 3,* 233–245.

Naar-King, S., Siegel, P. T., Smyth, M., & Simpson, P. (2003). An evaluation of an integrated health care program for children with special needs. *Children's Health Care, 32,* 233–243.

Ochieng, B. (2003). Minority ethnic families and family-centered care. *Journal of Child Health Care, 7,* 123–132.

O'Neil, M., & Palisano, R. J. (2000). Attitudes toward family-centered care and clinical decision making in early intervention among physical therapists. *Pediatric Physical Therapy, 12,* 173–182.

Parker, S. J., Zahr, L. K., Cole, J. G., & Brecht, M. L. (1992). Outcome after developmental intervention in the neonatal intensive care unit for mothers of preterm infants with low socioeconomic status. *Journal of Pediatrics, 120,* 780–785.

Patterson, J. M., & Hovey, D. L. (2000). Family-centered care for children with spe-

cial health needs: Rhetoric or reality? *Families, Systems and Health, 18*, 237–251.
Pless, I. B., Feeley, N., Gottlieb, L., Rowat, K., Dougherty, G., & Willard, B. (1994). A randomized trial of a nursing intervention to promote the adjustment of children with chronic physical disorders. *Pediatrics, 94*, 70–75.
Richards, J. S., Elliott, T. R., Cotliar, R., & Stevenson, V. (1995). Pediatric medical rehabilitation. In M. Roberts (Ed.), *Handbook of pediatric psychology* (2nd ed., pp. 703–722). New York: Guilford Press.
Rosenbaum, P., King, S., Law, M., King, G., & Evans, J. (1998). Family-centered service: A conceptual framework and research review. *Physical and Occupational Therapy in Pediatrics, 18*, 1–20.
Rosenbluth, L., Morehead, M. A., Grossi, M., Oliver, C. T., Uccellani, C., & Robinson, P. (1991). A model for evaluating the delivery of pediatric primary care services. *American College of Medical Quality, 6*, 2–8.
Scheirer, M.A. (1994). Designing and using process evaluation. In J. S. Wholey, H. P. Hatry, & K. E. Newcomer (Eds.), *Handbook of practical program evaluation* (pp. 40–68). San Francisco: Jossey-Bass.
Shelton, T. L. (1999). Family-centered care in pediatric practice: When and how? *Journal of Developmental and Behavioral Pediatrics, 20*, 117–119.
Shelton, T. L., Jeppson, E. S., & Johnson, B. H. (1987). *Family-centered care for children with special health care needs*. Washington, DC: Association for the Care of Children's Health.
Stein, R. E., & Jessop. D. J. (1984). Does pediatric home care make a difference for children with chronic illness?: Findings from the Pediatric Ambulatory Care Treatment study. *Pediatrics, 73*, 845–853.
Stein, R. E., & Jessop, D. J. (1991). Long-term mental health effects of a pediatric home care program. *Pediatrics, 88*, 490–496.
Thomas, R. B. (1987). Family adaptation to a child with a chronic condition. In M. H. Rose & R. B. Thomas (Eds.), *Children with chronic conditions; Nursing in a family and community context* (pp. 46–50). Orlando, FL: Grune & Stratton.
Turnbull, H. R., & Turnbull, A. P. (1985). *Parents speak out then and now* (2nd ed.). Columbus, OH: Merrill.
Van Riper, M. (1999). Maternal perceptions of family–provider relationships and well-being of families of children with Downs's syndrome. *Research in Nursing Health, 22*, 357–368.
Ware, J. E., Snyder, M. K., Wright, W. R., & Davies, A. R. (1983). Defining and measuring patient satisfaction with medical care. *Evaluation and Program Planning, 6*, 247–263.
Washington, K., & Schwartz, I. S. (1996). Maternal perceptions of the effects of physical and occupational therapy services on caregiving competency. *Physical and Occupational Therapy in Pediatrics, 16*, 33–54.
Williams, J., Sharp, B., Griebel, M. L., Knabe, M. D., Spence, G. T., Weinberger, N., Hendon, A., & Rickert, V. (1995). Outcome findings from a multidisciplinary clinic for children with epilepsy. *Children's Health Care, 24*, 235–244.
Woodside, J. M., Rosenbaum, P. L., King, S. M., & King, G. A. (2001). Family-centered service: Developing and validating a self-assessment tool for pediatric service providers. *Children's Health Care, 30*, 237–252.

10

Interventions to Support Families of Children with Traumatic Brain Injuries

SHARI L. WADE

Traumatic brain injury (TBI) is the most common cause of acquired disability in childhood (Kraus, Rock, & Hemyari, 1990). Recent epidemiological surveys indicate that 185–230 cases per 100,000 children below age 15 are admitted for TBI, with 10–15% of these cases involving more significant brain insult (Kraus, 1995). According to Division of Injury Control estimates, over 30,000 children per year in the United States sustain permanent disabilities due to traumatic injury.

The majority of children with moderate to severe injuries experience at least transient cognitive and behavioral impairment. Academic achievement, school performance, and adaptive abilities may also be impaired. Long-term outcomes range from complete recovery to severe physical, cognitive, and behavioral deficits, with the magnitude of deficits corresponding to the severity of the initial neurological insult (Fay et al., 1994). Longer term follow-up suggests that behavioral changes and emerging behavior problems represent the most persistent sequelae of TBI in children (Rutter, Chadwick, Shaffer, & Brown, 1980). In the 2 years following injury, a new psychiatric disorder (e.g., emotional disorders, disinhibited states, conduct disorders) develops in 10–21% of children with a mild TBI, and in 62–71% of children with a severe TBI, underscoring the importance of social and behavioral outcomes following TBI (Bloom et al., 2001; Fay et al., 1994; Fletcher, Ewing-Cobbs, Miner, Levin, & Eisenberg, 1990; Max et al.,

1998b; Rutter, 1981; Schwartz et al., 2003). These new psychiatric disorders cut across diagnostic categories and often involve personality changes marked by increased impulsivity and affective lability (Bloom et al., 2001; Max et al., 2000).

COMMON PSYCHOSOCIAL TREATMENT NEEDS

Several previous studies indicate that pediatric TBI creates significant stress for parents and families (Max et al., 1998; Rivara et al., 1992, 1996; Wade, Taylor, Drotar, Stancin, & Yeates, 1998; Wade et al., 2002). These data suggest that families with severe TBI experience persistent injury-related stress and burden during the first year postinjury. Families expressed varied needs following the acute hospitalization for pediatric TBI, including more information regarding the child's injury and possible sequelae; access to resources; and support–communication with those who have had similar experiences (Aitken, Mele, & Barrett, 2004; Hawley, Ward, Magnay, & Long, 2002: Marks, Sliwinski, & Gordon, 1993; Wade, Taylor, Drotar, Stancin, & Yeates, 1996). However, parents appeared to have more difficulty expressing their emotional and personal needs, despite obvious distress (Wade et al., 1996). The relevance of these findings for family interventions following TBI is twofold. First, it is possible to identify areas of heightened stress and burden following TBI, and thus to tailor interventions to address these needs. Second, the findings suggest that the needs of families are not currently being met by existing standard care, such as outpatient rehabilitation services or support groups.

Pediatric TBI has also been linked to elevated psychological symptoms and distress in family members (Rivara et al., 1992, 1996; Wade et al., 1998). In research following TBI in adults, distress has been shown to increase over time as a function of both the behavioral and personality changes in the injured adult and the psychological functioning of the family member prior to the injury (Brooks, 1991; Kreutzer, Gervasio, & Camplair, 1994). Prospective investigations have also documented continued family dysfunction among families of children with severe TBI 3 or more years postinjury (Rivara et al., 1996; Wade et al., in press). These findings suggest that pediatric TBI results in persistent caregiver and family distress in a subset of families despite available resources.

MODERATORS OF OUTCOME: WHO IS AT RISK?

Although a significant minority of parents experience persistent burden and distress, many families adapt successfully to the increased demands of the injury (Wade et al., 1998, 2002). Factors such as socioeconomic status, ethnicity, preinjury family resources and stresses, and initial response to the injury appear to moderate the impact of pediatric TBI on caregivers, placing some families at greater risk for long-term difficulties (Wade et al., 2001; Wade et al., 2004b; Yeates et al., 2002). Specifically, parents of children with severe TBI who had high levels of family stress and conflict coupled with low levels of family support at the time of the injury reported significantly more injury-related stress than parents of children with severe injuries who had low levels of stress and high levels of support. Thus, a supportive environment buffered the additional stress and burden typically associated with TBI. Similarly, individual differences in initial coping responses to the injury have been shown to contribute to parental distress (Wade et al., 2001). Specifically, acceptance and the use of humor contributed to fewer psychological symptoms following TBI, whereas both efforts to alter the situation by taking action (active coping) and denial resulted in higher levels of distress (Wade et al., 2001). Racial/ethnic differences in coping also appear to contribute to disparities in family outcomes (Yeates et al., 2002). This series of studies suggests that families without these risk factors might benefit from more limited intervention, such as access to information, anticipatory guidance, and support; in contrast, at-risk families may require more intensive, skills-building therapeutic strategies to facilitate their adaptation.

In Figure 10.1, which depicts a framework of family adaptation following pediatric TBI, the family's response to the injury and its immediate sequelae is mediated by the caregiver's appraisal of injury-related stressors and burdens. Stress results from a perceived imbalance between the demands of the situation and the resources available to meet these demands (Lazarus & Folkman, 1984). A range of environmental, intrapersonal, and interpersonal factors influence the caregiver's appraisal of the situation and directly affect parent/family adaptation. These factors include coping skills, social supports, financial resources, knowledge, chronic interpersonal stressors, and other life events. These risk and protective factors may intervene between TBI sequelae and family adaptation by (1) attenuating appraisals of stress and threat; (2) reducing the level or intensity of one's response to the stress; or (3) facilitating adaptive responses to stress, thereby reducing the likelihood of parent distress and family dysfunction. Although not depicted in Figure 10.1, this process repeats itself over time with increasing burden and distress contributing to subsequent appraisals of threat (Wade, Drotar, Taylor, & Stancin, 1995). Family and caregiver adaptation after TBI, and thus needs for intervention, vary as a function of these risk and protective factors.

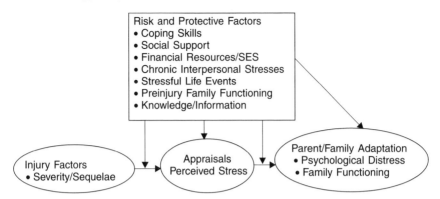

FIGURE 10.1. Model of influences on parent and family adaptation following TBI.

THE RELATIONSHIP BETWEEN FAMILY ADAPTATION AND THE CHILD'S PSYCHOLOGICAL RECOVERY

If specific family characteristics influence child outcomes following TBI, these factors can be targeted for intervention. Several prospective studies have demonstrated a relationship between the family environment and cognitive and behavioral outcomes among school-age children with TBI (Kinsella, Ong, Murtaugh, Prior, & Sawyer, 1999; Max et al., 1998b; Taylor et al., 1999; Yeates et al., 1997). In two related studies, Yeates et al. (1997) and Taylor et al. (1999) found that both poor premorbid and postinjury family functioning exacerbated the effects of the severe TBI on child functioning. Put differently, good family adjustment buffered the impact of TBI on child adaptation. Similarly, Kinsella and colleagues (1999) found a relationship between family factors at the time of the injury, such as single-parent status and psychological distress, and child behavioral symptoms at both 3 and 12 months following injury. In a study by Max et al. (1998b) poor preinjury family functioning, together with other premorbid family factors and injury severity, predicted the onset of novel behavioral disorders following TBI. In both of the latter investigations, the emergence of behavior problems was, in turn, predictive of postinjury family dysfunction. The findings by Kinsella et al. (1999) and Max et al. (1998b) are similar to those of Taylor and colleagues (1999), who found that (1) higher parent distress at 6 months predicted more child behavior problems at 12 months, when controlling for earlier behavior problems; and (2) conversely, more child behavior problems at 6 months predicted poorer family outcomes at 12 months, when controlling for earlier family adjustment. As depicted in Figure 10.2, these studies suggest that child recovery and family

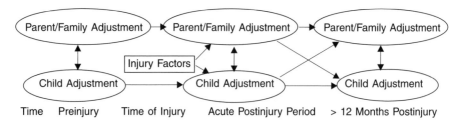

FIGURE 10.2. Relationship between parent and child adjustment following TBI.

adaptation exert reciprocal influences upon one another over time after an injury. Thus, family-centered interventions may provide a viable means for breaking this negative cycle, thereby improving both child and family outcomes.

CHALLENGES TO DEVELOPING EFFECTIVE INTERVENTIONS

Several issues contribute to the difficulty in conducting psychosocial interventions following pediatric TBI. First, the problems confronting children with TBI and their families are multifaceted and vary substantially across families (Rosenthal & Young, 1988; Wade et al., 1995). As a result, intervention models need to target multiple areas of vulnerability in a comprehensive intervention plan. Second, the family's needs are likely to change over the course of the child's recovery (Wade et al., 1995). For example, during the acute hospitalization, the family's primary concern is the child's survival. Many children receive no rehabilitation. For children receiving rehabilitation, the services are short-term and emphasize helping the child return to normal functioning at home and school. Only after the child returns home and resumes school do most families begin to come to terms with potentially persistent changes in the child (Max et al., 1998a). In fact, data suggest that the family's need for support and anticipatory guidance is likely to be greatest at the time when formal rehabilitation has ended. Family adaptation is an ongoing process influenced by the child's stage of recovery, as well as normal family development (e.g., sibling rebellion, birth of a child) and outside events (e.g., loss of a job, illness). Thus, any intervention must be individualized to take into account the family's stage of recovery and the stresses confronting it at that time.

Barriers to delivering family interventions must also be considered in developing effective treatments. Pediatric trauma and rehabilitation services are centralized in urban, university-affiliated hospitals, with inpatients drawn from broad geographic areas. Thus, returning to the rehabilitation facility for ongoing counseling may not be feasible. Moreover, regardless of whether the family lives in an urban or rural setting, local mental health providers and educators may lack requisite knowledge and expertise regarding the unique issues associated with TBI. Thus, services may be unavailable altogether, or families may be forced to travel prohibitively long distances to obtain them.

REVIEW OF AVAILABLE RESEARCH LITERATURE ON TREATMENT STRATEGIES

The literature reviewed thus far underscores the need for family-focused interventions to reduce psychiatric morbidity following pediatric TBI. Unfortunately, this clear need contrasts markedly with the current state of the art regarding empirically based, family-focused interventions. A recent National Institutes of Health (NIH) consensus panel decried the lack of psychosocial interventions for pediatric TBI, emphasizing the need for further efforts in this area (Agency for Health Care Policy and Research, 1999). The frameworks presented in Figures 10.1 and 10.2 suggest that there are several potential targets of interventions to facilitate family adaptation following pediatric TBI: (1) identified needs; (2) burden or symptoms arising from the injury (i.e., parental distress and child behavior problems); (3) risk and protective factors that influence outcomes; (4) parent–child interactions; or (5) some combination of the previous targets. The implications and advantages of each approach are discussed in turn.

Targeting Parent/Family Needs

Previous needs assessments, reviewed earlier, document parent needs for information, financial resources, and support (Aitken et al., 2004; Hawley et al., 2002; Marks et al., 1993). Thus, one approach to facilitating family adaptation is to address these identified needs. A major thrust of family-centered rehabilitation programs is responding to identified family needs (see Chapter 2 by Donders, this volume); however, there have been few randomized studies of the efficacy of providing information and support following pediatric TBI. Ponsford et al. (2001) examined the efficacy of providing an informational pamphlet regarding the symptoms of mild TBI and strategies for coping with these symptoms to children with mild TBI. Sixty-one children with mild TBI received the intervention and were seen at 1 week and 3 months postinjury. These children were compared to 58 children with mild TBI not receiving the intervention and two control groups of children with mild injuries not involving the head. The authors found that children receiving the informational pamphlet were less stressed, and had fewer behavioral and postconcussive symptoms overall than children with mild TBI not receiving the pamphlet. In a study with wives of adults with TBI, Rotondi, Sinkule, and Spring (2005) found high levels of satisfaction with a website providing information regarding TBI and an online peer support group.

Together, these studies provide tentative evidence that addressing needs for information and/or peer support can improve some outcomes. However, other studies have suggested a discrepancy between identified needs and levels of psychological distress following pediatric TBI (Wade et al., 1996). Moreover, a study by Singer and colleagues (1994), described below, found that informational support was associated with increasing rather than decreasing psychological distress. Thus, although identifying and addressing family needs is an important first step, it is unlikely to be sufficient for families with significant pre- or postinjury stressors.

Targeting the Symptoms/Outcomes

Because parent and child adaptation following TBI are closely related, interventions to improve either parent or child functioning are likely to contribute to improvements in the other individual as well. Singer and colleagues (1994) targeted parental anxiety and depression in parents of children with TBI using a structured stress management program involving self-monitoring, relaxation training, and cognitive modification. They compared this approach to an informational support group in a randomized trial involving nine families. Findings indicated that parents in the stress management group experienced a substantial reduction in both anxiety and depression following the intervention, whereas those in the informational support group actually reported an increase in anxiety and depression, suggesting that education alone is not sufficient to reduce symptoms. Unfortunately, the study sample was limited to only nine families, raising questions about the generalizability of the findings. Targeting symptoms is only likely to be successful if either the symptoms are primarily situational or the program also addresses any skills deficits (i.e., inadequate coping) underlying the symptom. Singer et al.'s stress management intervention falls into the latter category, in that teaching parents new strategies for responding to stressful situations is likely to alter both coping and symptoms.

Targeting the Moderators

Another approach to family intervention following pediatric TBI is to target the moderators of family adaptation, such as maladaptive coping or chronic interpersonal stresses. Problem-solving therapies are an example of a treatment approach that focuses on facilitating more effective coping. Training in problem-solving skills has been shown to be effective in reducing stress, negative affect, and depressive symptomatology in a wide range of clinical populations (D'Zurilla, 1986; Falloon, Boyd, & McGill, 1984; Nezu & Perri, 1989). Standard problem-solving skills interventions provide individuals with skills for coping with a stressful event or the daily hassles of life. In the case of TBI, caregivers are confronted with a wide range of new stressors that may tax existing coping resources or render them ineffective or maladaptive. A problem-solving framework may facilitate adaptation by equipping the individual with a new approach to these stressors. Depending on the situation, problem solving may lead to alternative "active" strategies for responding to the situation, or new ways of handling one's feelings. For example, in many cases, it may not be possible to return the injured child to his or her previous level of functioning. Thus, parental efforts directed toward this end may result in frustration and, ultimately, depression. However, if parents learn to come to terms emotionally with the changes in their child and to target potentially modifiable problems, they will experience a reduction in stress and subsequent distress.

Interventions that target potential moderators such as coping or interpersonal stressors are only likely to be effective if the parent or family has deficits in those areas. Thus, parents with good problem-solving skills are unlikely to show significant improvements following a problem-solving program. Moreover, standard problem-solving or skills-building approaches require tailoring to fit the needs of families following pediatric TBI. Nonetheless, the skills-building emphasis of these approaches holds merit for families at greatest risk for long-term difficulties following TBI.

Targeting the Interaction

Another approach to family intervention following pediatric TBI is to target the interaction between the parent and child. Family therapy approaches such as that outlined by Robin and Foster (1989) explicitly have the goal of reducing family conflicts by improving communication and eliminating dysfunctional interaction patterns. Likewise, the "positive everyday routines" outlined by Ylvisaker and Feeney (1998) emphasize clear communications between parent and child and structuring the environment to reduce problem situations. Although this approach has not been examined in controlled studies, the work by Ylvisaker and Feeney suggests that it holds promise for reducing problem behaviors. However, truly changing the interaction requires some level of participation from the child, which may not be possible with very young or very impaired children.

Comprehensive and/or Tailored Approaches

Given the multidimensional nature of family stress following TBI and the range of factors influencing family adaptation, comprehensive approaches targeting multiple risks, moderators, and/or outcomes might have the greatest efficacy. However, it is likely that the profile of individual needs and risk factors will vary widely, warranting a more individualized or tailored approach. For these reasons, I developed an intervention program integrating information regarding the cognitive and behavioral sequelae of TBI with family training in problem-solving skills, family communication, and antecedent behavior management approaches. The intervention is based on a modified transactional stress and coping model similar to that depicted in Figure 10.1 (Lazarus & Folkman, 1984). In addition to teaching problem-solving skills, the intervention targets parent–child interaction via training in communication skills. Training in antecedent behavior management strategies was targeted at reducing the child's behavior problems and facilitating parent–child interaction. Children with TBI also learned problem solving, communication, and self-management skills to address deficits arising from their injury.

The intervention consisted of a core of seven 90-minute, face-to-face sessions completed over a 6-month period. Table 10.1 outlines the session content for the seven core sessions. The sessions included parents and school-age children (children with TBI and siblings), and emphasized improving skills and communication in the entire family.

During the initial two sessions, family members (parents, injured children, and siblings) identified goals, learned the steps of the problem-solving framework (see Table 10.2), and implemented the problem-solving process with a goal identified by the family. Because family issues and concerns

TABLE 10.1. Family Problem-Solving Intervention Core Sessions

Session	Topic	Key features
1	Overview, identify goals	Learning about family, orientation to approach
2	Steps of problem solving	Reviewing steps, implement with easy problem
3	Cognitive changes	Identifying changes, strategies to reduce frustration
4	Behavior changes	Identifying changes, antecedent behavior management
5	Behavior/communication	More behavior management, communication skills
6	Crisis management/review	How to handle crises, family assets, and weaknesses
7	Planning for the future	Reviewing what works and planning for transitions

TABLE 10.2. The ABC's of the Problem-Solving Process

Step	What's involved
Aim	Individual or family identifies a detailed and specific goal to work on.
Brainstorm	The family comes up with as many solutions as possible to achieve the aim.
Choose	The family picks an option to implement after discussing the relative pluses and minuses of each option.
Do it	The family comes up with a detailed plan for how it will implement the option selected.
Evaluate	The family monitors when it tried the plan and whether or not it was successful.

vary widely, goals were not limited to problems arising from the injury. Session 2, and all subsequent sessions, included implementing the problem-solving process around a goal identified by the family.

Drawing upon previous work by Feeney and Ylivasker (1995; Ylvisaker & Feeney, 1998), the therapist devoted sessions 3–5 to providing didactic information regarding the cognitive and behavioral changes that may follow TBI and teaching the family antecedent behavior management strategies for addressing these difficulties. These strategies included creating positive behavioral momentum, giving the child choice and control, and eliminating environmental triggers to problem behaviors. Although we also discussed traditional rewards and punishments, the emphasis was on keeping things positive and heading off problems before they arise. During the fifth session, the therapist also introduced communication skills. In the sixth session, the therapist discussed crisis management (see Ylvisaker & Feeney, 1998), reviewed problem-solving, communication, and behavior management strategies, and identified unresolved stressors and difficulties. Based on the family's self-identified profile of needs, they received up to two individualized sessions per month during months 4 and 5 of the intervention. Modules for the individualized sessions included (1) managing behavior problems, (2) responding to siblings, (3) communicating with spouse–family members, (4) working with the school, and (5) stress management.

A randomized clinical trial of this intervention was completed with 37 families of children with moderate to severe TBI (Wade, Michaud, & Brown, in press). Consistent with hypotheses, significant group differences were found for the Child Behavior Checklist (CBCL) Internalizing Total and CBCL Anxiety/Depression and Withdrawal subscales. Corresponding effect sizes (η^2) were large, ranging from 0.17 to 0.21. Follow-up analyses revealed stronger group differences in child internalizing behaviors among children with less severe (GCS score > 12) and more recent injuries (time since injury less than 7 months). Among these subgroups, effect sizes were large (partial η^2 = 0.36–0.40), whereas the effect sizes for children with more severe and less recent injuries were small and not statistically significant. Similarly, larger treatment effects were observed among older (age ≥ 11 years) than among younger children, those whose fathers participated, and those with more educated mothers (more than a high school education).

Satisfaction data indicated that the program was successful and well received. All parents receiving the family problem-solving (FPS) intervention endorsed increased knowledge in program content areas, such as understanding their child's injury and awareness of strategies to improve attention and behavior. All parents reported that they understood and got along with their child better, while 83% of fathers and 65% of mothers reported feeling less stressed.

Taken together, the findings suggest that FPS holds promise as a structured intervention to facilitate family coping and improve child outcomes following TBI. However, they also underscored potential areas for improvement, such as the need for simplification of didactic materials and greater emphasis on involving fathers. Additionally, the intervention was delivered in the home for nearly half of the families who were unable to attend regular meetings at the hospital. The inability of many families to attend sessions consistently suggested a need to identify other approaches to delivering interventions to families.

Based on findings from the initial face-to-face study, I developed and piloted an online version of FPS. The intervention structure paralleled that of the face-to-face FPS, with seven biweekly core sessions providing training in problem solving, communication skills, and antecedent behavior management to all enrolled families. As in the face-to-face intervention, individualized sessions were conducted addressing the unique stressors and burdens of specific families, allowing us to provide an intervention that was both standardized and tailored to individual needs.

Each session of online FPS consisted of a self-guided online portion providing didactic content regarding the desired skill (i.e., problem solving), video clips showing individuals and families modeling the skill, and exercises and assignments giving the family an opportunity to practice the skill. The second part of each session involved a synchronous online appointment with the therapist to answer questions, review the exercises/worksheets, and implement the problem-solving process with a problem identified by the family.

A total of 19 participants in six families were recruited to participate in the online FPS feasibility project. Families completed 10.3 Web sessions (range = 7–12) and 10.1 synchronous videoconferences (range = 7–14) on average. Participating family members ranked the website and videoconferences as moderately easy to very easy to use (Wade, Wolfe, & Pestian, 2004c). Twelve of 19 participants (63%) preferred meeting online to meeting in person, noting perceived confidentiality and the convenience of accessing services within one's home. Perceptions of the helpfulness of the intervention were also high (Wade et al., 2004c). In addition to increased understanding of TBI, parents reported that the information gave them a sense of closure and helped them to feel less alone. All parents and siblings, and all but one child with TBI (94.7% of total), indicated that they would recommend the program to others. Again, the convenience of meeting within one's home was noted as a factor in perceptions of satisfaction.

Parents reported significant declines in psychological symptoms (depression and global psychiatric symptoms), parenting stress, and injury-related stress and burden from baseline to follow-up (Wade, Wolfe, Brown, & Pestian, 2005). Parents also reported improvements in child outcomes, as indicated by a significant decrease on the Antisocial Behavior scale of the Home and Community Social Behavior Scale. The findings suggest that children with TBI and their families can successfully use and benefit from an online intervention program to improve child and family adaptation. Given the range of prior computer experience among participants, the families' ability to independently complete the self-guided sessions supports the notion that a Web-based approach is feasible for parents of children with TBI. More importantly, our findings provide preliminary evidence that participation in such a program can substantially reduce parental burden and distress, as well as improve child behavior problems and conflicts with parents.

Taken together, findings from these studies suggest that treatments that incorporate components to target a variety of moderators and outcomes can successfully improve parent and child outcomes. However, these programs are relatively intensive and may not be necessary for families with good preinjury skills and functioning. Additionally, younger children or those with very severe deficits may be unable to participate in and benefit from the collaborative problem-solving process.

FUTURE DIRECTIONS

Treatment studies for families of children with TBI remain in their infancy. However, the handful of previous intervention studies reviewed earlier provides important directions for future investigators in this area. Because most of these approaches show some promise and target an important aspect of the family adaptation process, there can be no consensus about "evidence-based" practice at the present. However, given the diversity of preinjury family characteristics and child and family outcomes, it will be increasingly important to understand what works for whom. For example, interventions that place a heavy emphasis on didactics may be less effective for families with limited literacy or emotional (vs. cognitive) coping styles, whereas such families might respond well to peer support. Given the relatively small numbers of children available at a single site, multicenter collaborations will be essential to address this question.

Ease and accessibility should be important considerations for all future treatment studies. Today, all families experience a time crunch, and parents of children with a significant injury are likely to have even less available time than other parents. To be effective and doable in the real world, interventions will likely have to abandon traditional office or hospital-based sessions for more accessible alternatives. Studies by Rotondi et al. (2005) and Wade et al. (2004c, 2005) indicate that online models may be a viable alternative for many families. Home-based interventions, or those that are integrated into standard clinic visits, provide other possibilities.

Another important future direction for family interventions is to tailor them to the child's age and development level. Most studies include children ranging from early elementary school through adolescence. However, these children have very different cognitive abilities, and their parents face very different developmental and behavioral challenges. Again, through multicenter collaborations, we can begin to test different intervention approaches for different age groups. Young children and older adolescents have largely been neglected in previous interventions and warrant particular attention in future research.

Finally, although family-centered interventions for pediatric TBI are in their infancy, there is much we can learn from clinical trials in both child and adult psychology–psychiatry. For example, attention-deficit/hyperactivity disorder (ADHD) shares many features with behavioral sequelae of TBI, and secondary ADHD is a common diagnosis after injury (Max et al., 2004). Thus, the recent randomized clinical trials of treatments for ADHD may provide insights for subsequent interventions for pediatric TBI. Likewise, problem-solving therapies have been examined in randomized trials with a growing number of chronic illness populations, providing additional avenues for understanding their application to TBI. Subsequent research efforts will be most successful if they can benefit from advances in related areas of study. Ultimately, the greatest progress will be made through collaboration among centers and across disciplines.

REFERENCES

Agency for Health Care Policy and Research. (1999). *Rehabilitation for traumatic brain injury in children and adolescents* (Evidence Report No. 2, Suppl.; Publication No. 99-E025). Washington, DC: U.S. Government Printing Office.

Aitken, M. E., Mele, N., & Barrett, K. W. (2004). Recovery of injured children: Parent perspectives on family needs. *Archives of Physical Medicine and Rehabilitation, 85,* 567–573.

Bloom, D. R., Levin, H. S., Ewing-Cobbs, L., Saunders, A. E., Song, J., Fletcher, J. N., & Kowatch, R. A. (2001). Lifetime and novel psychiatric disorders after pediatric traumatic brain injury. *Journal of American Academy of Child and Adolescent Psychiatry, 40,* 572–579.

Brooks, D. N. (1991). The head-injury family. *Journal of Clinical and Experimental Neuropsychology, 13,* 155–188.

D'Zurilla, T. J. (1986). *Problem-solving therapy: A social competence approach to clinical intervention.* New York: Springer.

Falloon, I. R. F., Boyd, J. L., & McGill, C. W. (1984). *Family care of schizophrenia: A problem-solving approach to the treatment of mental illness* (pp. 207–284). New York: Guilford Press.

Fay, G. C., Jaffe, K. M., Polissar, N. L., Liao, S., Rivara, J. B., & Martin, K. M. (1994). Outcome of pediatric traumatic brain injury at three years: A cohort study. *Archives of Physical Medicine and Rehabilitation, 75,* 733–741.

Feeney, T. J., & Ylvisaker, M. (1995). Choice and routine: Antecedent behavioral interventions for adolescents with severe traumatic brain injury. *Journal of Head Trauma Rehabilitation, 10,* 67–86.

Fletcher, J., Ewing-Cobbs, L., Miner, M., Levin, H., & Eisenberg, H. (1990). Behavioral changes after closed head injury in children. *Journal of Consulting and Clinical Psychology, 58,* 93–98.

Hawley, C. A., Ward, A. B., Magnay, A. R., & Long, J. (2002). Children's brain injury a postal follow-up of 525 children from one health region in the UK. *Brain Injury, 16,* 969–985.

Kinsella, G., Ong, B., Murtaugh, D., Prior, M., & Sawyer, M. (1999). The role of the family for behavioral outcome in children and adolescents following traumatic brain injury. *Journal of Consulting and Clinical Psychology, 67,* 116–123.

Kraus, J. F. (1995). Epidemiologic features of brain injury in children: Occurrence, children of risk, causes and manner of injury, severity and outcomes. In S. H. Broman & M. E. Michel (Eds.), *Traumatic head injury in children* (pp. 22–39). New York: Oxford University Press.

Kraus, J. F., Rock, A., & Hemyari, P. (1990). Brain injuries among infants, children, adolescents, and young adults. *American Journal of Disorders in Childhood, 144,* 684–691.

Kreutzer, J. S., Gervasio, A. H., & Camplair, P. S. (1994). Primary caregivers' psychological status and family functioning after traumatic brain injury. *Brain Injury, 8,* 197–210.

Lazarus, R. S., & Folkman, S. (1984). *Stress, appraisal, and coping.* New York: Springer.

Marks, M., Sliwinski, M., & Gordon, W. A. (1993). An examination of the needs of families with a brain injured child. *Neurorehabilitation, 3,* 1–12.

Max, J. E., Castillo, C. S., Robin, D. A., Lindgren, S. D., Smith, W. L., Sata, Y., et al. (1998a). Predictors of family functioning following traumatic brain injury in children and adolescents. *Journal of the American Academy of Child and Adolescent Psychiatry, 37,* 83–90.

Max, J. E., Koele, S. L., Castillo, C. C., Lindgren, S. D., Arndt, S., Bokura, H., et al. (2000). Personality change disorder in children and adolescents following traumatic brain injury. *Journal of the International Neuropsychological Society, 6,* 279–289.

Max, J. E., Koele, S. L., Smith, W. L., Sato, Y., Lindgren, S. D., Robin, D. A., et al. (1998b). Psychiatric disorders in children and adolescents after severe traumatic brain injury: A controlled study. *Journal of American Academy of Child and Adolescent Psychiatry, 37,* 832–840.

Max, J. E., Lansing, A. E., Koele, S. L., Castillo, C. S., Bokura, H., & Schachar, R. (2004). Attention deficit hyperactivity disorder in children and adolescents following traumatic brain injury. *Developmental Neuropsychology, 25,* 159–177.

Nezu, A. M., & Perri, M. G. (1989). Social problem-solving therapy for unipolar depression: An initial dismantling investigation. *Journal of Consulting and Clinical Psychology, 57,* 408–413.

Ponsford, J., Willmott, C., Rothwell, A., Cameron, P., Ayton, G., Nelms, R., et al. (2001). Impact of early intervention on outcome after mild traumatic brain injury in children. *Pediatrics, 108,* 1297–1303.

Rivara, J. B., Fay, G., Jaffe, K., Polissar, N., Shurtleff, H., & Martin, K. (1992). Predictors of family functioning one year following traumatic brain injury in children. *Archives of Physical Medicine and Rehabilitation, 73,* 899–910.

Rivara, J. B., Jaffe, K. M., Polissar, N. L., Fay, G. C., Liao, S., & Martin, K. M. (1996). Predictors of family functioning and change 3 years after traumatic brain injury in children. *Archives of Physical Medicine and Rehabilitation, 77,* 754–764.

Robin, A. L., & Foster, S. L. (1989). *Negotiating parent–adolescent conflict: A behavioral–family systems approach.* New York: Guilford Press.

Rosenthal, M., & Young, T. (1988). Effective family intervention after TBI: Theory and practice. *Journal of Head Trauma Rehabilitation, 3,* 42–50.

Rotondi, A. J., Sinkule, J., & Spring, M. (2005). An interactive web-based intervention for persons with TBI and their families: Use and evaluation by female significant others. *Journal of Head Trauma Rehabilitation, 20,* 173–185.

Rutter, M. (1981). Psychological sequelae of brain damage in children. *American Journal of Psychiatry, 138,* 1533–1543.

Rutter, M., Chadwick, O., Shaffer, D., & Brown, C. (1980). A prospective study of children with head injuries: I. Description and methods. *Psychological Medicine, 10,* 633–645.

Schwartz, L., Taylor, H. G., Drotar, D., Yeates, K. O., Wade, S. L., & Stancin, T. (2003). Long-term postinjury-onset behavior problems following pediatric traumatic brain injury: Incidence, predictors, and correlates. *Journal of Pediatric Psychology, 28,* 251–263.

Singer, G. H. S., Glang, A., Nixon, C., Cooley, E., Kerns, K. A., Williams, D., et al. (1994). A comparison of two psychosocial interventions for parents of children with acquired brain injury: An exploratory study. *Journal of Head Trauma Rehabilitation, 9,* 38–49.

Taylor, H. G., Yeates, K. O., Wade, S. L., Drotar, D., Klein, S., & Stancin, T. (1999). Influences on first-year recovery from traumatic brain injury in children. *Neuropsychology, 13,* 76–89.

Wade, S. L., Borawski, E. A., Taylor, H. G., Drotar, D., Yeates, K. O., & Stancin, T.

(2001). The relationship of caregiver coping to family outcomes during the initial year following pediatric traumatic injury. *Journal of Consulting and Clinical Psychology, 69*, 406–415.

Wade, S. L., Drotar, D., Taylor, H. G., & Stancin, T. (1995). Assessing the effects of traumatic brain injury (TBI) on family functioning: Conceptual and methodological issues. *Journal of Pediatric Psychology, 20*, 737–752.

Wade, S. L., Michaud, L., & Brown, T. M. (in press). Putting the pieces together: A family problem-solving intervention for pediatric TBI. *Journal of Head Trauma Rehabilitation.*

Wade, S. L., Taylor, H. G., Drotar, D., Stancin, T., & Yeates, K. O. (1996). Childhood traumatic brain injury: Initial impact on the family. *Journal of Learning Disabilities, 29*, 652–661.

Wade, S. L., Taylor, H. G., Drotar, D., Stancin, T., & Yeates, K. O. (1998). Family burden and adaptation following traumatic brain injury (TBI) in children. *Pediatrics, 102*, 110–116.

Wade, S. L., Taylor, H. G., Drotar, D., Stancin, T., Yeates, K. O., & Minich, N. M. (2002). A prospective study of long-term caregiver and family adaptation following brain injury in children. *Journal of Head Trauma Rehabilitation, 17*, 96–111.

Wade, S. L., Taylor, H. G., Drotar, D., Yeates, K. O., Stancin, T., & Minich, N. M. (2004b). Interpersonal stressors and resources as predictors of caregiver adaptation following pediatric traumatic injury. *Journal of Consulting and Clinical Psychology, 72*, 776–784.

Wade, S. L., Taylor, H. G., Yeates, K. O., Drotar, D., Stancin, T., & Minich, N. M. (in press). Long-term parental and family adaptation following pediatric brain injury. *Journal of Pediatric Psychology.*

Wade, S. L., Wolfe, C. R., Brown, T. M., & Pestian, J. P. (2005). Putting the pieces together: Preliminary efficacy of a web-based family intervention for children with traumatic brain injury. *Journal of Pediatric Psychology, 30*, 437–442.

Wade, S. L., Wolfe, C. R., & Pestian, J. P. (2004c). A web-based problem solving intervention for families of children with traumatic brain injury. *Behavioral Research Methods and Instructional Computing, 36*, 261–269.

Yeates, K. O., Taylor, H. G., Drotar, D., Wade, S. L., Klein, S., Stancin, T., & Schatschneider, C. (1997). Pre-injury family environment as a determinant of recovery from traumatic brain injuries in school-age children. *Journal of the International Neuropsychological Society, 3*, 617–630.

Yeates, K. O., Taylor, H. G., Woodrome, S. E., Wade, S. L., Stancin, T., & Drotar, D. (2002). Race as a moderator of parent and family outcomes following pediatric traumatic brain injury. *Journal of Pediatric Psychology, 27*, 393–404.

Ylvisaker, M., & Feeney, T. (1998). *Collaborative brain injury intervention: Positive everyday routines.* San Diego: Singular.

11

Cognitive and Behavioral Rehabilitation

ROBERT W. BUTLER

The involvement of clinical psychologists and/or neuropsychologists in the rehabilitation treatment aspects of brain injury and developmental disabilities is a relatively recent phenomenon, particularly within the area of pediatrics. Traditionally, these professionals have played the role of evaluators and assessors: documenting the existence of neurocognitive deficits, establishing patterns and severity of dysfunction, and identifying treatment gains or progression of impairment. Over the past decade, however, psychologists are becoming increasingly involved in treatment. Brain injury rehabilitation in general is a well-established field, especially in regards to physiatry and speech/occupational therapy. Social workers have also played an important role in attempting to improve familial and behavioral functioning in individuals who have suffered developmental disabilities or deficits following an acquired insult to the central nervous system (CNS). In brain injury, these efforts typically occur within the inpatient setting during the acute phase of recovery. Outpatient treatment programs began to flourish in the late 1970s and early 1980s. Initially, these outpatient services were reasonably well funded by medical insurance companies. Unfortunately, in the early 21st century, this no longer appears to be the case. While inpatient treatment remains an important aspect of rehabilitation following a CNS insult, outpatient services have dwindled in accord with poor funding from medical insurance. This state of affairs has challenged the rehabilitation community to begin to offer more cost-effective treatment modalities. One can view this as detrimental to patient care, or, alternatively, as a charge to the development of brief but comprehensive treatment programs that will improve neurocognitive and behavioral functioning in the patient with a neurodevelopmental disability. The theoretical foundations of CNS rehabilitation can be considered to begin with the writings of Alexander Luria (1963). He posited that the brain is not a static organ. Luria recognized that after an acute insult to the CNS, there is a period of spontaneous recovery that typically extends 1 to 2 years. During this period of spontaneous recovery, it is believed that functional reorganization occurs within the brain, and that new neuronal pathways develop in order to compensate for terminally damaged neurons. Growing evidence within the field of brain injury clearly supports the likelihood of structural and functional changes in the brain associated with CNS rehabilitation (Levin & Grafman, 2000; Ogg et al., 2002; Laatsch, Pavel, Jobe, Lin, & Quintana, 1999; Laatsch, Thulborn, Krisky, Shobat, & Sweeney, 2004). Rehabilitation and cognitive remediation on an outpatient basis has traditionally involved efforts to stimulate the process of spontaneous recovery. Thus, the initial approaches to neurodevelopmental rehabilitation were very similar to a cognitive form of physical therapy: exercising the brain's abilities. As is elucidated in this chapter, this initial approach, while still relevant, has been significantly broadened to include the use of memory training, teaching metacognitive strategies, psychological treatments, and, particularly in the case of children and adolescents, interventions directed toward family members.

Not all neurocognitive deficits are associated with a brain insult, such as a traumatic injury or a chronic, poorly controlled seizure disorder. Children and adolescents with learning disability, attention-deficit/hyperactivity disorder (ADHD), Asperger syndrome, or other neurodevelopmental disorders frequently present with a constellation of neuropsychological impairment that cannot be attributed to an identified brain injury. It is, however, becoming increasingly apparent that the goals of workers in developmental disabilities and brain injury rehabilitation are frequently similar, particularly within the area of pediatrics. The need for increased communication between these professionals has become especially relevant given the aforementioned reduction of outpatient CNS rehabilitation services in childhood and adolescence. Essentially, the public school system has been tacitly given the task of brain injury rehabilitation for both populations: individuals with developmental disabilities and those who have an acquired brain injury. Correspondingly, this has left the educational system extremely overburdened and unprepared for a Herculean task. The point is, within childhood and adolescence, there needs to be more communication and cooperation between learning disability specialists, school psychologists, and brain injury rehabilitation psychologists and neuropsychologists.

The established approach to brain injury rehabilitation has been multidisciplinary, and this remains a valid methodology. Children who suffer trauma, and also those who experience unacquired neurodevelopmental disabilities, typically have more than one deficit. For example, the individual may suffer from language disturbances, visual–spatial processing deficits, and difficulties with self-control associated with frontal brain involvement. A treatment approach for such a patient would likely involve a speech pathologist, an occupational therapist, and a clinical psychologist or clinical neuropsychologist. However, there is an increasing appreciation that multidisciplinary services do not necessarily have to be administered "under one roof." With established communication advances such as e-mail and conference calling, the patient can receive therapies in various institutions/locations, and treating professionals can still interact as a close team. This reduces the financial burden of treatment. This chapter describes treatment efforts directed toward neurocognitive deficits in children and adolescents. Empirical studies in support of these approaches are presented. Most work in this area comes from attempts to improve the functioning of individuals who have suffered a traumatic brain injury, because this is the most common neurological complication in childhood–adolescence (Yeates, 2000). Exciting developments are also occurring in the pediatric hematology–oncology field. Thus, work with children and adolescents who have brain impairment associated with malignancies and their treatment is also described. An emphasis is placed on the importance of multimodal treatment. In addition to traditional brain injury rehabilitation approaches, it is believed that attention to other important psychological factors is equally needed. In accord, the need for effective psychotherapeutic interventions, and also directing treatment not only to the pediatric patient but also to family members, is described. I also discuss the necessity for early secondary education and vocational planning within the mid adolescence years. One of the major innovations in pediatric neurodevelopmental rehabilitation has been within the area of psychopharmacology. There has been an increasing recognition that medications, such as the stimulants, can play an important role in the rehabilitation process. Empirical evidence is summarized from this perspective.

NEURODEVELOPMENTAL TREATMENT IN REHABILITATION

A National Institutes of Health (NIH) Consensus Statement (1998) concluded that while research results remain somewhat equivocal, support exists for the use of cognitive rehabilitation methods with adults. The clinical efficacy of these intervention methods is also supported by an article documenting the effectiveness of remediation efforts to improve attention, memory, functional communication, and executive functioning in adults (Cicerone et al., 2000). Relatively less work has been directed toward the efficacy of these methods with children who are cognitively impaired (Sohlberg & Mateer, 2001), and much of the current evidence comes from case reports that provide limited documentation of improvements in attention, concentration, and academic functioning (Penkman, 2004).

While directly applying adult methods and techniques to the pediatric population is an inherently risky process, in my experience, many of the rehabilitation approaches developed for older individuals can be used with children and adolescents. The rehabilitation processes of massed practice, instruction in mnemonic strategies, cognitive-behavioral interventions to facilitate optimism and problem solving, instruction in metacognitive strategies that allow individuals to become more attuned to their own deficits and ways in which they can be managed, and attention to environmental issues, such as nutrition and sleep, all appear to have relevance for the pediatric population. An important caveat is that there is very little empirical evidence for the efficacy of these interventions with this population. It should be noted that very few randomized clinical trials of these methods have been conducted in either the adult or pediatric populations. Later in this chapter, I briefly describe the largest, to date, clinical trial of a multimodal rehabilitation approach with children and adolescents. At the time of the writing of this chapter, this clinical trial represents a very significant study of neurodevelopmental rehabilitation. There is clearly a need for more clinical trials, and multimodal intervention approaches will likely be the rule rather than the exception in effective rehabilitation. I now present evidence to support the use of various brain injury rehabilitation methods with children and adolescents.

Metacognitive strategies, that is, teaching individuals to monitor their own thinking, have received some of the strongest support in improving attentional processes in children with neurodevelopmental disabilities (Brett & Laatsch, 1998). Multimodal approaches, with or without metacognitive strategies, have been successful in reducing aggressive and disruptive behaviors, improving problem-solving skills, and decreasing cognitive deficits, and also have resulted in a high degree of parent and teacher satisfaction (Silver, Boake, & Cavazos, 1994; Slifer et al., 1997; Suzman, Morris, Morris, & Milan, 1997). These multimodal approaches introduce various combinations of behavior modification, rehearsed practice, cognitive-behavioral therapy, and parent training. Also applying a multimodal approach, Teichner, Golden, and Giannaris (1999) reported reductions in aggression in an adolescent with severe brain injury. The methods included contingency management, problem-solving skills training, social skills training, relaxation training, anger management, and also working with the adolescent's parents.

Psychological, behavioral, and psychiatric disturbances are frequently an outcome of brain impairment in childhood. A number of researchers have addressed the importance of these problems, in addition to attempting to improve cognition and academic functioning. Behavior therapy with pharmacological treatment has been shown to reduce aggressive behavior in children and adolescents who have experienced a traumatic brain injury (Kehle, Clark, & Jenson, 1996; Deaton, 1987). More detailed work on pharmacological interventions with children–adolescents who suffer attentional problems associated with CNS-related malignancies and their treatment is presented later in the chapter. Children and adolescents who experience a traumatic brain injury are at risk for social skills deficits and withdrawal. Socialization is a major component of quality of life, and initial attempts at improving functioning in this area are promising (Warschausky, Kewman, & Kay, 1999).

Baron and Goldberger (1993) have written about the importance of ecological, or environmentally based, interventions with children who have neurodevelopmental complications. Along with cognitive remediation, specific attention needs to be directed toward the child's environment in order to facilitate rehabilitation. Frequently, children will need extended time limits for examinations, the use of true–false and multiple-choice formats in testing rather than essay examinations, and encouragement to record classroom lectures for later review. Other ecological interventions recommended by the authors include using written handouts, in order to decrease demands for copying from the whiteboard, and substituting computers for handwritten assignments. An important point made by Baron and Goldberger is that while cognitive remediation can benefit many children who suffer a brain injury, one should not expect a return to baseline, preinjury status. Thus, alterations in environmental demands combined with rehabilitation are most likely to result in maximal therapeutic gains. Along with these changes and considerations, it has been my clinical experience that factors such as good nutrition, sleep patterns, and stimulation levels also need careful analysis. I encourage the reader to recall the last time he or she slept poorly for 2 to 3 nights, perhaps in conjunction with some jet lag and/or a decreased appetite. I suspect the recall of an incident such as this will be accompanied by memories of reduced mental efficiency/efficacy.

As noted earlier, rehabilitation efforts have been directed toward children and adolescents who have completed treatment for a malignancy and who subsequently experience resultant cognitive and learning disabilities. The two most common childhood cancers are the leukemias and brain tumors (Margolin & Poplack, 1997; Heideman, Packer, Albright, Freeman, & Rorke, 1997). These diseases and their associated treatments can result in a pattern of neurodevelopmental impairment that is very similar to that reported in children with nonverbal learning disabilities. More specifically, they tend to cause deficits in attention/concentration, nonverbal intelligence, visual–spatial processing, visual–motor integration, and socialization difficulties (Fletcher & Copeland, 1988; Ris & Noll, 1994; Butler, Hill, Steinherz, Meyers, & Finlay, 1994; Moleski, 2000).

In response to these established impairments, Butler (1998) described a treatment approach that combined massed practice, instruction in metacognitive strategies, and cognitive-behavioral psychotherapy applied to a single child participant who had experienced neurocognitive impairment associated with pediatric cancer. "Massed practice" refers to drill exercises that are designed to strengthen cognitive abilities, such as attention and information-processing speed. "Metacognitive strategies," as noted earlier, involve teaching individuals to be conscious of their own styles of thinking, and to incorporate the use of new thought methods and strategies that will result in superior performance. "Cognitive-behavioral psychotherapy" (Meichenbaum, 1977) is an intervention approach that recognizes the importance of self-thought and self-talk, and uses behavioral principles to strengthen appropriate positive internal dialogues. Thus, an individual is taught to avoid unproductive and irrational self-thinking, and to become one's "best coach" rather than one's own "worst enemy." These three methods, respectively, were selected from the fields of brain injury rehabilitation, educational psychology, and clinical psychology. The case study applied this innovative tripartite model for brain injury rehabilitation, and significant improvements in cognitive functions following the remediation process were reported.

As of this writing, the most comprehensive report of an intervention designed to improve neurocognitive functioning in pediatric cancer survivors has been published by Butler and Copeland (2002). This study described in greater detail the approach used in the aforementioned case study (Butler, 1998). Continuing to use the tripartite model, the authors applied brain injury rehabilitation training exercises. Techniques developed by Sohlberg and Mateer (1996), "attention process training" (APT), were administered to pediatric cancer survivors who had documented attentional dysfunction, in addition to other neuropsychological disturbances, such as delayed information-processing speed. These multidimensional exercises are designed to strengthen attentional abilities in the areas of sustained, selective, divided, and executive attentional control. The APT treatment exercises were combined with activities considered to be more intrinsically interesting to children. Various toys and games were selected that did have not only a significant attentional component but also stimulated active participation. These included games such as "Simon," and computer-administered exercises. An alternating rule was adopted in which an APT activity was maintained for approximately 15 minutes, at which time one of the more intrinsically interesting activities was then selected with the patient's input. Therapists would progress alternately in this manner. To maximize the participant's perception of progress and success, a 50–80% rule was adopted.

In order to maintain engagement in a single activity, the individual had to achieve at least 50% successful responding. When 80% successful responding was obtained, the exercises were advanced to the next level of difficulty.

Intensive instruction in metacognitive strategies was provided. Strategies were divided into three dimensions: task preparedness, on-task performance, and posttask behavior. Depending on the level of functioning of the participant, it was expected that at least 10–15 strategies be incorporated, preferably 15 or more. Individuals of younger age and with greater degrees of impairment may have been taught fewer than 10 strategies. These brain rehabilitation exercises were used to document the effectiveness of an individual strategy. An exercise was administered, a strategy was taught, and if improvement on the task was established, the strategy was incorporated into the participant's dictionary of metacognitive resources. Strategies were individualized for the patient, and the child's own terminology and language were used whenever possible. While a dictionary of metacognitive strategies exists (Butler & Copeland, 2002), therapists were encouraged to observe children–adolescents very closely in order to identify new potential strategies that would be effective for individual cognitive difficulties.

Cognitive-behavioral psychotherapeutic techniques and principles were also employed. Participants were initially instructed to talk out loud to themselves following the therapist's modeling. When appropriate successful dialogue patterns and structures were obtained, the individual was subsequently allowed to silently use his or her self-statements. These techniques were also applied to assist the children–adolescents in their ability to resist distraction. During this part of therapy, following modeling, the therapist served as a very active distractant to the participant, thus allowing for the verification of skills acquisition. Finally, close attention was directed toward the patients' own style of self-assessment. Appropriate, positive self-statements were encouraged and taught, and negative self-perceptions were challenged.

This cognitive remediation program (CRP) was administered as a team approach intervention. The team consisted of therapist and participant, as well as parents and teachers. Therapy was administered in an individualized manner, and treatment occurred over a 4- to 6-month period. The CRP consisted of 20 two-hour weekly sessions of therapy. The length of the intervention was based on traditional outpatient brain injury rehabilitation practice. Each week, parents were provided with the metacognitive strategies that had been taught in the session, and prompted to promote their use during homework and household chores at home. Parents were requested to ensure that teachers were familiar with all strategies, and teachers were contacted on a regular basis by the child–adolescent's therapist.

Based on a case control study, individuals who received the CRP exhibited significant improvement on a continuous performance test and also other measures of attention/concentration (Butler & Copeland, 2002). There was not, however, evidence to suggest that these benefits in neurocognitive functioning resulted in significantly improved arithmetic academic achievement. It was reported that potential problems regarding treatment generalizability would need to be addressed in order to promote success in this area. Nevertheless, there was evidence that benefits had been realized by most children–adolescents who received the CRP, and a more intensive, scientifically sophisticated design to assess effectiveness was recommended.

A randomized, multi-institutional, clinical trial of CRP for survivors of pediatric brain cancer and its treatments has recently been concluded. At the time of preparing this chapter, the analyses of the final data set are ongoing, and, unfortunately, results are not available for publication at this time. Our initial inspection of data comparing the CRP treatment group to a waiting-list control group indicates that participants who received cognitive remediation did exhibit significant increases in academic achievement. While not statistically significant, improvements on neurocognitive variables were all in the expected direction and approached statistical significance in many instances. Parents clearly viewed children who completed the CRP as having improved attentional functioning. Teacher perceptions were not as definitive, but these data are confounded by excessive occurrences of missing teacher reports, and also pre- and posttreatment reports from different teachers. At this time, my coinvestigators and I are extremely interested in addressing the question of who benefited maximally from the treatment program, and which individuals did not show significant gains. These analyses are likely to lead our group in appropriate directions for strengthening the treatment approach. Our clinical impressions suggest that familial factors are extremely important in this regard. Parents who missed treatment sessions, did not produce complete homework assignments on the part of their child, and were not effective in communicating metacognitive strategies to teachers appeared to be more likely to report that their child did not benefit from the CRP. These clinical impressions will need to be supported and verified by empirical data analysis. This clinical trial will provide critical information pertinent to these questions, primarily because of its randomized methodology. While we do not have empirical data on other pediatric populations with brain compromises, or on children who suffer from learning disabilities and other cognitive dysfunction not associated with an identified CNS insult, there is no a priori reason to believe that our techniques would not be effective with these children–adolescents. In fact, at the time of writing this chapter, I have begun applying our rehabilitation techniques to children–adolescents who have suffered a traumatic brain injury, and also those who are experiencing neurocognitive dysfunction with intractable epilepsy.

Few other published, available studies have evaluated cognitive-behavioral interventions for pediatric cancer survivors who experience learning difficulties. Moore and colleagues (2000) reported the results of a pilot study designed to improve arithmetic academic achievement. Their intervention involved 40–50 hours of math concept instruction, reflecting parallels to other neurodevelopmental populations. Results from this very preliminary pilot study suggest that the intervention group maintained stable academic achievement, while the comparison group declined in arithmetic performance over time. The approach used in this intervention appears to be consistent with traditional special education interventions, because the authors taught actual academic skills rather than implementing attempts to improve underlying neurocognitive functioning.

Kerns and Thomson (1998) investigated whether a compensatory memory device would improve neurocognitive functioning in an adolescent whose memory was severely impaired secondary to a brain tumor and its treatment. The patient was provided with a memory notebook assembled into several sections. These sections included not only note taking and planning but also orientation to time, person, and place. Training in the compensatory memory system involved three stages: acquisition, application, and adaptation. The patient was initially systematically trained in how to use the memory book. Next, role playing and teacher assistance were used in order to ensure adequate knowledge and use of the compensatory notebook. Finally, the adolescent was instructed to use the notebook on a daily basis and was supplied with a daily checklist to supplement the memory notebook. On pre- and post-testing, the patient, unfortunately, continued to demonstrate significantly impaired memory. Academic achievement, however, increased slightly when raw scores were evaluated. Qualitative improvement was observed. The authors reported that, most importantly, the patient continued to use the memory notebook over 1 year after the initial training phase. Teachers were surveyed, and none indicated difficulty with class attendance or timely completion of assignments and appropriate submission to the teacher. Thus, the compensatory memory system not only appeared to benefit this individual, but it was also successfully incorporated into her daily life.

While based only on one adolescent who suffered brain damage, the importance of this study is amplified by the description of the training methodology. Instruction must be an ongoing process with many individuals who suffer brain damage. Very few who experience cognitive-behavioral dysfunction return to their premorbid neuropsychological state. Most importantly, the study illustrates the need to expect, and to be reinforced by, small, but promising, steps toward improvement and reintegration.

The work of a child–adolescent is to attend school on a regular basis, learn, excel (we hope) in all studies, and, if needed, benefit from special services, such as individualized education plans. This latter point particularly applies to individuals with neurodevelopmental disabilities—congenital or acquired. As noted earlier, schools have increasingly been asked to assume the role as rehabilitation specialists for children and adolescents in this population. In addition to the necessity for individualized education plans and 504 considerations, it is important that school personnel be educated as to the specific needs of any individual student with a brain injury, and also to ensure a smooth integration into the academic environment following treatment for a CNS insult. Perhaps due to the chronic, progressive nature of brain dysfunction associated with many pediatric malignancies, much work on school reintegration has been conducted with this population.

It has been recommended that all pediatric oncology centers have a structured school re-entry program, one component of which is the education of the patient's teacher about childhood cancer and the specific signs, symptoms, and special needs associated with the pupil's treatment and treatment outcome (Leigh & Miles, 2002). This recommendation is likely appropriate for all causes of cognitive and behavioral deficits in childhood that have CNS involvement, acquired or inferred. Some special accommodations are obvious when needed; for example, allowing a patient with hemiparesis extra time to change classrooms. On the other hand, many neurological and neurocognitive deficits can be quite subtle, such as mild visual or hearing losses, or slowed visual–motor production. In addition, the neurocognitive status of the patient may not remain stable after the insult and/or its treatment has been completed. The onset of some deficits is delayed, and others are not evident until the ability is developmentally expected (Armstrong, Blumberg, & Toledano, 1999). One of the greatest dangers in not communicating these new problems to the patient's teachers is that the student's struggles in the classroom can be falsely attributed to a lack of motivation, attitude problems, daydreaming, or emotional maladjustment. On a very serious note, these tendencies to minimize school performance and cognitive declines can occasionally have dire consequences if the child–adolescent is suffering from a neurodegenerative disorder (Butler & Light, 2003).

Most commonly, simple classroom accommodations, such as reduced numbers of items on multiple-choice tests, preferential seating, limited course load, and decreased expectations for volume of homework, are oftentimes sufficient. The fact that most older children have multiple teachers in a school year, and that many, if not all, of these teachers will change with each school year, makes communication of the patient's special needs more difficult. Many children with CNS involvement will be classified as "other health impaired" by their local school systems as a means of accessing resources for their special needs. This is an important resource, because some states have very stringent requirements for learning disability-based individualized education plans.

As the adolescent with a neurodevelopmental disability approaches the termination of traditional high school education, concerns regarding postsecondary education become extremely relevant. Standard of care treatment for these adolescents is typically delivered by the school and includes therapies such as speech–language interventions, occupational therapy, special education, and school-based counseling and therapy. Adolescents who are provided individualized education plans and/or have been diagnosed as having mental retardation will continue to receive public school-based services for 2–3 years following the termination of their senior year in high school. At this time, however, for those young adults who have not been diagnosed as having mental retardation, federally funded services will soon end. While many individuals benefit from services over the childhood and adolescent years, brain injury rehabilitation often results in only modest improvements in functioning. Thus, those adolescents who are not likely to attend college are in need of early vocational planning, and a neuropsychological evaluation can be extremely important in assisting with effective placement. Therapies to improve vocational readiness are also needed to prepare the adolescent for eventual successful work performance.

The prospect of leaving school and entering into adult employment is somewhat intimidating for most students, but especially so for those who have a neurodevelopmental disability. For these adolescents, anticipation of this challenge can be daunting. Planning for this eventuality should begin early, perhaps even in middle school, depending on the degree of cognitive-behavioral involvement. If a student is not planning on attending college, or if this is not a viable option, the school district may have a work–study program with mentors in specific fields of work, and trial job placements with local employers. The high school student's enrollment in occupationally oriented vocational courses has important long-term implications according to a study conducted by the National Longitudinal Transition Study of Special Education Students (Blackorby & Wagner, 1997). This study demonstrated that those concentrating on vocational courses were less likely to drop out of high school and had a better chance of employment at a higher wage than students with disabilities whose coursework was restricted to academically oriented pursuits.

All patients should receive aptitude testing and vocational counseling if college is not a realistic option. Finally, these individuals should be provided information about study and work possibilities, and how to apply and interview for these opportunities. Patients with CNS impairment will likely benefit from working with a vocational counselor or coach who will ensure that the appropriate assessments are conducted, guide the student in finding placements for which to apply, and to participate in work hardening, as appropriate. Parents have a role in this domain as well. Key factors in students' success are the parent's encouragement of their child's–adolescent's learning, providing realistic expectations for performance, and being involved in school and community life (Henderson, 1994).

PSYCHOLOGICAL TREATMENT IN REHABILITATION

Psychotherapeutic interventions have long been recognized as essential to the cognitive and behavioral remediation process for patients, and also for their family members (Lezak, 1978). This work, however, has almost exclusively been conducted with adults, most commonly those having experienced a traumatic brain injury. While likely relevant for the pediatric population, research with children and adolescents has been surprisingly deficient.

Prigatano (1999) has written extensively on the importance and relevance of psychotherapeutic interventions for adults who have experienced a brain injury. Questions regarding why the injury occurred, whether persons regain normality, and how they can continue functioning following brain damage lend themselves well to supportive and explorative psychotherapy. Many children–adolescents experience neurocognitive deficits that impact on school performance, and this can result in very negative self-evaluations within the academic environment. This further amplifies the need for increased investigations on how psychotherapy can be of benefit to these individuals. One of the essential goals of psychotherapy with all patients involves exploration of, and instruction in, the most effective way of maximizing ones own self-interest (Prigatano, 1999). There are many different theories of how psychotherapeutic change occurs, with their respective techniques and approaches. Nevertheless, the overall goal is to reduce intrapsychic suffering and promote intra- and interpersonal adjustment, with presumed positive reverberations into the familial, vocational, and, especially with children and adolescents, academic arenas.

As noted earlier, most work has been conducted with adults following a brain injury. Nevertheless, Butler and Satz (1999) addressed the need for therapeutic interventions with children and adolescents who have suffered brain damage or involvement. In particular, it was deemed important to assess the possible presence of dysphoria and depression. Language functions are especially relevant with younger populations. Reduced facility with expressive speech and comprehension, combined with neuropsychological deficits, suggests that children are compromised in the ability for self-reflection and/or verbal expression of mood. While cognitive-behavioral therapy is frequently a very appropriate treatment for psychological disturbance, language delays and/or deficits may make this treatment modality difficult to apply. Nevertheless, it is my position that there is a strong psychotherapeutic component to cognitive and behavioral rehabilitation. At the very least, the therapeutic relationship begins to emerge when a patient and his or her family realize that the therapist has concerns regarding the individual's successful adjustment to life's challenges, be they educational, vocational, or inter- or intrapersonal. The aforementioned approach to cognitive remediation (CRP) with brain-injured cancer survivors is not only reasonably structured but also individualized. This is viewed as critical for optimal participant benefit. In short, while the therapist has an agenda, any unforeseen problem is "grist for the mill." If a patient arrives for therapy upset or perturbed, or if a parent points out a new problem area, this becomes a focus of psychotherapeutic intervention, in addition to the overall treatment plan.

Cognitive-behavioral, psychodynamic, and family therapy techniques have the potential for effectively supporting children–adolescents who are experiencing brain impairment. Behavioral approaches such as reinforcement and positive reframing are routinely used to help children and families in these populations. In addition, improvements in self-concept can be accomplished in a psychotherapeutic relationship, and in the interactions that occur within that framework (Altman, Briggs, Frankel, Gensler, & Pantone, 2002). For example, the child–adolescent has the therapist's full attention during a session, which implies that he or she is important. The therapist also redefines the child's identity by pointing out observed aspects or characteristics, such as "You did a fine job!"; "I see you are very careful in your work"; "I see you enjoy playing with other children"; "You are very articulate in expressing yourself." The child and therapist form a bond during psychotherapeutic sessions, out of which may emerge a student's new sense of self and others. Ideally, the child–adolescent adds new behaviors or ways of interacting with others that reflect improvement: increased confidence, self-direction, expressiveness, and organization.

PHARMACOLOGICAL TREATMENT IN REHABILITATION

The use of psychoactive medications to promote improved cognition and behavior in children and adolescents, particularly within the school environment, is well established. It is beyond the scope of this chapter to review the use of stimulant medications to accentuate attention and concentration, and improve behavioral control in the classroom. The reader is referred to an excellent text by Barkley (1997), which thoroughly reviews the nature of ADHD, and also addresses the beneficial effects that stimulant medications can have on attention and self-control in children–adolescents with this disorder. The application of these medications as an adjunct to cognitive and behavioral rehabilitation efforts, however, is a very new event. As of the writing of this chapter, only a handful of studies on pharmacological interventions in populations with neurodevelopmental disabilities, outside of the idiopathic attentional disorders, have been published. A number of studies conducted with pediatric cancer patients have documented acquired brain insults that influence patients' ability to attend and to concentrate accurately.

Given that attentional deficits, delayed information-processing speed, and processing efficacy are some of the most common neurocognitive impairments following not only pediatric oncology-related CNS insults but also many, if not most, neurodevelopmental insults, the potential benefits of stimulant medication become an attractive option. Methylphenidate hydrochloride (MPH) has been the classic medication used for children with attention deficit disorder (ADD), with and without hyperactivity (Brown, 1998; Brown, Dingle, & Dreelin, 1997). While newer forms of stimulant medications are being introduced into the market, MPH and its close molecular cousins remain a mainstay for the treatment of attentional difficulties for children and adults. MPH is a mixed dopaminergic–noradrenergic agonist that enhances function of the frontostriatal attentional network (Weber & Lutschg, 2002). Beneficial effects of MPH have been documented on measures of vigilance and sustained attention (Rapport, Denny, DuPaul, & Gardner, 1994), and also in hastening reaction time and improving learning (Brown, 1998). Thus, given that these are also some of the more common deficits observed in neurodevelopmental disabilities, it is intuitively enticing to expect that this medication would be effective in improving neurocognitive functioning and school performance in other children–adolescents with impairment.

Three studies have now been conducted using MPH as an intervention for childhood cancer survivors who have a documented attentional deficit associated with a brain insult. In a pilot study, DeLong, Friedman, Friedman, Gustafson, and Oakes (1992) reported that 8 out of 12 participants demonstrated a "good" response to MPH, 2 manifested a "fair" response, and 2 participants had a "poor" response. In a second pilot study, Torres et al. (1996) reported on six participants who had received cranial irradiation for brain tumors. No significant immediate or delayed benefits to the patients were reported. From a methodological perspective, the most sophisticated study has been reported by Thompson and coworkers (2001). This study investigated the effects of MPH using a randomized, double-blind trial with survivors of childhood cancer. Participants were over the age of 6, and had completed all treatment at least two years prior to entry into the study. Potential participants with a diagnosis of ADHD prior to the occurrence of the malignancy were excluded from the trial in an attempt to determine the influence of the medication on acquired brain dysfunction. Additionally, individuals being treated with other psychotropic medications were also excluded, as were those children with uncorrected endocrine difficulties or abnormal brain electrical activity. Thompson et al. reported significantly greater improvement following the administration of MPH when compared to a placebo condition on a continuous performance test of sustained attention. This was particularly salient in errors of omission. Reaction time remained unchanged, as did tendencies toward impulsivity. The two groups were not significantly different on measures of verbal and auditory learning.

Preliminary results suggest that pharmacological interventions may be appropriate and beneficial for some, if not many, survivors of childhood cancer, and brain damage associated with other forms of CNS injury, or idiopathic neurodevelopmental conditions. The increasing availability of newer medications that have fewer adverse side effects is especially encouraging for these populations. For example, a newer compound, Strattera, a selective norepinephrine reuptake inhibitor, has now been introduced as being potentially beneficial for the ADHD/ADD populations. Pharmacological advances are exciting, because side effects are decreasing, and direct targeting of critical neurotransmitters is becoming increasingly sophisticated. Cholinergic agonists, such as Provigil, may also be of clinical portent for pediatric patients who have neurodevelopmental involvement, and they have a mild side effect profile. These factors are particularly important, because, in our clinical experience, many parents of children without clinically apparent ADHD do not wish to avail themselves to the option of stimulant medication.

The use of pharmacokinetic agents as an adjunct to cognitive and behavioral brain injury rehabilitation interventions is viewed as a significant advance, and will, we hope, result in a synergistic interaction. Furthermore, pharmacological interventions become particularly attractive to families in rural areas, or to those who do not have the financial–insurance resources required for cognitive and behavioral interventions. While medications are likely to prove themselves as important components within neurodevelopmental rehabilitation, there also remain concerns. As of the writing of this chapter, considerable public concern and outcry has begun to appear associated with the use of antidepressant medications, primarily the selective serotonin reuptake inhibitors, with children and adolescents. In fact, the U.S. Food and Drug Administration has recently required drug manufacturing companies to place a warning label regarding the possibility of suicidal ideation and behavior associated with the use of these medications in pediatric patients. The upshot is that we need to conduct Phase III clinical trials on all of our interventions, and this methodology will not only allow for the documentation of effectiveness, but also will provide side effect profiles and identifiable risk factors. Although these are expensive endeavors, they are necessary in order to provide a systematic approach to continued advancements on the effectiveness of rehabilitation treatments.

CONCLUSIONS AND FUTURE DIRECTIONS

Over the past two decades, advances have occurred in the rehabilitation of neurocognitive and psychological functioning following a documented brain injury, and in children and adolescents with idiopathic developmental compromise. Not only should the child and his or her family receive habilitative and rehabilitative interventions, but the living environment can also be manipulated in order to maximize functioning. The use of behavioral interventions, cognitive-behavioral therapy, instruction in metacognitive strategies, social skills training, traditional brain injury rehabilitation techniques such as massed practice drills, and supportive and dynamic psychotherapeutic approaches all appear to be beneficial to the patient with brain dysfunction. Research on the effectiveness of cognitive remediation with children–adolescents is a fairly new and exciting field. There are clear indications that multimodal interventions in this population may be synergistic. From a methodological perspective, this suggests that additive approaches rather than dismantling clinical outcome designs may be the preferred experimental paradigm. Given that traumatic brain injury is the most common cause of brain dysfunction in children, the majority of studies to date have been conducted on this population, with isolated studies on children who have epilepsy, cancer, or have experienced a hypoxic episode. Recently, researchers who work with children and adolescents that have neurocognitive dysfunction associated with a malignancy are beginning to assume leadership roles in the area of cognitive remediation. This raises an important cooperative and collaborative question regarding obstacles in brain injury rehabilitation. Professionals in various fields, such as traumatic brain injury, neurodevelopmental disorders, oncology, epilepsy, and stroke, do not have common communication channels. There is a need for journals and societies that blend the needs of all pediatric rehabilitation specialists, and also invite insights from the cognitive neurosciences.

A potentially innovative addition to the development of interventions for pediatric cognitive deficits has been the documented evidence on the influence of family environment and resources following recovery from traumatic brain injury. The importance of family cohesiveness and stability in recovery from brain injury has long been recognized. As early as 1958, it was reported that children who suffered a traumatic brain injury and subsequently developed psychiatric disturbances had greater degrees of family pathology than those who did not experience a mental disorder (Harrington & Letemendia, 1958). Other researchers have further demonstrated the relationship between family pathology and behavioral difficulties among adult brain-injured patients (Lezak, 1978; Worthington; 1989). More currently, Yeates and colleagues (1997) have documented that chaotic and dysfunctional family environments have a significant adverse impact on both the neurological and neuropsychological recovery from traumatic brain injury among school-age children. This relationship appears to be valid even when severity of brain injury and other medical factors are experimentally controlled (Max et al., 1999). It appears that family burden, characterized by ratings from parents as to the negative impact of the child's injury to the family and also overall family adjustment, is a significant predictor of continued neurobehavioral symptoms following childhood traumatic brain injury (Yeates et al., 2001).

How might these findings be relevant to children–adolescents with neurocognitive problems of many different origins? One could speculate that the family environment is of equal or even greater importance in the treatment and recovery of a chronic neurodevelopmental condition than an acute event such as a traumatic brain injury. Educating parents to be advocates for their children by giving them sufficient information and support should be a component of any clinical intervention in this field. Parents with few financial and psychological resources are at a disadvantage in obtaining rehabilitation services for their children. These families also are likely to have heightened stress levels, and the existence of a "two-way clogged artery" becomes an appropriate analogy. There is no easy answer to problems surrounding the delivery of neurorehabilitative services to pediatric patients in need of remediation. Priorities, however, must be established, because the youth represent our future.

On a very exciting note, a number of researchers are directly addressing not only the need to provide family interventions but also the use of technologies such as Web-based networks, in order to allow maximal dissemination of clinical services. Wade and her colleagues have been developing family-based interventions, administered both individually and by Internet Web-based sources, designed to assist the cognitive remediation of children who have suffered a traumatic brain injury (Wade, Chapter 10, this volume; Wade, Wolfe, Brown, & Pestian, 2005). These advances will likely extend into neurodevelopmental, other brain injury, and learning disability areas. Active attempts are being made to ensure that families in rural areas have access to treatment services. As I noted earlier, systematic approaches to effective interventions with children and adolescents suffering deficits in academic achievement continue to be accomplished. Clinicians and researchers are committed to ensuring that all children and adolescents who require special assistance because of neurodevelopmental disorders receive appropriate intervention and rehabilitative services.

The field of brain injury rehabilitation, particularly in childhood, is approaching a crossroads. Growing concerns over the ecological validity of neuropsychological outcome measures are becoming apparent. For example, if a CRP results in significant improvement on a clinically administered neuropsychological test, such as a continuous performance test, what does this represent in terms of the child's or adolescent's real-world functioning? Within the school-age child population, rehabilitation specialists are extremely interested in improving the individual's ability to maintain attention over extended periods of time. This represents a primary and secondary academic environmental goal of great importance. It remains unclear how well our formal, standardized neuropsychological evaluations mirror a typical school day. Advances are being realized in this respect, and virtual reality technology is being applied to neuropsychological assessment, which may improve our ability to predict and improve classroom performance. This chapter has repeatedly emphasized financial issues, primarily centered about medical insurance reimbursement, and also the fact that our overburdened school systems are increasingly being expected to meet neurodevelopmental rehabilitation needs. I am an academically oriented clinical neuropsychologist, committed to developing brain injury rehabilitation programs that have documented effectiveness and are also financially feasible. This is, to say the least, a Herculean task. Nevertheless, through systematic clinical trials, increased interdisciplinary communication, and an appreciation for the fact that small improvements following remediation efforts are the rule as opposed to the exception, I believe that this field can maintain a spirit of optimism, excitement, and continued advancement.

ACKNOWLEDGMENTS

Portions of this chapter were written with the assistance of Donna R. Copeland and Raymond K. Mulhern. This work was supported by National Institute of Health/ National Cancer Institute Grant No. RO1 CA83936-01.

REFERENCES

Altman, N., Briggs, R., Frankel, J., Gensler, D., & Pantone, P. (2002). *Relational child psychotherapy.* New York: Other Press.

Armstrong, F. D., Blumberg, M. J., & Toledano, S. R. (1999). Neurobehavioral issues in childhood cancer. *School Psychology Review, 28,* 194–203.

Barkley, R. (1997). *ADHD and the nature of self-control.* New York: Guilford Press

Baron, I. S., & Goldberger, E. (1993). Neuropsychological disturbances of hydrocephalic children with implications for special education and rehabilitation. *Neuropsychological Rehabilitation, 3,* 389–410.

Blackorby, J., & Wagner, W. M. (1997). The employment outcomes of youth with learning disabilities: A review of findings from the National Longitudinal Transitional Study of Special Education Students. In P. J. Gerber & D. S. Brown (Eds.), *Learning disabilities and employment* (pp. 57–74). Austin, TX: Pro-Ed.

Brett, A. W., & Laatsch, L. (1998). Cognitive rehabilitation therapy of brain-injured students in a public high school setting. *Pediatric Rehabilitation, 2,* 27–31.

Brown, R. T. (1998). Short-term cognitive and behavioral effects of psychotropic medications. In R. T. Brown & M. Sawyer (Eds.), *Medications for school age children: Effects on learning and behavior* (pp. 29–61). New York: Guilford Press.

Brown, R. T., Dingle, A., & Dreelin, B. (1997). Neuropsychological effects of stimulant medication on children's learning and behavior. In C. R. Reynolds & E. Fletcher-Janzen (Eds.), *Handbook of clinical child neuropsychology* (pp. 539–572). New York: Wiley.

Butler, R. W. (1998). Attentional processes and their remediation in childhood cancer. *Medical and Pediatric Oncology,* (Suppl. 1), 75–78.

Butler, R. W., & Copeland, D. R. (2002). Attentional processes and their remediation in children treated for cancer: A literature review and the development of a therapeutic approach. *Journal of the International Neuropsychological Society, 8,* 113–124.

Butler, R. W., & Light, R. (2003). Late diagnosis of neurodegenerative disease in children: Agnosognosia by proxy. *Clinical Neuropsychologist, 17,* 374–382.

Butler, R. W., & Satz, P. (1999). Depression and its diagnosis and treatment. In K. Langer, L. Laatsch, & L. Lewis (Eds.), *Psychotherapy with the patient with neuropsychological impairment: A clinician's treatment resource.* Madison, CT: Psychological Press.

Butler, R. W., Hill, J. M., Steinherz, P. G., Meyers, P. A., & Finlay, J. L. (1994). The neuropsychological effects of cranial irradiation, intrathecal methotrexate and systemic methotrexate in childhood cancer. *Journal of Clinical Oncology, 12,* 2621–2629.

Cicerone, K. D., Dahlberg, C., Kalmar, K., Langenbahn, D. M., Malec, J. F., Bergquist, T. F., Felicetti, T., Giacino, J. T., Harley, J. P., Harrington, D. E., Herzog, J., Kneipp, S., Laatsch, L., & Morse, P. A. (2000). Evidence-based cognitive rehabilitation: Recommendations for clinical practice. *Archives of Physical Medicine and Rehabilitation, 81,* 1596–1615.

Deaton, A. V. (1987). Behavioral change strategies for children and adolescents with severe brain injury. *Journal of Learning Disabilities, 20,* 581–589.

DeLong, R., Friedman, H., Friedman, N., Gustafson, K., & Oakes, J. (1992). Methylphenidate in neuropsychological sequelae of radiotherapy and chemotherapy of childhood brain tumors and leukemia. *Journal of Child Neurology, 7,* 462–463.

Fletcher, J. M., & Copeland, D. R. (1988). Neurobehavioral effects of central nervous system prophylactic treatment of cancer in children. *Journal of Clinical and Experimental Neuropsychology, 10,* 495–538.

Harrington, J. A., & Letemendia, F. J. J. (1958). Persistent psychiatric disorders after head injuries in children. *Journal of Mental Science, 104,* 1205–1218.

Heideman, R. L., Packer, R. J., Albright, L. A., Freeman, C., & Rorke, L. (1997). Tumors of the central nervous system. In P. A. Pizzo & D. Poplack (Eds.), *Principles and practice of pediatric oncology* (3rd ed., pp. 633–681). Philadelphia: Lippincott-Raven.

Henderson, A. (1994). *A new generation of evidence: The family is critical to student achievement*. Washington, DC: National Committee for Citizens in Education.

Kehle, T. J., Clark, E., & Jenson, W. R. (1996). Interventions for students with traumatic brain injury: Managing behavioral disturbances. *Journal of Learning Disabilities, 29,* 633–642.

Kerns, K. A., & Thomson, J. (1998). Case study: Implementation of a compensatory memory system in a school age child with severe memory impairment. *Pediatric Rehabilitation, 2,* 77–87.

Laatsch, L., Pavel, D., Jobe, T., Lin, Q., & Quintana, J. C. (1999). Incorporation of SPECT imaging in a longitudinal cognitive rehabilitation therapy programme. *Brain Injury, 13,* 555–570.

Laatsch, L. K., Thulborn, K. R., Krisky, C. M., Shobat, D. M., & Sweeney, J. A. (2004). Investigating the neurobiological basis of cognitive rehabilitation therapy with fMRI. *Brain Injury, 18,* 957–974.

Leigh, L., & Miles, M. A. (2002). Educational issues for children with cancer. In P. A. Pizzo & D. G. Poplack (Eds.), *Principles and practice of pediatric oncology* (4th ed., pp. 1463–1475). Philadelphia: Lippincott-Raven.

Levin, H. S., & Grafman, J. (Eds.). (2000). *Cerebral reorganization of function after brain damage.* New York: Oxford University Press.

Lezak, M. D. (1978). Living with the characterological altered brain injured patient. *Journal of Clinical Psychiatry, 39,* 592–598.

Luria, A. R. (1963). *Restoration of function after brain injury.* New York: Pergamon.

Margolin, J. F., & Poplack, D. G. (1997). Acute lymphoblastic leukemia. In P. A. Pizzo & D. G. Poplack (Eds.), *Principles and practice of pediatric oncology* (3rd ed., pp. 409–462). Philadelphia: Lippincott-Raven.

Max, J. E., Roberts, M. A., Koele, S. L., Lindgren, S. D., Robin, D. A., Arndt, S., Smith, W. L., & Sato, Y. (1999). Cognitive outcome in children and adolescents following severe traumatic brain injury: Influence of psychosocial, psychiatric and injury-related variables. *Journal of the International Neuropsychological Society, 5,* 58–68.

Meichenbaum, D. (1977). *Cognitive-behavior modification: An integrative approach.* New York: Plenum Press.

Moleski, M. (2000). Neuropsychological, neuroanatomical, and neurophysiological consequences of CNS chemotherapy for acute lymphoblastic leukemia. *Archives of Clinical Neuropsychology, 15,* 603–630.

Moore, I. M., Espy, K. A., Kaufmann, P., Kramer, J., Kaemingk, K., Miketova, P., Mollova, N., Kaspar, M., Pasvogel, A., Schram, K., Wara, W., Hutter, J., & Matthay, K. (2000). Cognitive consequences and central nervous system injury following treatment for childhood leukemia. *Seminars in Oncology Nursing, 16,* 279–290.

National Institutes of Health Consensus Statement. (1998). *Rehabilitation of persons with traumatic brain injury* [Brochure]. Bethesda, MD: National Institutes of Health.

Ogg, R., Zou, P., White, H., Cooper, T., O'Grady, J., Butler, R., & Mulhern, R.

(2002). Attention deficits in survivors of childhood cancer: An fMRI study. *Journal of the International Neuropsychological Society, 8,* 494–495.

Penkman, L. (2004). Remediation of attention deficits in children: a focus on childhood cancer, traumatic brain injury and attention deficit disorder. *Pediatric Rehabilitation, 7,* 111–123.

Prigatano, G. P. (1999). *Principles of neuropsychological rehabilitation.* New York: Oxford University Press.

Rapport, M. D., Denny, C., DuPaul, G. J., & Gardner, M. J. (1994). Attention deficit disorder and methylphenidate: Normalization rates, clinical effectiveness, and response prediction in 76 children. *Journal of the American Academy of Child and Adolescent Psychiatry, 33,* 882–893.

Ris, M. D., & Noll, R. B. (1994). Long-term neurobehavioral outcome in pediatric brain tumor patients: Review and methodological critique. *Journal of Clinical and Experimental Neuropsychology, 16,* 21–42.

Silver, B. V., Boake, C., & Cavazos, D. I. (1994). Improving functional skills using behavioral procedures in a child with anoxic brain injury. *Archives of Physical Medicine and Rehabilitation, 75,* 742–745.

Slifer, K. J., Tucker, C. L., Gerson, A. C., Sevier, R. C., Kane, A. C., Amar, A., & Clawson, B. P. (1997). Antecedent management and compliance training improve adolescents' participation in early brain injury rehabilitation. *Brain Injury, 11,* 877–889.

Sohlberg, M. M., & Mateer, C. A. (1996). *Attention Process Training II (APT-II).* Puyallup, WA: Association for Neuropsychological Research and Development.

Sohlberg, M. M., & Mateer, C. A. (2001). *Cognitive rehabilitation: An integrative neuropsychological approach.* New York: Guilford Press.

Suzman, K. B., Morris, R. D., Morris, M. K., & Milan, M. A. (1997). Cognitive behavioral remediation of problem solving deficits in children with acquired brain injury. *Journal of Behavioral Therapy and Experimental Psychiatry, 28,* 203–212.

Teichner, G., Golden, C. J., & Giannaris, W. J. (1999). A multimodal approach to treatment of aggression in a severely brain-injured adolescent. *Rehabilitation Nursing, 24,* 207–211.

Thompson, S. J., Leigh, L., Christensen, R., Xioing, X., Kun, L. E., Heideman, R., Reddick, W. E., Gajjar, A., Merchant, T., Pui, C. H., Hudson, M. M., & Mulhern, R. K. (2001). Immediate neurocognitive effects of methylphenidate on learning-impaired survivors of cancer. *Journal of Clinical Oncology, 19,* 1802–1808.

Torres, C., Korones, D., Palumbo, D., Wissler, K., Vadasz, E., & Cox, C. (1996). Effect of methylphenidate in the postradiation attention and memory deficits in children. *Annals of Neurology, 40,* 331–332.

Wade, S. L., Wolfe, C., Brown, T. M., & Pestian, J. P. (2005). Putting the pieces together: Preliminary efficacy of a web-based family intervention for children with traumatic brain injury. *Journal of Pediatric Psychology, 30*(5), 437–442.

Warschausky, S., Kewman, D., & Kay, J. (1999). Empirically supported psychological and behavioral therapies in pediatric rehabilitation of TBI. *Journal of Head Trauma Rehabilitation, 14,* 373–383.

Weber, P., & Lutschg, J. (2002). Methylphenidate treatment. *Pediatric Neurology, 26,* 261–266.

Worthington, J. (1989). The impact of adolescent development on recovery from traumatic brain injury. *Rehabilitation Nursing, 14,* 118–122.

Yeates, K. O. (2000). Closed-head injury. In K. O. Yeats, M. D. Ris, & H. G. Taylor (Eds.), *Pediatric neuropsychology* (pp. 92–116). New York: Guilford Press.

Yeates, K. O., Taylor, H. G., Barry, C. T., Drotar, D., Wade, S. L., & Stancin, T. (2001). Neurobehavioral symptoms in childhood closed-head injuries: Changes in prevalence and correlates during the first year postinjury. *Journal of Pediatric Psychology, 26,* 79–91.

Yeates, K. O., Taylor, H. G., Drotar, D., Wade, S. L., Stancin, T., Klein, S., & Schatschneider, C. (1997). Pre-injury family environment as a determinant of recovery from traumatic brain injuries in school-age children. *Journal of the International Neuropsychological Society, 3,* 617–630.

12

Students with Acquired Brain Injury

Identification, Accommodations, and Transitions in the Schools

MARY R. HIBBARD
TAMAR MARTIN
JOSHUA CANTOR
ALBERTO I. MORAN

Children with acquired brain injury (ABI) are underidentified within the school system despite the fact that ABI is a high-incidence phenomenon (Ewing-Cobbs et al., 1997; Taylor et al., 2003; Yeates & Taylor, 2005). As a result, the needs of children with ABI may be misunderstood, ignored, or, at best, inadequately met beyond acute hospital care (Johnson & Rose, 2004). To complicate the issue, long-term educational implications of ABI often remain uncertain, since ABI occurs within the context of ongoing brain development (Klonoff, Clark, & Klonoff, 1995; Ylvisaker et al., 2001). If these children are to fulfill their educational potential, their ABIs need to be correctly identified, their academic progress needs to be monitored throughout their educational career, and accommodations need to be implemented when indicated to maximize academic success.

In this chapter, we review literature on the educational needs of students with ABI, the prevalence of pediatric ABI, reasons for lack of ABI identification within the schools, and the educational challenges presented by pediatric ABI. The importance of screening to enhance identification of ABI and the need for ongoing monitoring of potential psychological, cognitive, and behavioral challenges that can emerge post-ABI are stressed. We argue that current psychoeducational assessment must be expanded to include cognitive and qualitative, informal, functionally based classroom assessments. Accommodations based on these assessments should be proactively implemented. Issues related to key transition points within the child's school career are reviewed. We assume the reader to have a solid understanding of the neuroanatomy and neuropsychology of brain injury and the normal development of the brain during childhood. The reader is referred to Donders (Chapter 2, this volume, on traumatic brain injury) for additional information about challenges for children with ABIs.

PEDIATRIC ABI: A HIGH-INCIDENCE PHENOMENON

In this chapter, ABI is defined as a brain injury involving damage to the brain due to either an "external event," such as open or closed injury to the brain, or an "internal event," such as a cerebrovascular accident (Kraemer & Blancher, 1997). Although pediatric ABI is the major cause of permanent disability in children and adolescents (Guyer & Ellers, 1990; Kraus, Rock, & Hemyari, 1990; Snow & Hooper, 1994), the incidence of specific types of ABI varies widely. For example, pediatric-onset cerebrovascular accident (CVA) is a relatively "low" incidence phenomenon, since CVAs occur in only 2–3 children per 100,000 per year (Harding & Kleiman, 1996; Schoenberg, Mellinger, & Schoenberg, 1978). In contrast, traumatic brain injury (TBI) is the most frequent cause of pediatric ABI and the major cause of death and long-term disability in children (Hayman-Abello, Rourke, & Fuerst, 2002; Langlois, 2001). The Centers for Disease Control and Prevention estimate that over 430,000 children between birth and age 14 (Langlois, 2001) experience a TBI each year. These statistics underestimate the enormity of the problem for children (National Center for Injury Prevention and Control, 2003), because these numbers include only children who die, are hospitalized, or receive care in an emergency room (Kraus, 1995; Langlois, 2001). When mild TBI is included within these numbers, it has been estimated that 1 million children experience a TBI annually, with 80–90% of injuries classified as mild (Yeates & Taylor, 2005). Children with mild TBI often are not seen in emergency rooms or hospitalized, and many never receive formal medical interventions (Bryan, 1995; Ponsford, Willmott, Rothwell, et al., 2001). A small, yet significant, number of these children suffer persistent negative outcomes of the TBI. As a result, potential under-reporting of pediatric TBI is a serious public health problem (National Institutes of Health Consensus Panel, 1999), with specific implications for the educational setting.

IDENTIFICATION OF ABI IN EDUCATIONAL SETTINGS

Educational disability associated with brain injury is more prevalent than is normally assumed. The Individuals with Disabilities Education Act of 1990 (IDEA; Public Law 101-476; Federal Register, 1990) created a separate classification for students with brain injury over one decade ago. Despite a federal mandate, the number of students classified with ABI or TBI in the schools remains far below the estimated 1 million children experiencing a brain injury annually (Yeates & Taylor, 2005). For example, the Office of Special Education Programs of the United States Department of Education identified only 14,844 students classified with TBI (U.S. Department of Education, 2001) in the 2000–2001 academic year, a finding clearly discrepant from incidence reports of pediatric ABI on an annual basis (Cantor et al., 2004).

Lack of identification can arise from multiple sources: School personnel, children, and parents who may be unaware that an ABI has occurred; poor (or absent) transition services that may have existed between hospitals and schools; the "invisible" nature of brain injury compared to other physical disabilities; a lack of appreciation of potential consequences of ABI by family and health care providers; attempts to conceal the ABI (e.g., in cases of abuse); and potential lags in the presentation of symptoms postonset of the ABI (Cantor et al., 2004). Lack of identification of pediatric ABI may also reflect inadequate training of school personnel about what ABI is and how to assess and accommodate ABI-related cognitive and behavioral challenges in the classroom (Cantor et al., 2004; Cronin, 2001; Savage, 1991; Taylor et al., 2003). Differences in state-to-state interpretations of the eligibility requirements for classification of ABI may also account for lack of identification. For example, select states limit inclusion of students with TBI to those sustaining injuries caused by an "external force," thereby excluding students with other kinds of brain injuries from this classification (Clark, 1996).

Lack of proper identification of ABI can result in significant academic challenges for students. The potential scope and magnitude of a student's cognitive and learning difficulties post-ABI may be minimized, and the student may receive no accommodations, or conversely, be provided with inappropriate or inadequate accommodations in the classroom (Ponsford et al., 2001; Feeney & Ylvisaker, 1995; Savage, 1991; Taylor et al., 2003). For example, children with ABI may be misclassified as having an emotional disability. Academic interventions may be directed solely at behavioral problems, with cognitive problems misunderstood, misinterpreted, or ignored. Other children with ABI may be classified as having a learning disability, and receive functionally appropriate educational services despite the fact that their ABI remains unclassified (Ylvisaker, Jacobs, & Feeney,

2003). While incorrect classification is not necessarily a harbinger of ineffective service delivery (Ylvisaker et al., 2001), a correct classification can serve to alert school professionals to be watchful for potential late-onset educational challenges as a student matures (Hooper, Willis, & Stone, 1996; Taylor et al., 2003).

DEVELOPMENTAL CONSIDERATIONS FOR STUDENTS WITH ABI

In adults who experience an ABI, issues such as the severity of the injury, the diffuseness and/or localization of the injury (Harding & Kleiman, 1996), the level of pre-ABI functioning, and environmental resources (Ryan, LaMarche, Barth, & Boll, 1996) are important predictors of anticipated recovery and extent of community reintegration. While these factors are important to consider in recovery following pediatric ABI, additional developmental factors play key roles, including the age of the child at time of injury, the stage of brain development at time of injury, and the child's prior academic achievement (Farmer, Clippard, Luehr-Wiemann, Wright, & Owings, 1996; Ryan et al., 1996). Academic challenges are directly related to the "unfolding" of cognitive and behavioral impairments as students mature (Johnson & Rose, 2004). (The reader is referred to Donders, Chapter 2, this volume, for an in-depth review of developmental changes in brain structure as children mature to adulthood.)

The negative impact of ABI on a student's cognitive functioning has been documented across key developmental periods (i.e., infancy, preschool, school-age, and adolescence). Each developmental period produces a differing array of academic challenges for the student (Deaton & Waaland, 1994; De Pompei & Blosser, 1994; Kraemer & Blancher, 1997). During infancy and early toddlerhood, onset of an ABI may well disrupt the child's expected progress toward independence, self-determination, and social development (Lehr & Savage, 1990), and acquisition of expected expressive and receptive language skills (Ewing-Cobbs, Miner, Fletcher, & Levin, 1989). During the early elementary school years, onset of an ABI may disrupt a student's ability to acquire key academic skills of reading, spelling, writing, arithmetic, and basic reasoning. Adolescence is marked by a major reorganization of the brain, when the adolescent acquires the ability to think more abstractly, and use logic and reasoning to evaluate options and predict outcomes (Lehr & Savage, 1990). Parallel expectations of increased independence, autonomy, and peer interactions that accompany this normal brain development may be impacted in students experiencing an ABI during adolescents.

In younger children with an ABI, cognitive and behavioral abilities may actually worsen over the years postinjury rather than improving, as parents, teachers, and others predictably expect (Johnson & Rose, 2004; Koskiniemi, Kyykka, Nybo, & Jarho, 1995). Children who experience injuries early in life may perform relatively well during elementary school, only to experience "new" onset academic and social difficulties once as they enter middle school (Farmer & Peterson, 1995; Taylor et al., 2003; Ylvisaker et al., 2001). These new-onset academic and interpersonal difficulties reflect lags in self-regulation, problem solving, and social skills development secondary to frontal lobe dysfunction (Lord-Maes & Obrzut, 1996; Bryan, 1995; Eslinger, Grattan, Dinter, Schmidt, & Damasio, 1992). The negative impact of an ABI on a student's emotional and behavioral functioning is also significant. Neurobehavioral disorders associated with frontal lobe dysfunction are common. Primary symptoms include dysphoric mood, aggressive behaviors, and affective lability (Lord-Maes & Obrzut, 1996). Expression of these behavioral challenges post-ABI appears to be age-related. Younger children may display overactivity, difficulties with attention, and aggressiveness, while older children may display greater difficulties with impulse control and self-monitoring (Telzrow, 1987).

The long-term impact of pediatric ABI has been highlighted by findings of Klonoff and colleagues (Klonoff, Low, & Clark, 1977; Klonoff et al., 1995) who initially evaluated students with a range of ABI severity at 5 years postinjury and follow-up 23 years later. At the initial assessment 5 years after injury, most students (76%) showed improvement on neuropsychological testing. However, almost one-fourth of the children (24%) exhibited continued impaired cognitive performance (Klonoff et al., 1977). At 23-year follow-up, 31% of these individuals continued to report subjective ABI complaints suggesting that symptoms endure into adulthood (Klonoff et al., 1995). Thus, onset of pediatric brain injury may create lifelong challenges.

CHALLENGES IN EDUCATIONAL SETTINGS FOR STUDENTS WITH ABI

The vast majority of students return to school for continued "habilitation" regardless of ABI severity (Farmer & Peterson, 1995; Hawley, 2003). Following other physical illnesses, return to school is often viewed by families and school personnel as an indication of the students having made a "full recovery." In ABI, "physical recovery" is often noted. However, this often dramatic physical recovery may fuel unrealistic expectations of parents and educators alike about a parallel recovery of the student's cognitive and behavioral functions (Johnson, 1992). Several authors (Lord-Maes & Obrzut, 1996; Taylor & Alden, 1997) argue that the act of returning to school should not be viewed as an acceptable index of "recovery" for students after ABI. This is particularly true for students with more severe ABI, who often present with greater cognitive, behavioral and, emotional challenges upon school re-entry (Donders & Ballard, 1996; Gil, 2003; Hayman-Abello et al., 2002). Furthermore, their cognitive and behavioral challenges are most likely to increase rather than decline over the course of their subsequent school years (Koskiniemi et al., 1995). These increasing cognitive and behavioral difficulties often result in a corresponding increase in the need for special education, or related services, and potential grade repetition (Goldstein & Levin, 1985).

Studies of long-term academic outcome following ABI provide support for these impressions. At 2 years post-ABI onset, Hawley (2003; Hawley, Ward, Magnay, & Long, 2002) found that students with more severe injuries presented proportionately greater difficulties in completing schoolwork and had greater discipline problems and more personality changes (21% of those with mild injuries; 46% of those with moderate injuries, and 69% of those with severe injuries). Special education needs were highest in students with severe injury (28%). However, a number of students with moderate and mild injuries (3 and 8%, respectively) also required special education services. When contrasted with noninjured children, students with ABI, regardless of severity, demonstrated more frequent behavioral and anger-control issues. Emotional changes, including depression and anxiety, were common.

Although students with mild ABI are most likely to make a good functional recovery, and by implication, a good academic recovery, some researchers argue that the extent of recovery following mild ABI may be overestimated (e.g., Bijur & Haslum, 1995; Fay, Jaffe, & Polissar, 1993, Prior, Kinsella, Sawyer, Bryan, & Anderson, 1994). Indeed, some children with mild ABI exhibit cognitive and behavioral challenges similar to those with severe ABI as they age (Boll, 1983; Levin, Ewing-Cobbs, & Fletcher, 1989; Hawley et al., 2002; Ponsford et al., 2001). Thus, pediatric ABI places all students, regardless of the initial severity of the injury, at risk of emergent cognitive, physical, and behavioral challenges as they mature. These ABI-related challenges can interfere with students' educational success and ultimate capacity to learn relative to preinjury levels (Catroppa & Anderson, 2002).

EXPANSION OF PSYCHOEDUCATIONAL ASSESSMENTS FOR STUDENTS WITH ABI

Schools are federally mandated to provide services to students with ABI who either meet criteria for placement or require classroom accommodations under Section 504 of the Individuals with Disabilities Act of 1990 (IDEA Public Law 101-476; Federal Register, 1990) (Semrud-Clikeman, 2001). Placement needs and/or accommodations for these students should be dictated by solid familiarity with the general features of ABI (Ylvisaker et al., 2001), and derived from expanded psychoeducational assessment of the student's cognitive abilities, as well as qualitative assessments of the student's cognitive and behavioral functioning within the school and classroom setting.

To date, cognitive assessment has traditionally been viewed as the domain of the neuropsychologist (Lord-Maes & Obrzut, 1996) rather than school-based assessment teams. Only a small percentage of children (usually those with more severe ABIs) typically undergo cognitive testing as part of a neuropsychological assessment. Most assessments are completed prior to school re-entry. These evaluations provide a valued "baseline" of post-ABI cognitive abilities, augment traditional psychoeducational assessments findings, and assist with planning school re-entry (Farmer et al., 1996). However, children are rarely seen for neuropsychological re-evaluations to determine changes or plateaus in their cognitive recovery over time. Thus, "baseline" neuropsychological assessments soon become outdated in their ability to quantify changes in cognitive or behavioral functioning as a student matures. Typically, students with less severe brain injuries are rarely referred for neuropsychological evaluation; hence, a cognitive and behavioral baseline is lacking. As a result, the actual consequences of a student's brain injury may remain underappreciated (Boll, 1983).

Within the school setting, psychoeducational assessment traditionally has been limited to intelligence testing (Sattler, 1988) and assessment of academic achievement. However, neither IQ nor achievement tests by themselves are sufficient to determine the impact of brain injury or extent of recovery after brain injury (Farmer & Peterson, 1995). While traditional psychoeducational measures used in assessing students with other learning disabilities can be utilized (Ylvisaker et al., 2001), it has been argued that psychoeducational assessment needs to be expanded to include both standardized and informal qualitative assessments of cognitive processing and learning abilities that may be selectively impacted by ABI (Farmer & Peterson, 1995; Donders & Minnema, 2004).

The adequacy of intelligence testing as an indicator of cognitive abilities following ABI has been questioned by a number of education researchers. More specifically, intelligence quotients can overestimate actual cognitive functioning and abilities in the classroom (Lezak, 1995). Stable verbal intellectual abilities (due to good recovery of previously learned skills after injury) may inadvertently create false-positive expectations (Bigler, Clark, & Farmer, 1996; Ewing-Cobbs et al., 1997). While reduced intellectual abilities (Banich, Levine, Kim, & Huttenlocher, 1990; Farmer & Peterson, 1995; Johnson, 1992) can readily be identified by school-based professionals, educational assessors often fail to consider or assess the multifactorial nature of IQ subtests and the negative impact of impairments in sequencing, perceptual planning, processing speed, fluency, and/or abstraction on overall performance (Farmer & Peterson, 1995; Johnson, 1992). Thus, IQ testing may, by itself, not be sensitive enough to uncover learning difficulties (Semrud-Clikeman, 2001), and too narrow to provide information required for developing focused educational interventions for children with ABI (D'Amato & Rothlisberg, 1996). It has been argued that psychoeducational evaluations need to incorporate assessment of cognitive domains most frequently impacted by ABI, including learning capacity and speed of processing (Hoffman, Donders, & Thompson, 2000; Donders & Minnema, 2004), language, memory, attention, reasoning, abstract thinking, judgment, problem solving, sensory, perceptual, and motor abilities (Dalby & Obrzut, 1991; Farmer & Peterson, 1995).

Given the complexity and diversity of cognitive deficits and strengths observed in students after ABI and the potential for delayed onset of cognitive and academic challenges as these students mature, we recommend ongoing monitoring of students' cognitive functioning. In students with ABI who present with academic challenges at time of school re-entry, we recommend an initial cognitive assessment and periodic reassessment of cognitive strengths and weaknesses across the students' school careers. While the appropriate frequency of retesting has been debated (Savage, 1991; Semrud-Clikeman, 1999), more frequent reassessments during the initial 5 years postinjury have been recommended. In our experience, reassessments must continue throughout the students' academic lives, with testing paralleling anticipated shifts in school curricula when cognitive demands on students are significantly increased (i.e., in fourth grade, at transition from grammar to middle school, at transition from middle school to high school, and prior to high school graduation). Students with milder injuries may not initially present with academic challenges. With these students, schools typically opt for a "wait and see" approach, preferring to delay any accommodations or testing referrals until a student exhibits academic failure. For these students, we recommend qualitative (informal) assessments of their classroom behaviors (see below) on a yearly basis for the duration of their school careers. Referral for cognitive testing should be initiated when academic challenges initially emerge, so as to prevent and/or contain academic failure for the student.

INFORMAL QUALITATIVE ASSESSMENTS FOR STUDENTS WITH ABI

Informal qualitative assessments can enrich the understanding of students' functional abilities as related to their underlying cognitive challenges post-ABI (Semrud-Clikeman, 2001; Ylvisaker et al., 2005). These qualitative assessments permit evaluation of students' strengths and weaknesses. Perhaps most crucial to academic success, this approach to hypothesis testing provides an understanding of how students learn; as well as what they know (Semrud-Clikeman, 2001). Individualized assessments typically utilize input obtained from the student, his or her family, pertinent rehabilitation professionals, and school staff who knew the student both pre- and postinjury (Harrington, 1990; Smith & Tyler, 1997). Information can be gathered through use of interviews, functional scales, and/or observations of the student's environment, classroom dynamics, and peer relationships (Farmer & Peterson, 1995). Informal qualitative assessments can focus on a wide variety of student-specific abilities, such as attention span, frustration tolerance, level of fatigue, need for routine, ability to navigate within the school setting, confusion as to expectations, amount of time required for processing of new information, consistency of performance across classrooms, and best learning strategies (Harrington, 1990). Thus, informal qualitative assessments serve as excellent tools with which to gather data about the impact of a student's cognitive challenges on his or her classroom behaviors, the impact of classroom milieu on the student's behaviors, and the social and motivational factors needed to enhance the student's learning abilities. These qualitative assessments can also be used to evaluate the effectiveness of selected classroom strategies, to monitor changes in a student's behaviors over time, to track consistency of classroom approaches across settings, and/or to determine needed refinements in classroom accommodations (Ylvisaker et al., 2003). Information obtained from qualitative assessments should be combined with standardized psychoeducational evaluation data to facilitate the development of an effective educational plan, implementation of needed interventions and strategies, and selection of accommodations for a given student.

For students with ABI presenting with academic challenges in the classroom, we recommend that informal qualitative assessments of students' classroom functioning be completed several times during the academic year and repeated yearly for the remainder of the their academic careers. The information derived from these qualitative assessments can assist classroom personnel in rapidly shifting educational approaches as necessary, even before a formal individualized education plan (IEP) or 504 plan (Ewing-Cobbs & Fletcher, 1990; Farmer & Peterson, 1995) is revised. Data from these informal qualitative assessments also serve to inform school-based assessment teams as to the timing and nature of repeated cognitive evaluations for the student. For students who do not present academic challenges, we recommend qualitative assessments of classroom abilities at least yearly. These assessments serve to monitor changes in academic or behavioral functioning proactively as the student matures. Any alterations (i.e., academic decline, inability to learn new concepts, alterations in behaviors, etc.) should alert teaching staff to consider whether ABI-related lags in cognitive development underlie these academic changes for the student. When indicated, timely referral for focused cognitive testing will assist with planning needed accommodations.

EXPANDED ROLES FOR SCHOOL-BASED ASSESSMENT TEAMS

Regardless of progress, plateau, or decline in cognitive performance for students with ABI, the school psychologist is well positioned to monitor and evaluate students' cognitive progress in the school setting (Farmer & Peterson, 1995; Walker, Williams, & Cobb, 1999). Farmer and Peterson (1995) argue that school psychologists need to assume a neuropsychological orientation within their assessments. For psychoeducational assessments to be more useful, expansion of school psychologists' assessments to include multiple domains of cognitive functioning (e.g., arousal, perception, attention, processing speed, fluency, memory, and executive functioning) are necessary. The psychologist should place findings within a developmental framework and contrast them to the student's level of skills prior to ABI (Ewing-Cobbs & Fletcher, 1990; Harrington, 1990; Johnson, 1992; Semrud-Clikeman, 2001).

Semrud-Clikeman (2001) argues that the school assessment team (i.e., psychologist, speech pathologist, occupational therapist, and special education evaluator) can employ many cognitive and functional tools that are already within the scope of their training to evaluate a student's learning abilities and cognition. She provides a list of measures commonly utilized by psychologists and other professionals who traditionally are members of the school-based assessment team. These tools can be used to assess cognition functioning in areas such as memory, executive functioning, attention, language, visual–motor and motor performance, and behavior (see Semrud-Clikeman, 2001, Table 5.4, pp. 66–70). Other researchers argue that school-based assessment teams may be ill-prepared to provide cognitive assessments necessary for targeted program planning for children after brain injury (Ponsford et al., 2001; Walker et al., 1999). Additional training of school-based assessors in cognitive and informal qualitative assessment techniques is necessary (Ylvisaker et al., 2001). With appropriate training, it is anticipated that school-based assessors can expand their traditional role to case managers, consultants, and counselors for students with ABI, their families, and teaching staff (Walker et al., 1999). Finally, it is our opinion that school-based assessors must assume a key role in ensuring that teachers across classroom settings, between grades, and between school buildings remain cognizant of any given student's ABI. This approach will ensure that all school-based staff are aware of the potential for delayed academic challenges for a student, which in turn will permit more timely implementation of needed classroom accommodations to minimize potential academic failure (Semrud-Clikeman, 2001).

EDUCATIONAL PLANNING FOR STUDENTS WITH ABI

Planning of educational accommodations varies with the severity of each student's injury. As many as 20% of students with ABI require some educational services during their school career (Boyer & Edwards, 1991; Kinsella et al., 1997; Semrud-Clikeman, 2001; Taylor et al., 2003). For children with more severe ABIs, educational services can range from individual instruction (both at home and institutional settings) to support-oriented, contextually sensitive behavioral and cognitive accommodations in the general education classroom (Ylvisaker et al., 2003). Students with more severe ABIs are more likely to require special educational services. Rosen and Gerring (1986) reported that a significant proportion of students with severe ABI required home instruction, were unable to return to school, and/ or required institutional placement. Of those students who did return to school, 11% required a reduced or modified school program and 20% attended special education programs. Only 18% of these students did not require special education services (Rosen & Gerring, 1986).

For students with severe ABI, educational accommodations are typically based on an IEP and revised on an ongoing basis. Students with milder ABI may require accommodations within the general education setting. Since these students are not eligible for special education services, their educational accommodations are best met under Section 504 of the Individuals with Disabilities Act of 1990 (Federal Register, 1990; Farmer et al., 1996).

When designing instructional programming for students with ABI, collaborative involvement of families is crucial. Educational outcomes have been associated with the adequacy of family functioning both before and after the onset of a child's brain injury (Taylor, Yeates, Wade, Drotar, Klein, & Stancin, 1999). For example, families that were dysfunctional before a student's injury may remain dysfunctional after the injury, or become more dysfunctional over time (Rivera et al., 1993), and families that were underinvolved in their child's education prior to the student's injury may have difficulty seeking needed supports after the injury (Taylor et al., 1999). Placement and accommodations may also be complicated by conflicting needs and requests of the family. For example, during the initial phases of school re-entry, families may be unaware of the immediate or delayed effects of an injury (e.g., in students with mild ABI). Conversely, families may equate a return to school with a return to normalcy and may not want their children classified with an ABI within the school. In these instances, students with ABIs may return to school without services. On the other end of the continuum, parents of children with more severe ABIs may expect support similar to that provided within a rehabilitation setting, and place excessive pressure on the school to provide similar services (Savage & Carter, 1991). In order to promote positive family involvement in the student's educational planning process (Braga & Campos da Paz, 2000; De Pompei & Blosser, 1994; Wayland, Burns, & Cockrell, 1993), assessment of the adequacy of family support both pre- and postinjury is suggested. When indicated, additional support for families to assist with transition back to school may be beneficial.

Todis, Glang, and Fabry (1997) identified additional factors that may contribute to problematic educational planning for students with ABIs. System issues, including dwindling resources, resistance to change, outdated techniques, and the lack of expertise by educators in providing appropriate accommodations, may contribute to a school's difficulty in responding flexibly to the varying needs of students with ABIs and their families. Additional teacher training has been suggested to increase levels of teacher confidence in both use of informal (qualitative) assessments and application of cognitive-behavioral techniques in the classroom setting (Ylvisaker et al., 2001).

EDUCATIONAL INTERVENTIONS FOR STUDENTS WITH ABI

Pediatric ABI has been viewed as too diverse a disability category to support general statements such as "intervention/teaching strategy X works/ does not work" for this group of students (Farmer & Peterson, 1995; Taylor et al., 2003; Ylvisaker et al., 2001). Children with ABI, like all students, learn best in a setting that provides clear instruction, adequate practice, consistent and clear feedback, and ongoing assessment. Effective teaching techniques, including varying teaching methods, emphasizing the student's best modality of learning, providing an overview and outline of steps involved in a task, initiating tasks one step at a time, using repetition and review, teaching to saturation, providing demonstrations, remaining flexible, and keeping expectations realistic, are good classroom practices for all students but are essential for students with ABI (Farmer & Peterson, 1995; Telzrow, 2001).

Additional models of classroom instruction have also been suggested. For example, Madigan, Hall, and Glang (1997) argue for the use of Direct Instruction, a systematic instructional approach designed for building and maintaining a student's cognitive skills, with an emphasis on the use of small-group instruction and frequent responding by students within an active, participation-oriented classroom. For additional information and a detailed description of instructional design and delivery practices, see Engelmann, Carnine, and Steely (1992), Kameenui and Simmons (1990) and Madigan et al. (1997). Ylvisaker and colleagues (2001) recommend use of several instructional strategies found to be effective in varied populations of students, with and without disabilities, to address the educational needs of students with ABI. These instructional strategies are listed in Table 12.1. Selection of a given strategy should be dictated by the presenting ABI characteristics of a given student.

Ylvisaker and colleagues (2001) also recommend integrated educational, behavioral, and social interventions that have been shown to be effective for students with and without disabilities. These integrated approaches are presented in Table 12.2. Selection of the appropriate approaches for students with ABI, again, is dependent upon the presenting academic challenge(s).

Both instructional approaches and interventions offer useful hypotheses and reasonable intervention choices for teachers in the classroom setting. Findings from psychoeducational assessments and informal classroom observations should inform selection of instructional approaches taken, with informal classroom observations utilized to monitor their efficacy within the classroom setting.

REHABILITATION WITHIN THE SCHOOL SETTING FOR STUDENTS WITH ABI

While children with ABI return to school for "habilitation" (Farmer & Peterson, 1995; Hawley, 2003), students with more severe injuries may require focused "rehabilitation" in order to regain previously acquired academic skills and abilities. Thus, school-based learning following pediatric ABI may require the dual processes of "habilitation" and "rehabilitation." Rehabilitation needs to focus on both relearning of academic abilities impacted by the ABI and introduction of compensatory approaches to address residual deficits. Selection of specific rehabilitation tasks are student-dependent and typically derived from information obtained from psychoeducational–cognitive assessments and informal classroom observations (Dennis, Wilkenson, Koski, & Humphreys, 1995). In our experience, students with more severe injuries typically require focused rehabilitation efforts directed at improving their functioning in the areas of attention, memory, executive functioning, and behavioral control.

Semrud-Clikeman (2001) recommends techniques utilized in rehabilitation for adults with brain injuries (e.g., Mateer, Kerns, & Eso, 1996; Sohlberg & Mateer, 1989), as well as cognitive-behavioral approaches utilized for children with attention deficits (Braswell & Bloomquist, 1991) and those with impulsivity (Kendall & Braswell, 1993). The goals of these

TABLE 12.1. Research-Based Instructional Strategies Related to Characteristics of Many Students with TBI

TBI characteristic	Instructional strategy	Description
Fluctuating attention; decreased speed of processing	Appropriate pacing	Delivering material in small increments and requiring responses at a rate consistent with a student's processing speed increases acquisition of new material.
Memory impairment (associated with need for errorless learning)	High rates of success	Acquisition and retention of new information tends to increase with high rates of success.
High rates of failure; organizational impairment; inefficient learning	Task analysis and advance organizational support	Careful organization of learning, tasks, including systematic sequencing of teaching targets and advance organizational support, increases success.
Inefficient learning; inconsistency	Sufficient practice and review (including cumulative frequent review)	Acquisition and retention of new information is increased with review.
Inefficient feedback loops; implicit learning of errors	Errorless learning combined with corrective feedback when errors occur	Students with severe memory and learning problems benefit from errorless learning. When errors occur, learning is enhanced when those errors are followed by nonjudgmental corrective feedback.
Possibility of gaps in the knowledge base	Teaching to mastery	Learning is enhanced with mastery at the acquisition phase.
Frequent failure of transfer; concrete thinking and learning	Facilitation of transfer/ generalization	Generalizable strategies and general case teaching (wide range of examples and settings) increase generalization.
Inconsistency; unpredictable recovery	Ongoing assessment	Adjustment of teaching based on ongoing assessment of students' progress facilitates learning.
Unusual profiles; unpredictable recovery	Flexibility in curricular modification	Modifying the curriculum facilitates learning in special populations.

Note. From Ylvisaker et al. (2001). Copyright 2001 by Aspen Publishers, Inc. Reprinted by permission.

TABLE 12.2. Integrated Approaches to Educational, Behavioral, and Social Interventions That Have a Research Base and Are Applicable to Many Students with TBI

TBI characteristic	Approach	Description
New learning needs; impaired strategy behavior; impaired organizational functioning	Metacognitive/ strategy intervention	Organized curricula designed to facilitate a strategic approach to difficult academic tasks, including organizational strategies; validated for adolescents with and without specific learning disabilities (Pressley et al., 1995; Schumaker & Deshler, 1992)
Decreased self-awareness; denial of deficits	Self-awareness/ attribution training	Facilitation of students' understanding of their role in learning; validated for students with learning difficulties (Borkowski, Chan, & Muthukrishna, in press)
Weak self-regulation related to frontal lobe injury; disinhibited and potentially aggressive behavior	Cognitive-behavioral modification	Facilitation of self-control of behavior; validated with adolescents with ADHD and aggressive behavior (Robinson, Smith, Miller, & Brownell, 1991)
Impulsive behavior; inefficient learning from consequences; history of failure; defiant behavior; initiation impairment; working memory impairment	Positive, antecedent-focused behavior supports	Approach to behavior management on the antecedents of behavior (in a broad sense); validated in developmental disabilities and with some TBI subpopulations (Carr, Horner, & Turnbull, 1999)
Frequent loss of friends; social isolation; weak social skills	Circle of friends	A set of procedures designed to support students' social life and ongoing social development; validated in developmental disabilities and TBI (Forest & Lusthaus, 1989; Glang, Singer, & Todis, 1997)

Note. From Ylvisaker et al. (2001). Copyright 2001 by Aspen Publishers, Inc. Reprinted by permission.

interventions are to increase the students' independence in learning and to expand their ability to generalize learning to new situations (Semrud-Clikeman, 2001).

In older students, rehabilitation efforts may be directed at helping students relearn executive functioning skills, for example, problem solving (Gentner, Loewenstein, & Thompson, 2003) or abstraction (Gentner et al.,

2003; Hershkowitz, Schwarz, & Dreyfus, 2001), that may have been negatively impacted as a result of the ABI. These students may also need to relearn select elements of academics skills in reading, spelling, writing, and/or mathematics (e.g., Madigan et al., 1997; Semrud-Clikeman, 2001). Behavioral challenges that interfere with learning may also necessitate referral to the school psychologist or social worker. Behavioral interventions should be directed at development of alternative coping strategies and identification of potential precipitants of inappropriate behavior.

Several authors propose that rehabilitation should be directed at specific cognitive domains impaired by the ABI. For example, Kraemer and Blancher (1997) suggest that educational techniques and strategies for students with ABI be organized around the student's presenting cognitive impairments in attention, orientation, information processing, organization and planning, memory and learning, reasoning, problem solving, sensory–motor function and behavior (see Kraemer & Blancher, 1997, Table I, pp. 22–24). Semrud-Clikeman (2001) also emphasizes the need for specific accommodations for challenges in attention, memory, social skills, and cognitive processing post-ABI. In our experience, most students with ABI require help in learning to use external organizers (i.e., a daily planner or personal data assistant [PDA] device), to compensate for their memory and organization difficulties. These compensatory tools are essential for students in middle and high school, and often must be taught to students prior to entry into middle school. In our experience, rehabilitation strategies can be taught by most school-based professionals (e.g., the school psychologist, the educational specialist, the resource room teacher, and the occupational or the speech therapist). However, it is important to identify a targeted school professional that has primary responsibility to assist the student in relearning these generic learning building blocks. Finally, to enhance learning and generalization of compensatory tools, students should be encouraged to use compensatory tools within all classroom settings, with teachers serving as facilitators of their use.

TRANSITION PLANNING FOR STUDENTS WITH ABI

Students with more severe ABIs often require ongoing transition planning throughout their school careers, with challenges emerging at each core transition point viewed within the developmental perspective of normal (and therefore expected) brain development (Bergland, 1996). Prior research has focused on two primary transitions: at point of re-entry back to the school from rehabilitation settings (Kraemer & Blancher, 1997; Farmer & Peterson, 1995; Farmer et al., 1996) or in preparation for high school graduation (Lehr & Savage, 1990).

Several reintegration strategies have been recommended to ease school re-entry for the student with more severe ABIs. These strategies include maintenance of a neuropsychological orientation when assessing the returning student, use of a multidisciplinary team approach to assess and plan school-based interventions, use of frequent and ongoing evaluation of the student's overall adjustment, and use of contextual assessments to round out educational planning (Farmer & Peterson, 1995). A transitional IEP, created by both school personnel and rehabilitation staff at the time of the student's discharge from rehabilitation (Savage, 1991) will require frequent revisions during the initial phases of school re-entry due to the often dynamic nature of early recovery for these students (Farmer & Peterson, 1995). To ease re-entry back to the school setting, school-based consultation by the rehabilitation staff and/or a pediatric neuropsychologist may be beneficial (Lash & Scarpino, 1993).

A second transition period discussed in the pediatric ABI literature is that leading up to graduation from school (Lehr & Savage, 1990). For students injured early in childhood, adolescence may be a particularly difficult time period, since it presents additional challenges for the student with already lagged cognitive and social skills development. As a result, transition planning for these students is often difficult. Planning should be initiated as early in the student's high school years as possible (Koskiniemi et al., 1995). Schools typically need to provide a comprehensive program that includes academic support, community-based education focused on independent living, employment and life skills, and age-appropriate peer activities, in order for the student to acquire the skills necessary for a successful adult life (Ylvisaker, Feeney, & Urbanczyk, 1993). Early networking to develop resources for postsecondary school planning (i.e., community college, vocational rehabilitation services) may facilitate this transition (Ylvisaker et al., 2001).

In our experience, students may have their academic needs well met in a given school setting, only to lose gains made in the classroom at the time of transfer to another class or school building, due to lack of adequate communication of school staff. Thus, it is argued that additional points of transition planning should be considered for *all* students with ABI and provided across the students' school careers. These additional transition points occur when a student moves from grade to grade, from school to school, and from school to adulthood. It is at these points that effective communication and collaboration among the students, their families and school personnel are essential. The students' needs and preferences, actual level of functioning (Smith & Tyler, 1997), and approaches to classroom instruction that were effective (as well as ineffective) should be communicated to the new school staff that will be working with the student.

In students with more severe ABIs, these transition points are often fraught with difficulty and therefore necessitate increased communication of staff and close monitoring of the student's adjustment in the new academic setting. Supports that were judged unnecessary earlier in a student's academic program may be indicated as the student matures and is faced with greater cognitive challenges (Ylvisaker et al., 2001). Transition planning for postsecondary education should be considered for students with less severe ABI when their academic and/or behavioral challenges may limit their choice of long-term academic and career plans.

Given the need for ongoing transition services for students with ABI, a case management model has been recommended (Ylvisaker et al., 2001). In our experience, case management services appear to work most effectively when provided by the school system itself, with a school-based professional identified as the "coordinator" of the student's transitional services. The coordinator serves as the primary liaison between the student, his or her family, and the school-based team. Key roles of the coordinator may include orienting school staff from year to year about ABI (Ylvisaker & Feeney, 1998), review of needed accommodations for a student within the classroom, and assistance in the successful implementation (or continuation) of needed classroom accommodations. In consultation with the school-based staff, the coordinator may work with other staff to augment classroom interventions or rehabilitation (e.g., a resource room teacher begins to work with the student on use of a PDA to improve memory or organizational skills; the school psychologist begins to explore behavioral issues with the student). Thus, similar to assessment after ABI, accommodations after ABI need to be broadly based, require the involvement of a multidisciplinary team, and need to be revised as needed given the shifts in the student's academic and behavior challenges.

FUTURE DIRECTIONS

Pediatric ABI may result in lifelong challenges for children, their families, and school professionals who work with these students. Ylvisaker and his colleagues (2001) propose a series of recommendations for future research and policy in pediatric ABI in the areas of epidemiology, assessment, transition, instructional and behavioral interventions, training and support of teachers and families, and system change. We propose the following additional suggestions aimed at enhancing academic success for students with ABI:

1. *Systematic screening for ABI is recommended to enhance identification of students with ABI in the educational system.* Screening should involve history taking regarding ABI events (e.g., CVAs, blows to the head re-

sulting in altered mental status, hypoxic events, exposure to neurotoxins, etc.) and symptoms (e.g., cognitive difficulties, behavioral problems, etc.). Systematic screening will decrease the number of students who remain unidentified and serve to establish realistic estimates of the number of students with ABI in the education system. Ultimately, screening should serve to correct the misperception that ABI is a "low" incidence phenomenon. The definition of ABI for screening purposes should be standardized across states to include both "internal" and "external" etiologies. Three levels of screening are recommended: (1) screening for ABI in all students at entry (or transfer) to a new school system; (2) yearly screenings thereafter to identify new onset or secondary ABIs during the prior year (Ylvisaker et al., 2005); and (3) screening for ABI in all students referred for special education services.

2. *Expansion of psychosocial assessments to include cognitive assessment for students with ABI.* When students with ABI are referred for educational services, an initial cognitive assessment is recommended, with repeat assessments of cognitive abilities at times of major expected developmental change (e.g., fourth grade, prior to starting middle school, prior to starting high school, and prior to graduation). Repeat assessments allow for monitoring of plateau or decline in cognitive functioning as the student matures, and serve to direct needed revisions and additions to educational plans and classroom accommodations. Training of school psychologists and other assessment team members is indicated to enhance comfort with use of these cognitive measures.

3. *Students with ABI who are not presenting academic challenges should be monitored yearly for potential lags in academic abilities.* For all students who have experienced an ABI, informal qualitative assessments should be utilized within the classroom setting for the duration of their school career. The purpose of these assessments is to identify proactively emergence of delayed academic challenges secondary to the ABI. Referral for assessment of cognitive functioning should be initiated when academic challenges are noted.

4. *Classroom teachers need to be empowered to collect and integrate informal, qualitative assessment findings into their classroom approaches for students with ABI.* The school-based assessment team needs to empower teachers with tools to evaluate ways that a student's cognitive and behavioral functioning impact his or her classroom performance. These assessment findings need to inform selection of classroom interventions for each student, with follow-up assessments utilized to evaluate efficacy of these approaches. Consultation with a pediatric neuropsychologist is suggested as a means of capacity building at the local school level.

5. *Embedding cognitive and behavioral accommodations within instructional strategies will serve to maximize a student's ability to learn in*

the classroom setting. Knowledge of cognitive and behavioral accommodations to address challenging behaviors in the classroom will empower teachers across settings to provide the consistent support needed for the student to succeed in school. Expanded training for teachers about these issues is indicated.

ACKNOWLEDGMENTS

This research was supported by the National Institute on Disability and Rehabilitation Research, United States Department of Education (Grant No. H133B980013), to the Department of Rehabilitation Medicine, Mount Sinai School of Medicine.

REFERENCES

Banich, M. T., Levine, S. C., Kim, H., & Huttenlocher, P. (1990). The effects of developmental factors on IQ in hemiplegic children. *Neuropsychologia, 28,* 35–47.

Bergland, M. M. (1996). Transition from school to adult life: Key to the future. In A. L. Goldberg (Ed.), *Acquired brain injury in childhood and adolescents* (pp. 171–194). Springfield, IL: Thomas.

Bigler, E. D., Clark, E., & Farmer, J. (1996). Traumatic brain injury: 1990 update. *Journal of Learning Disabilities, 29,* 512–513.

Bijur, P. E., & Haslum, M. (1995). Cognitive behavioral and motoric sequelae of mild head injury in a national birth cohort. In S. H. Broman & M. E. Michel (Eds.), *Traumatic head injury in children* (pp. 147–164). New York: Oxford University Press.

Boll, T. J. (1983). Minor head injury in children: Out of sight, not out of mind. *Journal of Clinical Child Psychology, 12,* 74–80.

Borkowski, J. G., Chan, K. S., & Muthukrishna, N. (in press). A process-oriented model of metacognition: Links between motivation and executive functioning. In G. Shraw (Ed.), *Issues in measurement of metacognition.* Lincoln, NB: University of Nebraska Press.

Boyer, M. G., & Edwards, P. (1991). Preparing educational professionals for meeting the needs of students with traumatic brain injury. *Journal of Head Trauma Rehabilitation, 6,* 73–82.

Braga, L. W., & Campos da Paz, A. (2000). Neuropsychological pediatric rehabilitation. In A. L. Christensen & B. Uzzell (Eds.), *International handbook of neuropsychological rehabilitation* (pp. 283–295). New York: Kluwer Academic/Plenum Press.

Braswell, L., & Bloomquist, M. L. (1991). *Cognitive-behavioral therapy with ADHD children: Child, family, and school interventions.* New York: Guilford Press.

Bryan, T. (1995). The social competence of students with learning disabilities over time: A response to Vaughn and Hogan. *Journal of Learning Disabilities, 27,* 304–308.

Cantor, J. B., Gordon, W. A., Schwartz, M. E., Charatz, H. J., Ashman, T. A., & Abramowitz, S. (2004). Child and parent responses to a brain injury screening questionnaire. *Archives of Physical Medicine and Rehabilitation, 85*, S54–S60.

Carr, E. G., Homer, R. H., Tumbull, A. P., et al. (1999). *Positive behavior support for people with developmental disabilities: A research synthesis.* Washington, DC: American Association of Mental Retardation.

Catroppa, C., & Anderson, V. (2002). Recovery in memory function in the first year following TBI in children. *Brain Injury, 16*, 369–384.

Clark, E. (1996). Children and adolescents with traumatic brain injury: Reintegration challenges in educational settings. *Journal of Learning Disabilities, 29*, 549–560.

Cronin, A. F. (2001). Traumatic brain injury in children: Issues in community function. *American Journal of Occupational Therapy, 55*, 377–84.

D'Amato, R. C., & Rothlisberg, B. A. (1996). How education should respond to students with traumatic brain injury. *Journal of Learning Disabilities, 29*, 670–683.

Dalby, P. R., & Obrzut, J. E. (1991). Epidemiological characteristics and sequelae of closed head-injured children: A review. *Developmental Neuropsychology, 7*, 35–68.

Deaton, A. V., & Waaland, P. (1994). Psychosocial effects of acquired brain injury. In R. C. Savage & G. G. F. Wolcott (Eds.), *Educational dimensions of acquired brain injury* (pp. 239–255). Austin, TX: Pro-Ed.

Dennis, M. C., Wilkenson, M., Koski, L., & Humphreys, R. P. (1995). Attention deficits in the long term after childhood head injury. In S. Broman & M. E. Michel (Eds.), *Traumatic head injury in children* (pp. 165–187). New York: Oxford University Press.

De Pompei, R., & Blosser, J. L. (1994). The family as collaborator for effective school reintegration. In R. C. Savage & G. Wolcott (Ed.), *Educational dimensions of acquired brain injury* (pp. 489–506). Austin, TX: Pro-Ed.

Donders, J., & Ballard, E. (1996). Psychological adjustment characteristics of children before and after moderate to severe traumatic brain injury. *Journal of Head Trauma Rehabilitation, 11*, 67–73.

Donders, J., & Minnema, M. T. (2004). Performance discrepancies on the California Verbal Learning Test—Children's Version (CVLT-C) in children with traumatic brain injury. *Journal of the International Neuropsychology Society, 10*, 482–488.

Engelmann, S., Carnine, D., & Steely, D. (1992). Making connections in mathematics. In D. Carnine & E. Kameeui (Eds.), *Higher order thinking: Designing curriculum for mainstreamed students* (pp. 75–106). Austin, TX: Pro-Ed.

Eslinger, P. J., Grattan, L. M., Dinter, D., Schmidt, B., & Damasio, A. R. (1992). Developmental consequences of childhood frontal lobe damage. *Archives of Neurology, 49*, 764–769.

Ewing-Cobbs, L., & Fletcher, J. M. (1990). Neuropsychological assessment of traumatic brain injury in children. In E. D. Bigler (Ed.), *Traumatic brain injury* (pp. 107–128). Austin, TX: Pro-Ed.

Ewing-Cobbs, L., Fletcher, J. M., Levin, H. S., Francis, D. J., Davidson, K., & Miner, M. E. (1997). Longitudinal neuropsychological outcome in infants and preschoolers with traumatic brain injury. *Journal of the International Neuropsychological Society, 3,* 581–591.

Ewing-Cobbs, L., Miner, M. E., Fletcher, J. M., & Levin, H. S. (1989). Intellectual, motor, and language sequelae following closed head injury in infants and preschoolers. *Journal of Pediatric Psychology, 14,* 531–547.

Farmer, J., & Peterson, L. (1995). Pediatric traumatic brain injury: Promoting successful school reentry. *School Psychology Review, 24,* 230–243.

Farmer, J. E., Clippard, D. S., Luehr-Wiemann, Y., Wright, E., & Owings, S. (1996). Assessing children with traumatic brain injury during rehabilitation: Promoting school and community reentry. *Journal of Learning Disabilities, 29,* 532–548.

Fay, G. C., Jaffe, K. M., & Polissar, N. L. (1993). Mild pediatric traumatic brain injury: A cohort study. *Archives of Physical Medicine and Rehabilitation, 74,* 895–901.

Federal Register. (1990). Individuals with Disabilities Education Act. Public Law No. 101-476, 104 Stat. 1103 (October 30, 1990).

Feeney, T., & Ylvisaker, M. (1995). Choice and routine: Antecedent behavioral interventions for adolescents with severe traumatic brain injury. *Journal of Head Trauma Rehabilitation, 10,* 67–86.

Forest, M., & Lusthaus, E. (1989). Promoting educational equality for all students: Circles and maps. In S. Stainback, W. Stainback, & M. Forest (Eds.), *Educating all students in the mainstream of regular education.* Baltimore, MD: Paul H. Brookes Publishing.

Gentner, D., Lowenstein, J., & Thompson, L. (2003). Learning and transfer: A general role for analogical encoding. *Journal of Educational Psychology, 95,* 393–405.

Gil, A. M. (2003). Neurocognitive outcomes following pediatric brain injury: A developmental approach. *Journal of School Psychology, 41,* 337–353.

Glang, A., Singer, G. H. S., & Todis, B. (1997) *Children with acquired brain injury: The school's response.* Baltimore, MD: Paul H. Brookes Publishing.

Goldstein, F., & Levin, H. S. (1985). Intellectual and academic outcome following closed head injury in children and adolescents: Research strategies and empirical findings. *Developmental Neuropsychology, 1,* 195–214.

Guyer, B., & Ellers, B. (1990). Childhood injuries in the United States. *American Journal of Diseases of Children, 144,* 649–652.

Harding, J. A., & Kleiman, M. D. (1996). Cerebrovascular disorders. In E. S. Batchelor & R. S. Dean (Eds.), *Pediatric neuropsychology. Interfacing assessment and treatment for rehabilitation* (pp. 163–210). Boston: Allyn & Bacon.

Harrington, D. E. (1990). Educational strategies. In M. Rosenthal, E. R. Griffith, M. R. Bond, & J. D. Miller (Eds.), *Rehabilitation of the adult and child with traumatic brain injury* (2nd ed., pp. 476–492). Philadelphia: Davis.

Hawley, C. A. (2003). Reported problems and their resolution following mild, moderate and severe traumatic brain injury amongst children and adolescents in the UK. *Brain Injury, 17,* 105–129.

Hawley, C. A., Ward, A., Magnay, A., & Long, J. (2002). Children's brain injury: A postal follow up of 525 children from one health region in the UK. *Brain Injury, 16,* 969–985.

Hayman-Abello, S. E., Rourke, B. P., & Fuerst, D. R. (2002). Psychosocial status after pediatric brain injury: A subtype analysis using the Child Behavior Checklist. *Journal of the International Neuropsychological Society, 9,* 887–898.

Hershkowitz, R., Schwarz, B., & Dreyfus, T. (2001). Abstraction in context: Epistemic actions. *Journal for Research in Mathematics Education, 32,* 195–222.

Hoffman, N., Donders, J., & Thompson, E. (2000). Novel learning abilities after traumatic head injury in children. *Archives of Clinical Neuropsychology, 15,* 47–58.

Hooper, S. R., Willis, W. G., & Stone, B. H. (1996). Issues and approaches in the neuropsychological treatment of children with learning disabilities. In E. S. Batchelor & R. S. Dean (Eds.), *Pediatric neuropsychology: Interfacing assessment and treatment for rehabilitation* (pp. 211–248). Boston: Allyn & Bacon.

Johnson, D. A. (1992). Head injured children and education: A need for greater delineation and understanding. *British Journal of Educational Psychology, 62,* 404–409.

Johnson, D. A., & Rose, D. (2004). Prognosis, rehabilitation and outcome after inflicted brain injury in children—A case of professional developmental delay. *Pediatric Rehabilitation, 7,* 185–193.

Kameenui, E. J., & Simmons, D. (1990). The effect of task alternatives on vocabulary knowledge: A comparison of students with and without learning disabilities. *Journal of Learning Disabilities, 23,* 291–297.

Kendall, P. C., & Braswell, L. (1993). *Cognitive behavioral therapy for impulsive children* (2nd ed.). New York: Guilford Press.

Kinsella, G. J., Prior, M., Sawyer, M., Ong, B., Murtagh, D., Eisenmajer, R., et al. (1997). Predictors and indicators of academic outcome in children 2 years following traumatic brain injury. *Journal of the International Neuropsychological Society, 3,* 608–616.

Klonoff, H., Clark, C., & Klonoff, P. S. (1995). Outcomes of head injuries from childhood to adulthood: A twenty-three year follow-up study. In S. H. Broman & M. E. Michael (Eds.), *Traumatic head injury in children* (pp. 219–234). New York: Oxford University Press.

Klonoff, H., Low, M. D., & Clark, C. (1977). Head injuries in children: A prospective five year follow-up. *Journal of Neurology, Neurosurgery, and Psychiatry, 40,* 1211–1219.

Koskiniemi, M., Kyykka, T., Nybo, T., & Jarho, L. (1995). Long-term outcome after severe brain injury in preschoolers is worse than expected. *Archives of Pediatric and Adolescent Medicine, 149,* 249–254.

Kraemer, B. R., & Blancher, J. (1997). An overview of educationally relevant effects, assessment and school reentry. In A. Glang & G. H. Singer (Eds.), *Students with acquired brain injury: The school response* (pp. 3–31). Baltimore: Brookes.

Kraus, J. F. (1995). Epidemiological features of brain injury in children: Occurrence, children at risk, causes and manner of injury, severity, and outcomes. In S. H. Broman & M. E. Michael (Eds.), *Traumatic head injury in children* (pp. 22–39). New York: Oxford University Press.

Kraus, J. F., Rock, A., & Hemyari, P. (1990). Brain injuries among infants, children, adolescents, and young adults. *American Journal of Diseases of Children, 144,* 684–691.

Langlois, J. (2001). *Traumatic brain injury in the United States: Assessing outcomes in children.* Atlanta: National Center for Injury Prevention and Control, Centers for Disease Control and Prevention.

Lash, M., & Scarpino, C. (1993). School reintegration for children with traumatic brain injuries. *NeuroRehabilitation, 3,* 13–25.

Lehr, E., & Savage, R. (1990). Community and school integration from a developmental perspective. In J. Kreutzer & P. Wehman (Eds.), *Community integration following traumatic brain injury* (pp. 301–310). Baltimore: Brookes.

Levin, H. S., Ewing-Cobbs, L., & Fletcher, J. (1989). Neurobehavioral outcome of mild head injury in children. In H. Levin, H. M. Eisenberg, & A. L. Benton (Eds.), *Mild head injury* (pp. 189–213). New York: Oxford University Press.

Lezak, M. D. (1995). *Neuropsychological assessment* (3rd ed.). New York: Oxford University Press.

Lord-Maes, J., & Obrzut, J. E. (1996). Neuropsychological consequences of traumatic brain injury in children and adolescents. *Journal of Learning Disabilities, 29,* 609–617.

Madigan, K. A., Hall, T. E., & Glang, A. (1997). Effective assessment and instructional practices for students with ABI. In A. Glang & G. H. Singer (Eds.), *Students with acquired brain injury: The school's response* (pp. 123–160). Baltimore: Brookes.

Mateer, C. M., Kerns, K. A., & Eso, K. L. (1996). Management of attention and memory disorders following traumatic brain injury. *Journal of Learning Disabilities, 29,* 618–632.

National Center for Injury Prevention and Control. (2003). *Report to Congress on Mild Traumatic Brain Injury in the United States: Steps to prevent a serious public health problem.* Atlanta: Centers for Disease Control and Prevention.

National Institute of Health. (1999). Development Panel on Rehabilitation of Persons with Traumatic Brain Injury. Consensus conference. Rehabilitation of Persons with Traumatic Brain Injury. *Journal of the American Medical Association, 282*(10), 974–983.

Ponsford, J., Willmott, C., Rothwell, A., Cameron, P., Ayton, G., Nelms, R., et al. (2001). Impact of early intervention on outcome after traumatic brain injury in children. *Pediatrics, 108,* 1297–1303.

Pressley, M., et al. (1995). *Cognitive strategy instruction that really improves children's academic performance* (revised ed.). Cambridge, MA: Brookline Books.

Prior, M., Kinsella, G., Sawyer, M., Bryan, D., & Anderson, V. (1994). Cognitive and psychosocial outcome after head injury in children. *Australian Psychology, 29,* 116–123.

Rivera, J., Jaffe, K., Fay, G., Polisser, N., Martin, K., Shurtleff, H., & Liao, S. (1993). Family functioning and injury severity as predictors of child functioning one year following traumatic injury. *Archives of Physical Medicine and Rehabilitation, 74,* 1047–1055.

Robinson, T. R., Smith, S. W., Miller, M. D., & Brownell, M. T. (1999). Cognitive behavior modification of hyperactivity–impulsivity and aggression: A meta-analysis of school-based studies. *Journal of Educational Psychology, 91,* 195–203.

Rosen, C. D., & Gerring, J. P. (1986). *Head trauma educational reintegration.* San Diego: College Hill Press.

Ryan, T. V., LaMarche, J. A., Barth, J. T., & Boll, T. J. (1996). Neuropsychological consequences and treatment of pediatric head trauma. In E. S. Batchelor & R. S. Dean (Eds.), *Pediatric neuropsychology: Interfacing assessment and treatment for rehabilitation* (pp. 117–138). Boston: Allyn & Bacon.

Sattler, J. M. (1988). *Assessment of children* (3rd ed.). San Diego: Author.

Savage, R. C. (1991). Identification, classification, and placement issues for students with traumatic brain injuries. *Journal of Head Trauma Rehabilitation, 6,* 1–9.

Savage, R. C., & Carter, R. R. (1991). *Head injury: A family matter.* Baltimore: Brookes.

Schoenberg, B. S., Mellinger, J. F., & Schoenberg, D. G. (1978). Cerebrovascular disease in infants and children: A study of incidence, clinical features, and survival. *Neurology, 28,* 763–768.

Schumaker, J. B., & Deshler, D. D. (1992). Validation of learning strategy interventions for students with learning disabilities: Results of a programmatic research effort. In B. Y. L. Wong (Ed.), *Contemporary intervention research in learning disabilities: An international perspective.* New York: Springer-Verlag.

Semrud-Clikeman, M. (1999). Psychosocial aspects of neurological impairments in children. In V. Schwean & D. Sakolfske (Eds.), *Handbook of psychosocial characteristics of exceptional children* (pp. 299–328). New York: Plenum Press.

Semrud-Clikeman, M. (2001). *Traumatic brain injury in children and adolescents: Assessment and interventions.* New York: Guilford Press.

Smith, H., & Tyler, T. R. (1997). Choosing the right pond: The impact of group membership on self-esteem and group-oriented behavior. *Journal of Experimental Social Psychology, 33,* 146–170.

Snow, J. H., & Hooper, S. R. (1994). *Pediatric traumatic brain injury.* Thousand Oaks, CA: Sage.

Sohlberg, M. M., & Mateer, C. A. (1989). *Introduction to cognitive rehabilitation: Theory and practice.* New York: Guilford Press.

Taylor, H. G., & Alden, J. (1997). Age-related differences in outcomes following childhood brain insults: An introduction and overview. *Journal of International Neuropsychological Society, 3,* 555–567.

Taylor, H. G., Yeates, K. O., Wade, S. L., Drotar, D., Klein, S. K., & Stancin, T. (1999). Influences on first-year recovery from traumatic brain injury in children. *Neuropsychology, 13,* 76–89.

Taylor, H. G., Yeates, K. O., Wade, S. L., Drotar, D., Stancin, T., & Montpetite, M. (2003). Long-term educational interventions after traumatic brain injury in children. *Rehabilitation Psychology, 48,* 227–236.

Telzrow, C. (1987). Management of academic and educational problems in head injury. *Journal of Learning Disabilities, 20,* 536–545.

Telzrow, C. (2001). Interim alternative educational settings school district implementation of IDEA 1997 requirements. *Education and Treatment of Children, 24,* 72–98.

Todis, B., Glang, A., & Fabry, M. A. (1997). Family school child: A qualitative study of the school experiences of students with ABI. In A. Glang & G. Singer (Eds.),

Students with acquired brain injury: The school's response (pp. 33–72). Baltimore: Brookes.

U.S. Department of Education. (2001). *Twenty-fourth annual report to Congress on the implementation of the Individuals with Disabilities Education Act.* Washington, DC.

Walker, N., Williams, B., & Cobb, H. (1999). Training of school psychologists in neuropsychology and brain injury: Results of a national survey of training programs. *Child Neuropsychology, 5,* 137–142.

Wayland, P. K., Burns, C., & Cockrell, J. (1993). Evaluation of needs of high and low income families following pediatric traumatic brain injury. *Brain Injury, 7,* 135–146.

Yeates, K. O., & Taylor, G. (2005). Neurobehavioral outcomes of mild head injury in children and adolescents. *Pediatric Rehabilitation, 8,* 5–16.

Ylvisaker, M., Adelson, P. D., Braga, L. W., Burnett, S. M., Glang, A., Feeney, T. J., Moore, W., Rumney, P., & Todis, B. (2005). Rehabilitation and ongoing support after pediatric TBI: Twenty years of progress. *Journal of Head Trauma Rehabilitation, 20*(1), 95–109.

Ylvisaker, M., & Feeney, T. J. (1998). School reentry after traumatic brain injury. In M. Ylvisaker (Ed.), *Traumatic brain injury rehabilitation: Children and adolescents* (2nd ed., pp. 369–387). Boston: Butterworth Heinemann.

Ylvisaker, M., Feeney, T. J., & Urbanczyk, B. (1993). Developing a positive communication culture for rehabilitation: Communication training for staff and family members. In N. Scmidt (Ed.), *Staff development and clinical intervention in brain injury rehabilitation* (pp. 57–85). Gaithersburg, MD: Aspen.

Ylvisaker, M., Jacobs, H., & Feeney, T. (2003). Positive supports for people who experience behavioral and cognitive disability after brain injury: A review. *Journal of Head Trauma Rehabilitation, 18,* 7–32.

Ylvisaker, M., Todis, B., Glang, A., Urbanczyk, B., Franklin, C., De Pompei, R., et al. (2001). Educating students with TBI: Themes and recommendations. *Journal of Head Trauma Rehabilitation, 16,* 76–93.

13

Social Integration of Children with Physical Disabilities

PAMELA J. THOMAS
SETH WARSCHAUSKY

Social integration refers to the level and quality of participation within social networks, including dyadic relationships with peers and larger social networks, such as neighborhoods and school settings. It extends beyond access to the physical environment to access to the social roles and experiences typically available to a specific peer group. It is well documented that children with disabilities are at greater risk for poor social integration than their physically healthy peers (Bohnert, Parker, & Warschausky, 1997; Finset, Dyrnes, Krogstad, & Berstad, 1995; Galski, Tompkins, & Johnston, 1998; Janusz, Kirkwood, Yeates, & Taylor, 2002; Warschausky, Cohen, Parker, Levendosky, & Okun, 1997). The social integration of children with disabilities and their healthy or typically developing peers is affected by many of the same factors, such as social skills, parent involvement, and community access. However, challenges unique to the population of children with disabilities, such as stigma and cognitive or mobility impairments, may combine to make the process of becoming and staying social integrated more difficult.

Community and school environments have an impact on the level and quality of children's social experiences. Children with neurodevelopmental disorders, typically falling into the multiple disabilities, orthopedic impairments, and traumatic brain injury classifications, make up approximately 3.6% of the population of students in American classrooms (Office of Special Education Programs, 2002). These students with low-incidence disabilities are less likely to spend the majority of their school day in the regular education classroom than students with other disabilities. Children are more likely to be fully included in all aspects of the school setting if they exhibit basic social skills (Mancini, Coster, Trombly, & Heeren, 2000). Full participation in school, in turn, provides greater opportunities for meaningful interaction with peers.

"Community participation" or "integration," defined as involvement in structured and unstructured nonschool leisure activities, is an important avenue for the development of social relationships. Children with physical disabilities are at risk for lower community participation than their peers without disabilities. Research indicates that these children engage in fewer and in a more restricted range of leisure activities (Brown & Gordon, 1987; Meijer, Sinnema, Bijstra, Mellenbergh, & Wolters, 2000). Level of community participation is a stronger predictor of social contact than intellectual impairment or severity of disability (Hammal, Jarvis, & Colver, 2004).

Studies have examined the relations between level of community participation and specific factors, such as disability severity and family support, but to date no multifactorial studies have been conducted as part of a larger conceptual framework. King and colleagues (2003) propose a promising conceptual model in which community participation is achieved via the multidimensional influence of factors such as environmental barriers, family supports, and child characteristics (e.g., cognitive functioning) (Figure 13.1).

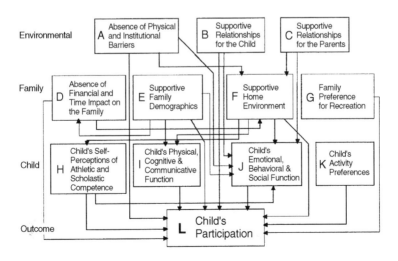

FIGURE 13.1. A model of factors affecting the participation of children with disabilities.

COMMON PSYCHOSOCIAL TREATMENT NEEDS

The relationship between community participation and social functioning probably is bidirectional; participation in a variety of social or community settings with peers provides opportunities for children to interact with and thus strengthen their friendships. In turn, having a close friend may increase community participation, because children are more likely to participate in activities with their friends (Patterson & Blum, 1996).

Research indicates that compared with their typically developing peers, children with neurodevelopmental disorders have less contact with peers, fewer friends in their social networks, less validation and caring in their best-friend relationships, and poorer social skills (Dixon & Warschausky, 2004). Children with a history of brain injury clearly are at risk for impaired social skills and relative isolation (Bohnert et al., 1997; Janusz et al., 2002). Similarly, studies have shown that children with visible physical disabilities are at risk for social adjustment problems, experiencing more rejection and bullying, and having fewer friends than physically healthy peers (Bell & Morgan, 2000; Yude, Goodman, & McConachie, 1998). The factors that contribute to social isolation and the interventions designed to bolster social functioning are the focus of this chapter.

Stigma

Much has been written about the role of stigmatization in the social environment of children with visible physical disabilities or illnesses (Schuman & LaGreca, 1999). The term "stigmatization" describes a cognitive process that involves first identifying a salient, usually negative characteristic about a person that makes him or her different from others in a particular environment, and then overgeneralizing the influence of this characteristic on the total person.

The behavioral manifestation of this cognitive process varies but involves differential treatment in the form of victimization, teasing, or coddling; children with disabilities may be relegated to the role of victim or mascot. The child who acquires a disabling injury may already have a well-developed impression about disability and what a child or adult with a disability can or cannot do. Furthermore, the effects of stigma may operate through parents. Mothers' levels of perceived stigma are associated with the amount of contact their children have with peers. Children of mothers who perceive a high degree of stigma in their environments spend less time with peers (Green, 2003). In effect, if parents are protecting themselves from negative interactions with others, the results can be less social contact and support for themselves and their children.

Children report preferences for playmates without disabilities when presented with hypothetical situations regarding interactions with children with disabilities, such as using crutches or wheelchairs, or having a facial cleft (Nabors & Keyes, 1997). However, social preferences are dependent upon the type of disability and type of hypothetical play task. Harper (1999), for example, found that children in wheelchairs are less frequently chosen for activities that involve physical activity. Conflicting findings were reported by Nabors and Larson (2002), who conducted a study in which they presented children with line drawings of typically developing children and children in wheelchairs, along with a script that described either the child's physical condition or his or her abilities and interests. Contrary to the investigators' hypotheses, the study participants did not indicate a preference for the pictures of children who were not using wheelchairs. These inconsistencies suggest the need to move beyond the use of hypothetical scenarios to *in vivo* research methods that provide an assessment of actual rather than hypothetical perceptions and social behavior.

Social Information Processing and Social Competence

Studies of child characteristics that predict social functioning include an extensive literature on social information processing (SIP). Measures of SIP have been shown to predict interpersonal behavior and social status among children who do not have neurodevelopmental conditions. For example, children with aggressive conduct tend to generate aggressive solutions to social problems (Dodge, Laird, Lochman, & Zelli, 2002). SIP models have placed increasing emphasis on the effects of underlying cognitive factors such as processing speed, attention, and memory on development of SIP skills (e.g., (Crick & Dodge, 1994; Wallander & Hubert, 1987).

To the extent that the components of SIP differ in cognitive demands or underlying mechanisms, there may be differing effects of specific cognitive impairments on social problem solving. Using steps from the Crick and Dodge (1994) model of SIP by way of example, encoding social cues may be adversely affected by impairments in aspects of attention or visuoperceptual functions. Selecting a goal for social behavioral response could be dependent upon aspects of memory, causal analysis, and inferential abilities. Learned passivity associated with childhood disability may have its most detrimental effect on goal selection. Specifically, diminished sense of self-efficacy may affect the types of goals formulated for a social scenario. On the other hand, deficits in key domains such as executive functions may have adverse effects on multiple aspects of social cognition and behavior.

Initial studies of SIP in children with neurodevelopmental conditions provide qualified support for the applicability of current models. Children with neurodevelopmental conditions generate less assertive solutions and choose lower level strategies for solving social problems (Dixon & Warschausky, 2004; Janusz et al., 2002; Warschausky, Argento, & Hurvitz, 2003; Warschausky et al., 1997). The few studies that have examined social problem solving (SPS) as a predictor of social functioning have suggested complex associations between multidimensional social cognitions and different aspects of social functioning (Janusz et al., 2002). In a recent study of children who sustained traumatic brain injury (TBI), Yeates and colleagues (2004) showed that executive functions and pragmatic language predict social outcomes, with little evidence that SPS mediates those influences. Recent findings have highlighted the complexities of the nature of pragmatic impairments associated with TBI (Dennis, Purvis, Barnes, Wilkinson, & Winner, 2001; Turkstra, McDonald, & De Pompei, 2001).

The evidence of risk for passivity in children with neurodeveopmental conditions suggests reciprocal interactions between the person with a disability and his or her social environment, as illustrated in Figure 13.2.

In this model, children with disabilities, particularly those with neurological impairment, have difficulty generating or selecting assertive strategies to solve social dilemmas (e.g., entering an ongoing peer activity). The combination of a passive approach to social situations in addition to social stigma often results in fewer social contacts for children with disabilities. There is some evidence that, compared to their typically developing peers, children with congenital neurodevelopmental conditions have fewer friends and less contact with peers (Dixon & Warschausky, 2004). Interestingly, self-reported size of social networks in children with TBI does not differ from those of noninjured peers (Bohnert et al., 1997). Lack of social interactions would diminishes the opportunity to hone social skills such as assertiveness, which, when combined with peer stigmatization, could contribute to relative social isolation.

INTERVENTION STRATEGIES

There is a paucity of studies that examine intervention strategies for facilitating the social integration of children with physical disabilities in general, and neurodevelopmental disorders specifically. Treatment approaches have focused on intervening at the level of the child with the disability, for example, by teaching prosocial skills such as assertive communication, or addressing behaviors that impede interaction with peers. Other types of interventions address the perceptions and behaviors of peers. Unfortunately, few programs are evidence-based.

Children with neurodevelopmental conditions and physical impairments are at high risk for specific neuropsychological impairments. Social intervention programs may be inappropriate for children with neurodevelopmental disorders, because most programs are designed for persons with

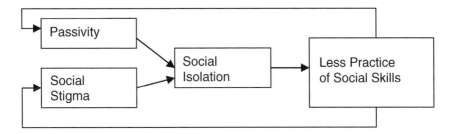

FIGURE 13.2. Person–environment interactions and social functioning.

presumed intact cognition or those with significant cognitive impairment, such as mental retardation (Warschausky, Kewman, & Kay, 1999). Programs tailored to meet the specific needs of children with neurodevelopmental disorders would present needed content in a "cognitively accessible" manner (e.g., utilizing instructional techniques that address executive dysfunction, processing speed, or memory impairments).

Social Skills Interventions

Social skills programs, delivered in groups or individually, are a popular method of intervening with children who exhibit problematic social behaviors, typically targeting those on either end of the aggression–withdrawal continuum. These interventions often focus on teaching various aspects of problem solving and communication, utilizing methods such as coaching, modeling, and/or reinforcement. Meta-analytic and review studies of social skills interventions suggest that, overall, programs are moderately effective in improving outcomes such as social competence (Moote, Smyth, & Wodarski, 1999; Schneider, 1992). Major shortcomings of social skills or social competence training programs are the lack of maintenance and generalization of skills. While children frequently exhibit social gains during the intervention, they often do not maintain those gains, nor are they able to generalize skills from the programs to everyday situations.

Studies that focus specifically on social skills outcomes for children with physical disabilities are scarce. Typically, the studies that do exist are uncontrolled multiple- or single-case designs (Kehle, Clark, & Jenson, 1996). Similar to the research on social skills programs with typically developing children, results have shown improvements in social functioning, suggesting that social skills programs designed specifically for children with disabilities have the potential to improve social functioning, though maintenance of skills after the program ends remains a concern (King et al., 1997). Barakat, Kunin-Batson, and Kazak (2003) evaluated the effectiveness of a manual-based social skills training group intervention for children treated for brain tumors. Their results indicated improvement in child- and parent-reported social competence from baseline to 9 months after intervention. The authors recommend that future studies employ a randomized design, using a sample size with sufficient power to detect treatment effects. In contrast, Kim (2003) conducted a study of assertiveness training with visually impaired children and adolescents using a manual-based program and randomized controlled design. Upon completion of the training, there were no differences in assertiveness scores between those who received the training and a comparison group. The negative findings may have stemmed, at least in part, from limited statistical power. No long-term follow-up assessment was conducted.

The study of social skills interventions traditionally has focused on identifying the best approach or technique (e.g., cognitive-behavioral vs. social learning). Yet recent evidence suggests that the most effective programs are multimodal or use a combination of approaches. In order to address the specific needs of children with physical disabilities, many of whom have concomitant cognitive impairments, we need to move to the evaluation of specific techniques within general approaches that are most appropriate for children with disabilities. The unique combination of physical and cognitive impairments affects the core social skills curriculum and requires specific maintenance and generalization strategies applied in a child's natural environment (King et al., 1997).

Classroom Interventions

Given the amount of time that children are in school, this milieu has great potential to affect social functioning. Teachers are critical facilitators for both curricular and social inclusion. In inclusive classrooms, which consist of children with and without disabilities, children with disabilities often are passive recipients of social gestures rather than initiators (Evans, Salisbury, Palombaro, Berryman, & Hollywood, 1992; Hanline, 1993). Evans and colleagues (1992) found that physically healthy students related to the students with disabilities in a parental manner (i.e., providing assistance, reprimanding) rather than in a reciprocal friendship manner. The interactions between the students with and without disabilities were positive, and the students with disabilities were included, per se, but the social roles ascribed to them were restricted. True inclusion means that the child with a disability has access to the full range of social roles in his or her social environment.

Snell and Janney (2000) have compiled a bevy of suggestions for facilitating social inclusion of students with disabilities in the classroom. While not specific to children with physical impairments, these recommendations emphasize the importance of teachers in the inclusion process and highlight the need for a multilevel approach, implemented at classroom and broader school environment levels. The foci of these interventions are the skills of the child with the disability, as well as the attitudes and perceptions of their peers. Recommendations include direct adult facilitation of interactions, the establishment of peer support, including instructional pairings or groups, and social skills instruction. Again, many of these approaches are not evidence-based, so it is not clear how to match specific child characteristics with interventions. It is perhaps for this reason that research findings support the simultaneous use of several techniques.

Children without disabilities benefit from support in interacting with their peers with disabilities. Participation in programs aimed at promoting familiarity and inclusion leads to acceptance by peers. Favazza, LaRoe, and Odom (1999) described a classroom-based intervention focused on the typically developing peers of children with disabilities. This intervention consisted of storytime and discussion involving books about children with disabilities, structured play with children with disabilities, and storytime and discussion at home with the students' families. A study of this intervention revealed that children who had experiences with disability, either through the stories or direct play, had higher levels of acceptance of their peers with disabilities, while the acceptance ratings of children who did not have such exposure remained constant (Favazza, Phillipsen, & Kumar, 2000).

Practices such as teacher modeling of appropriate interactions for all students and utilizing classwide peer tutoring are also effective in increasing social interactions between children with and without disabilities (Salisbury, Galluccu, Palombaro, & Peck, 1995). Hunt, Alwell, Farron-Davis, and Goetz (1996) found that a program designed to promote inclusion was successful in increasing the occurrence of reciprocal interactions between children with and without disabilities. Typically developing children who have had more personal contact with children with disabilities report more positive preferences for playmates with disabilities. In addition, children are more supportive when they have been educated about the particular illness–injury of their classmate (Chekryn, Deegan, & Reid, 1986) and demonstrate more positive behavioral intentions toward children with disabilities when they are exposed to programs that promote acceptance (Morgan, Bieberich, Walker, & Schwerdtfeger, 1998). These results support the concept that inclusion of children with physical disabilities in general education settings must be accompanied by teacher support.

Classroom-based programs may utilize a team approach, such as the Building Friendships program, that involves collaboration between the child, his or her parent, school staff, and peers. The team creates and implements an action plan that includes specific social goals and strategies (Cooley, Glang, & Voss, 1997). Goals and strategies are identified, and an action plan is developed and implemented. The team meets periodically throughout the intervention, and the action plan is reviewed and modified as necessary. The Building Friendships program has been studied with small samples of children with TBI (Glang, Todis, Cooley, Wells, & Voss, 1997; Van Horn, Levine, & Curtis, 1992). The students participating in the program experienced initial increases in social contact, though social gains that resulted from the program were not maintained over time (Glang et al., 1997). This highlights the need for programs that focus on maintenance of skills, as well as creating change in peer attitudes and perceptions. This also points to the need to focus on building relationship quality rather than focusing on quantity of social contact or peers.

Emerging Approaches

Peer Mentoring

Peer mentoring in children and adolescents has been used successfully to improve academic performance (Rohrback, Fantuzzo, Ginsburg-Block, & Miller, 2003), promote social inclusion (Hughes et al., 1999), and teach social skills (Muscott & O'Brien, 1999) in samples of children with and without disabilities. A recent meta-analysis of research studies on mentoring (Dubois, Holloway, Valentine, & Cooper, 2002) and the National Mentoring Partnership's Elements of Effective Practice in Mentoring (2003) provide valuable resources in developing mentoring interventions. Previous results indicate that positive outcomes for children in mentoring programs are predicted by (1) ongoing training for mentors, (2) structured activities for mentor–mentee dyads, (3) clear expectations for frequency of contact between mentors and mentees, (4) parental involvement, and (5) monitoring of overall program implementation.

Community Participation

At Thames Valley Children's Centre (a regional children's rehabilitation centre located in Ontario, Canada), several new programs have been developed using the Life Needs Model of pediatric service delivery as a planning tool, including a self-discovery and transition assistance program for adolescents and young adults (Youth En Route) (King et al., 2002; King, Tucker, Baldwin, & LaPorta, 2004). This program reflects an ecological–experiential approach to transition planning for youth with disabilities (King, Baldwin, Currie, & Evans, 2004).

Youth En Route is an individualized program that prepares and supports youth in transitioning into their communities after high school. The program embodies the Life Needs Model's goal of enabling and supporting youth to participate in their communities. The program has a broad perspective and reflects the belief that opportunities for participation lead to other outcomes, such as enhanced skills and successful engagement in desired adult roles. The program reflects the view that it is important to provide youth with employment opportunities, preparation for postsecondary education, and leisure and recreation opportunities. The services encompassed in this program support self-discovery, skills development, and community experiences. Youth are supported, through a coaching model, to develop their own goals and life plans, and family and other community members are supported to facilitate the implementation of these goals. Supports are provided to families, including information on youth development and on the spectrum of available community supports and services. Parent-to-parent sharing opportunities also are offered. An initial evaluation study measured clients' self-determination skills, sense of autonomy, and community participation prior to and 1 year following their initiation into the program, and found significant pre–post differences in all areas (Evans, Baldwin, & McDougall, 2004a, 2004b).

Parent-Focused Interventions

Our recent work has examined the social facilitation methods employed by parents of children with and without disabilities (Dixon & Warschausky, 2004). Findings indicate that children with disabilities had lower social functioning than the typically developing control group. Parents of both groups reported similar usage of structured social situations for their children, such as taking their children to public places (e.g., parks) or enrolling them in groups or clubs (e.g., Scouts). Where the two groups differ is in the extent to which they arranged informal or unstructured social situations for their children, with parents of typically developing children utilizing this method more than parents of children with disabilities. It is difficult to arrange informal contact when children do not have many close friends. Furthermore, parents may be hesitant to allow their children with physical disabilities to go to a friend's home and be in the care of a parent who does not understand their care needs. These findings may have important implications for interventions that focus on parenting. Parents should be encouraged and assisted in broadening social activities to include informal, unstructured contact with peers whenever possible.

CONCLUSIONS AND FUTURE DIRECTIONS

Most of the research on social interventions has been developed and conducted using samples of typically developing children. The majority of these programs report initial success but variability in maintenance of gains over time. The social interactions that naturally occur as part of an intervention delivered in group format are beneficial, even though the intervention may not specifically address the individual needs of each group member. There is at least as much, if not more, variability in needs within groups of children with physical disabilities as there is among typically developing children. That said, interventions could target common psychological needs of children with physical disabilities, including addressing social isolation, stigma, and passivity, as well as specific social problem-solving difficulties associated in part with neuropsychological status. Multimodal interventions both to develop social skills and to address stigmatization by changing perceptions of peers hold promise for improving the social functioning of children with disabilities. The clinician who is interested in creating or administering social skills interventions is encouraged to include a focus on assertiveness skills training, individualized to meet the specific needs of each participant. Furthermore, a team approach is likely to tap into the strengths and resources of the various levels of influence on social functioning (i.e., the child, and his or her home, school, and community environments). Evaluation of these interventions, using well-controlled longitudinal designs, will help tease out specific predictors and directions of influence.

ACKNOWLEDGMENTS

Completion of this chapter was supported by U.S. Department of Education grants, including Office of Special Education Programs model demonstration project (No. H324M020077), field-initiated project (No. H324C0020026), and initial career award (No. H324N010010), and by a National Institute on Disability and Rehabilitation field-initiated project award (No. H133G000038).

REFERENCES

Barakat, L. P., Kunin-Batson, A., & Kazak, A. E. (2003). Child health psychology. In A. M. Nezu & C. M. Nezu (Eds.), *Handbook of psychology: Health psychology* (Vol. 9, pp. 439–464). New York: Wiley.

Bell, S. K., & Morgan, S. B. (2000). Children's attitude and behavioral intentions toward a peer presented as obese: Does a medical explanation for the obesity make a difference? *Journal of Pediatric Psychology, 25*, 137–145.

Bohnert, A. M., Parker, J. G., & Warschausky, S. A. (1997). Friendship and social adjustment of children following a traumatic brain injury: An exploratory investigation. *Developmental Neuropsychology, 13*, 477–486.

Brown, M., & Gordon, W. (1987). Impact of impairment on activity patterns of children. *Archives of Physical Medicine and Rehabilitation, 68*, 828–832.
Chekryn, J., Deegan, M., & Reid, J. (1986). Normalizing the return to school of the child with cancer. *Journal of the Association of Pediatric Oncology Nurses, 3*, 20–24, 34.
Cooley, E. A., Glang, A., & Voss, J. (1997). Helping children with ABI build friendships. In A. Glang, G. H. S. Singer, & B. Todis (Eds.), *Students with acquired brain injury: The school's response* (pp. 255–275). Baltimore: Brookes.
Crick, N. R., & Dodge, K. A. (1994). A review and reformulation of social information-processing mechanisms in children's social adjustment. *Psychological Bulletin, 115*, 74–101.
Dennis, M., Purvis, K., Barnes, M. A., Wilkinson, M., & Winner, E. (2001). Understanding literal truth, ironic criticism and deceptive praise following childhood head injury. *Brain and Language, 78*, 1–16.
Dixon, P., & Warschausky, S. (2004). *Parent facilitation of social integration for children with neurological conditions.* Paper presented at the American Psychological Association, Honolulu, HI.
Dodge, K. A., Laird, R., Lochman, J. E., & Zelli, A. (2002). Multidimensional latent-construct analysis of children's social information processing patterns: Correlations with aggressive behavior problems. *Psychological Assessment, 14*, 60–73.
Dubois, D. L., Holloway, B. E., Valentine, J. C., & Cooper, H. (2002). Effectiveness of mentoring programs for youth: A meta-analytic review. *American Journal of Community Psychology, 30*, 157–197.
Evans, J., Baldwin, P., & McDougall, J. (2004a). *An evaluation study of the Youth En Route Program.* Paper presented at the Ontario Association of Children's Rehabilitation Services, Richmond Hill, Ontario, Canada.
Evans, J., Baldwin, P., & McDougall, J. (2004b). *Youth En Route: An evaluation of an individualized transition program.* Manuscript submitted for publication.
Evans, I. M., Salisbury, C. L., Palombaro, M. M., Berryman, J., & Hollywood, T. M. (1992). Peer interactions and social acceptance of elementary-age children with severe disabilities in an inclusive school. *Journal of the Association for Persons with Severe Handicaps, 17*, 205–212.
Favazza, P. C., LaRoe, J., & Odom, S. L. (1999). *Special friends: A manual for creating accepting environments.* Boulder, CO: Roots and Wings.
Favazza, P. C., Phillipsen, L., & Kumar, P. (2000). Measuring and promoting acceptance of young children with disabilities. *Exceptional Children, 66*, 491–508.
Finset, A., Dyrnes, S., Krogstad, J. M., & Berstad, J. (1995). Self-reported social networks and interpersonal support 2 years after severe traumatic brain injury. *Brain Injury, 2*, 141–150.
Galski, T., Tompkins, C., & Johnston, M. V. (1998). Competence in discourse as a measure of social integration and quality of life in persons with traumatic brain injury. *Brain Injury, 12*, 769–782.
Glang, A., Todis, B., Cooley, E., Wells, J., & Voss, J. (1997). Building social networks for children and adolescents with traumatic brain injury: A school based intervention. *Journal of Head Trauma Rehabilitation, 12*, 32–47.
Green, S. E. (2003). "What do you mean 'what's wrong with her?' ": Stigma and the

lives of families of children with disabilities. *Social Science and Medicine, 57*, 1361–1374.

Hammal, D., Jarvis, S. N., & Colver, A. F. (2004). Participation of children with cerebral palsy is influenced by where they live. *Developmental Medicine and Child Neurology, 46*, 292–298.

Hanline, M. F. (1993). Inclusion of preschoolers with profound disabilities: An analysis of children's interactions. *Journal of the Association for Persons with Severe Handicaps, 18*, 28–35.

Harper, D. C. (1999). Presidential address: Social psychology of difference: Stigma, spread and stereotypes in childhood. *Rehabilitation Psychology, 44*, 131–144.

Hughes, C., Guth, C., Hall, S., Presley, J., Dye, M., & Byers, C. (1999). "They are my best friends": Peer buddies promote inclusion in high school. *Teaching Exceptional Children, 31*, 32–37.

Hunt, P., Alwell, M., Farron-Davis, F., & Goetz, L. (1996). Creating socially supportive environments for fully included students who experience multiple disabilities. *Journal of the Association for Persons with Severe Handicaps, 21*, 53–71.

Janusz, J. A., Kirkwood, M. W., Yeates, K. O., & Taylor, H. G. (2002). Social problem-solving skills in children with traumatic brain injury: Long-term outcomes and prediction of social competence. *Child Neuropsychology, 8*, 170–194.

Kehle, T. J., Clark, E., & Jenson, W. R. (1996). Interventions for students with traumatic brain injury: Managing behavioral disturbances. *Journal of Learning Disabilities, 29*, 633–642.

Kim, Y.-I. (2003). The effects of assertiveness training on enhancing the social skills of adolescents with visual impairments. *Journal of Visual Impairment and Blindness, 97*, 285–297.

King, G., Tucker, M. A., Baldwin, P., & LaPorta, J. (2004). *Bringing the Life Needs Model to life: Implementing a service delivery model for pediatric rehabilitation.* Manuscript submitted for publication.

King, G., Tucker, M. A., Baldwin, P., Lowry, K., LaPorta, J., & Martens, L. (2002). A Life Needs Model of pediatric service delivery: Services to support community participation and quality of life for children and youth with disabilities. *Physical and Occupational Therapy in Pediatrics, 22*, 53–77.

King, G. A., Baldwin, P. J., Currie, M., & Evans, J. (2004). Planning successful transitions from school to adult roles for youth with disabilities. *Children's Health Care, 34*(3), 195–216.

King, G. A., Law, M., King, S., Rosenbaum, P., Kertoy, M., & Young, N. (2003). A conceptual model of the factors affecting the recreation and leisure participation of children with disabilities. *Physical and Occupational Therapy in Pediatrics, 23*, 63–90.

King, G. A., Specht, J. A., Schultz, I., Warr-Leeper, G., Redekop, W., & Risebrough, N. (1997). Social skills training for withdrawn unpopular children with physical disabilities: A preliminary evaluation. *Rehabilitation Psychology, 42*, 47–60.

Mancini, M. C., Coster, W. J., Trombly, C. A., & Heeren, T. C. (2000). Predicting elementary school participation in children with disabilities. *Archives of Physical Medicine and Rehabilitation, 81*, 339–347.

Meijer, S. A., Sinnema, G., Bijstra, J. O., Mellenbergh, G. J., & Wolters, W. H. G.

(2000). Social functioning in children with a chronic illness. *Journal of Child Psychology and Psychiatry, 41*, 309–317.

Moote, G. T., Smyth, N. J., & Wodarski, J. S. (1999). Special skills training with youth in school settings: A review. *Research on Social Work Practice, 9*, 427–465.

Morgan, S. B., Bieberich, A. A., Walker, M., & Schwerdtfeger, H. (1998). Children's willingness to share activities with a physically handicapped peer: Am I more willing than my classmate? *Journal of Pediatric Psychology, 23*, 367–375.

Muscott, H. S., & O'Brien, S. T. (1999). Teaching character education to students with behavioral and learning disabilities through mentoring relationships. *Education and Treatment of Children, 22*, 373–390.

Nabors, L., & Keyes, L. (1997). Brief report: Preschoolers' social preferences for interacting with peers with physical differences. *Journal of Pediatric Psychology, 22*, 113–122.

Nabors, L., & Larson, E. R. (2002). The effects of brief interventions on children's playmate preferences for a child sitting in a wheelchair. *Journal of Developmental and Physical Disabilities, 14*, 403–413.

National Mentoring Partnership. (2003). *Elements of effective practice*. Alexandria, VA: Author.

Office of Special Education Programs. (2002). *Twenty-Fourth Annual Report to Congress on the implementation of the Individuals with Disabilities Education Act*. Washington, DC: U.S. Department of Education, Office of Special Education Programs.

Patterson, J., & Blum, R. (1996). Risk and resilience among children and youth with disabilities. *Archives of Pediatric and Adolescent Medicine, 150*, 692–698.

Rohrback, C., Fantuzzo, J., Ginsburg-Block, M., & Miller, T. (2003). Peer-assisted learning interventions with elementary school students: A meta-analytic review. *Journal of Educational Psychology, 95*, 240–257.

Salisbury, C. L., Galluccu, C., Palombaro, M. M., & Peck, C. A. (1995). Strategies that promote social relations among elementary students with and without severe disabilities in inclusive schools. *Exceptional Children, 62*, 125–137.

Schneider, B. (1992). Didactic methods for enhancing children's peer relations: A quantitative review. *Clinical Psychology Review, 12*, 363–382.

Schuman, W. B., & La Greca, A. M. (1999). Social correlates of chronic illness. In R. T. Brown (Ed.), *Cognitive aspects of chronic illness in children* (pp. 289–311). New York: Guilford Press.

Snell, M. E., & Janney, R. (2000). *Social relationships and peer support*. Baltimore: Brookes.

Turkstra, L. S., McDonald, S., & De Pompei, R. (2001). Social information processing in adolescents: Data from normally developing adolescents and preliminary data from their peers with traumatic brain injury. *Journal of Head Trauma Rehabilitation, 16*, 469–483.

Van Horn, K. R., Levine, M. J., & Curtis, C. L. (1992). Developmental levels of social cognition in head injured patients. *Brain Injury, 6*, 15–28.

Wallander, J. L., & Hubert, N. C. (1987). Peer social dysfunction in children with developmental disabilities: Empirical basis and a conceptual model. *Clinical Psychology Review, 7*, 203–221.

Warschausky, S., Argento, A. G., & Hurvitz, E. B. M. (2003). Neuropsychological status and social problem-solving in children with congenital or acquired brain dysfunction. *Rehabilitation Psychology, 48*, 250–254.

Warschausky, S., Cohen, E., Parker, J. G., Levendosky, A., & Okun, A. (1997). Social problem solving skills of children with traumatic brain injury. *Pediatric Rehabilitation, 1*, 77–81.

Warschausky, S., Kewman, D. G., & Kay, J. B. (1999). Empirically supported psychological and behavioral therapies for children with THI. *Journal of Head Trauma Rehabilitation, 14*, 373–383.

Yeates, K. O., Swift, E., Taylor, H. G., Wade, S. L., Drotar, D., Stancin, T., et al. (2004). Short- and long-term social outcomes following pediatric traumatic brain injury. *Journal of the International Neuropsychological Society, 10*, 412–426.

Yude, C., Goodman, R., & McConachie, H. (1998). Peer problems of children with hemiplegia in mainstream primary schools. *Journal of Child Psychology and Psychiatry, 39*, 533–541.

14

Empirically Based Interventions for Children with Autism

ELAINE CLARK
LORA TUESDAY-HEATHFIELD
DANIEL OLYMPIA
WILLIAM R. JENSON

Data presented in the 23rd Report to Congress in 2000 showed a 189% increase in the number of individuals diagnosed with autism between 1994 and 2000, and recent prevalence figures put the rate at 6 out of 1,000 individuals for the full autistic spectrum, and 3.4 out of 1,000 for individuals whose functioning is more limited, for example, those who have severe intellectual impairments (Yeargin-Allsopp et al., 2003). A sizable literature has been amassed over the past 20 or more years about autism spectrum disorders (ASDs), including literature that pertains to the efficacy of treatments. However, there is still a lot to be learned about the most effective ways to treat the core symptoms of autism and the associated problems. Research on long-term outcomes continues to show that individuals with autism, even those at the higher end of the spectrum, do very poorly as adults. In fact, the vast majority do not have academic, vocational, or social successes. As adults, these individuals are not working regular paying jobs, are not living on their own, and report having few or no friends. Several of the core features of autism that prevent these individuals from having the quality of life they deserve include social and communication impairments, and unusual behaviors, such as inflexible adherence to routines, rituals, and stereotypies (Howlin, Goode, Hutton, & Rutter, 2004).

The complex nature of the disorder will likely require complex, multiple-treatment modalities that have a solid research base. Unfortunately, many of the interventions that are used today do not have this level of support (e.g., TEACCH [Treatment and Education of Autistic and Related Communication Handicapped Children], naturalistic behavior analytic methods, drug therapies such as risperidone), or have little or no support (e.g., vitamin B, sensory integration therapy, patterning, Fast ForWord, secretin, and facilitated communication) (Green, 2004). The only intervention for which there has been substantial scientific evidence of effectiveness is intensive, early applied behavioral analysis (ABA; e.g., Anderson & Romanczyk, 1999; Eikeseth, Smith, Jahr, & Eldevik, 2002; Green, 1996a). Although researchers have found that ABA can be extremely effective in helping children to improve their behaviors, increase their social interactions, and attain academic success (e.g., placement in regular classrooms), the studies to date indicate that the treatment must be implemented early (e.g., before age 5, and preferably by age 2 or 3) and must be intensive, that is, at least 27 hours a week for 2 years (Green, 1996a; Smith, Groen, & Wynn, 2000). Unfortunately, many children with ASD are not identified when they are 2 or 3 years of age, and there are relatively few ABA-trained professionals to provide the services. Many researchers, however, including Green (1996b), argue that only interventions that have been scientifically validated by multiple investigators (e.g., ABA) should be used. This, however, becomes challenging given the multifaceted nature of many interventions and the multiple factors that need to be considered when implementing treatments, including the specific characteristics of the child (e.g., cognitive and communication ability), the setting in which the treatment is to be implemented, and the skills of the interventionist. To this end, it is critical that professionals learn as much as possible about a variety of interventions, and what research support they have received.

In the meantime, it is critical that professionals not deprive children of receiving the interventions that have been shown to be effective, such as ABA, by using poorly (or un-) supported treatments. Professionals must be knowledgeable about various treatment options and the research base that supports these, in order to help educate parents and educators about ways to discriminate between interventions that are empirically validated and those that are not (Freeman, 1997; Rogers, 1998). Our intent in this chapter is to provide professionals with some of this information. Readers should keep in mind, however, that the literature on intervention techniques for autism is extensive and ranges from anecdotal reports and case studies to well-controlled empirical investigations. Researchers interested in the efficacy of interventions for ASD often focus their studies on social interaction or functional communication skills deficits, or behavioral excesses such as aggression, self-injury, and perseverative behaviors. What follows is a summary of intervention strategies that have empirical support and show promise in ameliorating some of these disabling effects.

OVERVIEW OF SOCIAL SKILLS DEFICITS AND TREATMENTS

Children with ASD typically have delays, deficits, or atypical characteristics in their social relationships and social interactions with others. Even children with high-functioning autism face challenges in processing the social cues necessary for appropriate interactions and have difficulty forming and maintaining friendships. These atypical social skills are considered the classic feature of autism across the entire spectrum and lifespan (Sigman, 1994). From a young age, children with autism may avoid eye contact, may not actively seek physical comfort from caregivers, and may show delays in joint attention, sharing of emotions, and reciprocal social play. Overall, the social interactions of children with ASD are characterized by fewer social initiations, fewer responses to the initiations of others, and shorter bursts of interaction (McConnell, 2002). These are serious concerns given the research demonstrating that a lack of successful social interaction skills can inhibit the development of intelligence, language, and other related skills considered critical to normal childhood development (Garrison-Harrell & Kamps, 1997). Social interaction deficits can also lead to social isolation, mental health problems, and difficulty maintaining employment and living independently.

Researchers have devoted substantial efforts toward the design and evaluation of interventions that encourage the development of social competencies among children with autism. Successful interventions range from direct social skills training to collateral improvements in social relatedness as a result of pharmacological treatment, such as tetrahydrobiopterin (Fernell et al., 1997) and naltrexone (Williams, Allard, Sears, Dalrymple, & Bloom, 2001). Based in part on a recent meta-analysis (Miller, 2005), interventions demonstrating significant improvements in reciprocal social interaction skills for individuals with ASD are peer-mediated and related skills interventions, with mixed results for structured environment interventions and direct social skills instruction (see Table 14.1).

Peer-Mediated Interventions

Peer-mediated interventions target the typically developing peers of children with ASD by increasing peers' social initiations and interactions, and using peer tutoring. Peer-mediated interventions have shown promising and robust outcomes across a wide range of social behaviors. For example, peer-mediated interventions have been used to increase communicative ex-

TABLE 14.1. Empirically Supported Interventions for Children with Autism

	Social interaction skill deficits
Peer-mediated interventions	• Prompt, reinforce peers to initiate (e.g., playing, asking questions) or respond to target child's initiations. • Pair target child with peer tutor for academic instruction. • Pair peer buddy with target child.
Related skills interventions	• Teach communication or language skills (e.g., picture activity schedule, asking questions). • Teach specific play skills (e.g., game or activity).
Structured environment interventions	• Increase preferred activities or predictability of activities. • Introduce structure to activities (e.g., play groups or objects).
Direct skills instruction	• Pivotal response training. • Prompt, reinforce specific social skill (e.g., social problem solving). • Group social skills training or social scripts. • Self-monitoring of social behaviors (e.g., responding).
	Functional communication skill deficits
ABA interventions	• Discrete trial training. • Reinforce communication attempts. • Direct instruction of communication behavior.
Functional equivalence training	• Teach, reinforce functional communication skill (verbal or nonverbal) that serves same function as problematic behavior.
Structured environment interventions	• Pivotal response training. • Visual activity schedules.
Alternative communication interventions	• Symbolic communication systems (e.g., Picture Exchange Communication Systems [PECS]). • Sign language and total communication training. • Electronic speech output devices (e.g., Voice Output Communication Aids).
	Aggression, self-injury, self-stimulatory behaviors
Positive behavioral interventions	• Shaping, extinction, and antecedent control. • High-probability demands (behavioral momentum). • Positive attention, tangibles, and edibles. • Differential reinforcement of other behavior or alternative behavior.

(*continued*)

TABLE 14.1. (*continued*)

Communication interventions	• Simple verbal directives (e.g., "stop"). • Teach appropriate, alternative communicative behavior (e.g., PECS). • Pivotal response training.
Aversive interventions	• Time-out, noxious substance. • Response cost, overcorrection. • Movement suppression "time-out."

changes (Goldstein & Ferrell, 1987), reciprocal interactions (McGee, Almeida, Sulzer-Azaroff, & Feldman, 1992), and rates of social interaction (Goldstein, Kaczmarek, Pennington, & Shafer, 1992). Odom et al. (1999) provided evidence of improved social interactions of children with disabilities, including those with ASD, and longer maintenance of treatment gains compared to other treatments. In addition, peer-mediated interventions can reduce unwanted challenging behaviors as a function of increased social interactions (Lee & Odom, 1996).

Although peer-mediated interventions have demonstrated strong treatment effects across a number of studies, intervention strategies, and children, it is critical that these interventions focus on maintenance and generalization of treatment effects to untrained peers and across environments. Despite positive results for children with ASD, peer-mediated interventions typically focus on improving the social responding of children with ASD to their peers' initiations, with limited evidence of corresponding increases in the social initiations of children with ASD, which minimizes the potential for treatment generalization and maintenance.

Related Skills Interventions

Increases in social interaction have been demonstrated as a result of training in related but dissimilar skills, such as interventions designed to enhance play skills (Thorp, Stahmer, & Schreibman, 1995). A corresponding line of research suggests that matching games and activities to the perseverative behaviors of children with autism results in increased rates of social interaction (Baker, Koegel, & Koegel, 1998). Collateral increases in social interaction also have been observed with language interventions, such as teaching children with ASD to ask questions (Koegel, Camarata, Valdez-Menchaca, & Koegel, 1998). Related skills interventions seem to result in increased social interactions by maximizing the contact between children with autism and their more socially competent peers, thereby increasing social opportunities, enhancing the likelihood of social development, and possibly increasing the reinforcement value of social interactions with peers. Related skills interventions, especially those aimed at generalized or pretend play, however, are more often included as components of a more comprehensive intervention, not a stand-alone treatment (McConnell, 2002).

Structured Environment Interventions

The literature suggests a relationship between increasing the structure of environments and the social interaction skills of children with ASD. These interventions include modifying the structure of an activity, an individual's daily schedule, or a child's exposure to peer groups. In one of the more prevalent environmental interventions, pivotal response training, the child with autism is taught a "pivotal" or critical social skill, such as initiating, that can have a broad impact on social skills development (e.g., Koegel & Frea, 1993). Greater social interaction has been found to occur when activities are highly structured (DeKlyen & Odom, 1989), and when activities and materials are predictable (Ferrara & Hill, 1980). Although increasing a child's access to developmentally integrated play groups results in increased initiations by peers, corresponding increases in reciprocal social interaction by children with ASD have not been demonstrated (Myles, Simpson, Ormsbee, & Erickson, 1993). Increasing access to integrated play groups following direct social skills instruction or peer-mediated social skills interventions, however, has been shown to promote the maintenance and generalization of social interaction skills (Strain & Schwartz, 2001). Unfortunately, despite positive findings, the effects of structured environment interventions alone are inconsistent across studies, specific strategies, and children, but have been successfully incorporated into more comprehensive interventions. Consequently, structured environment interventions are viewed as requisite, but not sufficient, in promoting social interaction in children with ASD (McConnell, 2002).

Direct Social Skills Instruction Interventions

Interventions designed specifically to enhance social skills through direct instruction and/or reinforcement procedures include instructional strategies to improve social problem solving, direct teaching of specific social skills, adult-mediated prompting, reinforcement procedures that "prime" social responses (e.g., behavioral momentum), and self-monitoring. A recent review of research suggests that children with ASD can be trained to initiate and maintain social interactions, and that these skills generalize to interactions with siblings in the home environment (Pollard, 1998). However, Pollard concludes that direct social skills interventions are often limited in that the focus is on prerequisite skills, such as initiations, rather than on sustaining complex social interactions. McConnell (2002) suggests that because social interactions do not have a strong reinforcement value for children with ASD, the long-range effectiveness of these interventions may be limited without the addition of explicit generalization strategies and/or external reinforcers. For example, more comprehensive interventions that combine direct social skills training and reinforcement during free play (e.g., Gonzalez-Lopez & Kamps, 1997) have resulted in positive social skills gains for children with ASD. However, the identification of the key intervention components to combine with direct social skills training to ensure their success have not yet been delineated.

OVERVIEW OF COMMUNICATION DEFICITS AND TREATMENTS

Functional communication skills are among of the strongest predictors of developmental outcome for children with ASD (Venter, Lord, & Schopler, 1992). In fact, a number of studies have found that limited speech skills by the age 5 or so are strongly predictive of a poor outcome in adulthood (Howlin et al., 2004). Many children with autism never acquire expressive language, and those who do often lack the speech necessary for effective communication (e.g., difficulty with pragmatics and use of language within a social context) (Grossman, Carter, & Volkmar, 1997). Children with high-functioning autism usually develop speech at a typical age-appropriate rate; however, these children often experience communication difficulties due to deficits resulting in literal interpretations of language and inappropriate social comments.

Interventions designed specifically to enhance the communication skills in children with ASD range from targeting nonverbal communicative responses and single-word utterances to complex language interactions (see Table 14.1 for examples). In fact, with intense language interventions, there is evidence that approximately 75–90% of children with ASD can develop expressive speech (Mastergeorge, Rogers, Corbett, & Solomon, 2003). Based on the premise that most children with ASD can learn to speak, many believe that verbal communication training should be the first choice of communication interventions. In fact, the National Research Council (2001) concludes that functional, spontaneous communication should be the primary focus of early education for children with ASD. Treatment strategies designed to enhance the communication skills of children with ASD that have some empirical support include applied behavior analysis, functional equivalence training, structuring environments, and alternative communication strategies (e.g., sign language, symbolic communication, augmentative communication).

ABA Interventions

Applied behavior analysis techniques that focus on increasing the speech and language skills of children with ASD are well known and have considerable empirical support. Lovaas, Newsome, and Hickman (1987) describe these techniques as "discrete trial training," in which the focus is on enhancing oral speech rather than on other forms of communication using discrete teaching trials in which a trainer provides a stimulus, and the child is provided with a consequence based on whether the response is correct or incorrect. Behavioral techniques such as prompting, fading, shaping, chaining, and task analysis are also utilized. The initial goal of training is verbal imitation, with a gradual fading of verbal prompts and training progresses to more complex language skills, such as a social greeting. Discrete trial training has been demonstrated to increase language skills and to improve cognitive ability and behavior (Lovaas et al., 1987). Due to its directive, repetitive teaching style, however, discrete trial training has been criticized as being too dependent on specific adult directives, and language gains fail to generalize across settings (and individuals) (Goldstein, 2002).

Functional Equivalence Training Interventions

Functional equivalence communication training stems from the hypothesis that challenging behaviors serve a communicative function (Carr & Durand, 1985). Individuals with severe disabilities, including those with ASD, often exhibit communication deficits, which thereby limit the amount of control they have over their immediate environments and their day-to-day lives. The goal of functional equivalence training is to teach specific communication skills that serve the same function for the individual as the challenging behaviors. Additionally, this same concept can be applied in a preventive fashion, in that by teaching functional communication skills to individuals with ASD at an early age, the development of challenging behaviors may be prevented. There is considerable empirical support that teaching communication skills that are functionally equivalent results in a reduction of a variety of undesirable behaviors, such as aggression, and self-injury (e.g., Bird, Dores, Moniz, & Robinson, 1989). Additionally, functionally equivalent communication skills typically are taught in the individual's natural environment, which aids in the maintenance and generalization of skills gains.

Structured Environment Interventions

By structuring the learning environment, incidental teaching opportunities are increased in order to enhance communication skills within the natural environments for children with ASD. Interventions based in naturalistic environments have gained increasing support due to the enhanced generalization of communication skills in comparison to discrete trial training. For example, placing a desired toy out of reach may increase the child's motivation to initiate a request for the item (e.g., "car"), thereby providing a teaching opportunity, such as an adult prompting or modeling an expanded communication (e.g., "want car"). Obtaining the desired toy then serves as a natural reinforcer rather than having an adult deliver a social or tangible reinforcer (e.g., sticker) that may be unrelated to the task. Structured environment interventions allow for learning opportunities to be child-initiated rather than relying on adult-led instruction, and also occur within the child's natural routines and environments instead of drill and practice sessions. In pivotal response training, for example, rather than teaching a child to emit a specific communication response, such as labeling, "pivotal" communication skills, such as requesting, that are targeted within the natural environment can be applied across persons and settings.

Another common structured environment intervention used for children with ASD is the use of picture or word schedules designed to increase the predictability and understanding of the sequence of activities at school and at home (Quill, 1997). This visually augmented language input can be either pictorial or text-based, or a combination of the two. The reasoning behind the use of visual schedules is that they capitalize on visual–spatial processing skills, often a strength for children with ASD, while minimizing auditory processing, which is frequently a weakness. Activity schedules are also conducive to teaching individuals to make choices. For example, a selection of picture or text cues that represent different activities can be used to provide a choice, and once the individual indicates a preference, the activity is added to the activity schedule, and the individual engages in the chosen activity (McClannahan & Krantz, 1999). Although these types of structured environment interventions result in communication skills that are more spontaneous and easier to generalize (Delprato, 2001), they rely heavily on spontaneous communication opportunities and the motivation of the child. Therefore, communication skills interventions may first need to begin with discrete trial training for children with ASD who have no or low rates of initiation (Mastergeorge et al., 2003).

Alternative Communication Interventions

Alternative communication interventions include symbolic communication strategies, assistive communication devices, and sign language. All of these interventions are designed to provide a means to communicate functionally nonverbally, particularly for children with ASD who do not develop oral speech. The most well-known symbolic communication strategy used to teach functional communication skills to individuals with ASD is the Picture Exchange Communication System (PECS), which combines the use of picture symbols with ABA methods such as prompting, shaping, and differential reinforcement. PECS teaches children to initiate requests, to respond to questions, and to make comments using black-and-white or color drawings that represent an array of communicative phrases (e.g., "I want"), and items and activities in the environment to encourage self-initiated referential communication (Bondy & Frost, 2001). To date, there are very few empirical studies that demonstrate the efficacy of PECS with children who have autism; however, it is widely used with this population due to its ease of use and prevalent anecdotal reports of rapid skills acquisition and the development of spoken language. Improvements in both spontaneous and imitative speech, along with collateral outcomes, such as increases in social–communicative behavior and decreases in problem behaviors following PECS training, have been empirically supported (e.g., Charlop-Christy, Carpenter, Le, LeBlanc, & Kellet, 2002). Improved research methods, such as well-controlled study designs and replication of studies, are clearly needed in order to determine the overall efficacy of PECS for children with ASD.

Assistive devices designed to augment oral communication include portable electronic speech output devices and symbol boards. These devices are used to supplement a child's existing oral language or as an alternative to using one's voice as the primary modality for communication. Speech output devices produce synthetic or digitized speech when an individual makes a selection from a variety of graphic symbols used to represent a particular message. Research indicates that individuals with ASD can be taught to use such devices when they are matched to the individual's specific needs, such as skill level (Durand, 1999), and there is a match between environmental demands and the abilities of the intended listeners (Mirenda, 2003). It is believed that the immediate voice output of electronic speech devices may serve as a reinforcer to the individual with ASD who is using the device, thereby serving to increase communication skills. Although research to date is limited, studies indicate that assistive devices can be successfully used by children with autism and show some promise as a means to increase communicative interactions.

Using sign language training to increase the communication skills of individuals with ASD has had mixed results in the literature. The principles of operant conditioning are used extensively in the sign language training process; however, the majority of studies include complex treatment packages that make it difficult to attribute gains to any one particular intervention component. Since many children with autism who are nonverbal appear to have difficulty understanding spoken language, signing, which is a more visual form of communication, may be more accessible to them. Parents and teachers can mold or manually prompt a child's hands into appropriate sign configurations. Total communication involves sign language paired with oral speech, and many believe that this pairing will better facilitate natural speech development in children with autism (Goldstein, 2002). Schlosser and Lee (2000) found that approaches such as manual signing were significantly more effective than aided approaches with regard to acquisition of skills, although there was no difference in the generalization or maintenance of skills. Several researchers have found total communication training to be effective in teaching basic receptive and expressive vocabulary skills to children with ASD (Mirenda, 2003). In spite of these results, there is some evidence that sign language and total communication training are contraindicated for children with ASD, due to the prevalence of fine motor difficulties in this population. Sign language and total communication interventions also have inherent limitations, in that respondents are required to know the child's signs in order for communication to be effective, and children with ASD often have difficulty imitating others (Rogers, Bennetto, McEvoy, & Pennington, 1996).

OVERVIEW AND TREATMENTS FOR RESTRICTED AND REPETITIVE BEHAVIORS, SELF-STIMULATORY AND SELF-INJURIOUS BEHAVIORS, AND AGGRESSION

By definition, individuals with ASD display restricted, stereotypical behaviors, that is, encompassing interests that are abnormal in intensity and focus, and inflexible adherence to nonfunctional routines and rituals, motor mannerisms, and persistent preoccupations with parts or sensory qualities of objects (American Psychiatric Association, 2000). These behaviors are observed in individuals at both ends of the autism spectrum, including those with Asperger syndrome (Ozonoff & Rogers, 2003). Self-stimulation, self-injury, and aggression, on the other hand, are reported less often among individuals with high-functioning autism, and found more often among individuals with marked intellectual impairments (Borthwick-Duffy, 1994; Lainhart, 1999; Lewis & Bodfish, 1998) and deficits in communication and social skills (Koegel, Koegel, & Surratt, 1992).

Regardless of where a person is along the spectrum, these behaviors have been found to significantly interfere with learning, social interactions, and vocational outcomes (Howlin et al., 2004; Iwata, Zarcone, Vollmer, & Smith, 1994; Rosenthal-Malek & Mitchell, 1997), and many of these behaviors can increase a person's chance of being hospitalized or institutionalized (Dekeyzer, 2004; Symons, Koppekin, & Wehby, 1999). This is especially true of children who are self-injurious (e.g., who display head banging) and overtly aggressive (e.g., who assault others or destroy property). Dekeyzer (2004), in fact, found that of a sample of children with ASD, 81% who were receiving inpatient psychiatric treatment were admitted for assault and/or property destruction. Self-stimulation, though not necessarily harmful (physically), does interfere with educational and social outcomes, and is seen at very high rates. Malone (1996) believes that nearly all children with ASD engage in some type of repetitive and purposeless (voluntary) motor movements, such as body rocking, hand flapping, or object twirling. These behavioral excesses are thought to be associated with underlying deficits from autism (e.g., poor social judgment, frustration over miscommunications, and lack of awareness of feelings) (e.g., Schopler, 1994; Schopler & Mesibov, 1994); however, the most effective treatments are behavioral (Green, 2004). (See Table 14.1 for examples).

Prior to the 1990s reinforcements and punishments were frequently studied; however, since that time, there have been more investigations of stimulus- and instruction-based interventions (Horner, Carr, Strain, Todd, & Reed, 2002). A review of the research, however, shows that interventions employed still range from extreme aversive procedures or punishments (e.g., movement suppression) (Van Houten & Rolider, 1988) to nonaversive interventions such as choice making and positive behavioral support (Becker-Cottrill, McFarland, & Anderson, 2003). Although psychotropic medication has become increasingly popular in treating these behaviors, especially aggression (Campbell & Cueva, 1995), there is limited support to date for drugs beyond the effects of behavioral interventions. Drug therapies are not discussed in this chapter (see Sweeney, Forness, & Levitt, 1998, for a review of drugs commonly used in autism treatment).

Aversive Interventions

Aversive intervention techniques often include time-out, the use of noxious substances, response cost, overcorrection, and movement suppression time-out. These types of interventions have been shown to be effective in reducing aggressive behaviors displayed by individuals with ASD (see Connelly, 2004); however, the use of aversive interventions is not without controversy. The controversy typically centers on the ethics of using aversive techniques, that is, using methods that might undermine the rights and dignity of an individual. According to two recently conducted meta-analytic studies, however, aversive methods appeared to be the least effective in treating aggression and self-stimulatory behaviors compared to nonaversive techniques (Heathfield et al., 2004).

Nonaversive or Positive Interventions

A number of nonaversive approaches to treating behavioral excesses associated with ASD that have been developed use operant conditioning techniques such as shaping, extinction, manipulating environmental antecedents, using high probability demands, and applying different schedules of positive reinforcement (Lancioni & Hoogeveen, 1990). Positive reinforcements have been found to be particularly effective in treating self-stimulation and aggression (e.g., Heathfield et al., 2004; Houlihan, Jacobson, & Brandon, 1994; Romano & Roll, 2000). These methods include positive attention and edibles (Adelinis, Piazza, & Goh, 2001), choice making (DeLeon, Fisher, Herman, & Crosland, 2000; Peck-Peterson, Caniglia, & Royster, 2001), differential reinforcement of alternative behaviors, and differential reinforcement of other behaviors (Paisey, Fox, Curran, Hooper, & Whitney, 1991). Communication-based treatments, also considered nonaversive, have also been shown to reduce aggression by teaching children socially appropriate communications (Braithwaite & Richdale, 2000; Cafiero, 2001; Connelly, 2004).

FUTURE RESEARCH DIRECTIONS

In order to ensure the most effective intervention, practitioners need to consider carefully the empirical basis for the treatment and the methods used to select treatment options. For example, functional behavior assessment (FBA) has often been used to select interventions for children with ASD (e.g., Peck-Peterson et al., 2001; Reese, Richman, Zarcone, & Zarcone, 2003); however, recent research has called into question the utility of FBA after examining 150 studies of school-based interventions based on this procedure (Gresham et al., 2004). Gresham and his colleagues found that FBA was no more effective than interventions in which these assessments were not included. It is not clear at the present time what specific advantages or disadvantages are associated with FBA in developing effective interventions for individuals with ASD. Research, however, has demonstrated more clearly the efficacy of functional analyses to select interventions, including ABA. In fact, research shows that functional analyses and ABA are likely to remain as critical tools for intervening with a variety of problem behaviors associated with ASD.

Although a number of interventions for ASD are described in the literature (scientific and other), in most cases, empirical support is insufficient, or the results are mixed. Furthermore, many of the studies have serious methodological flaws, making the results difficult to interpret and treatment decisions uncertain. A review of the autism literature suggests that several problems have not been addressed and there are common methodological problems. This includes failure to describe adequately the specific features of the ASD being studied, lack of random assignment to treatment groups, failure to describe treatment components, and a lack of attention to issues of maintenance, generalization, and treatment integrity. For example, oftentimes, researchers omit important information regarding individual characteristics of study participants. A meta-analysis completed at the University of Utah that examined the effectiveness of interventions for aggressive behavior with children who have ASD revealed that over 40% of the published literature had no data concerning the cognitive ability of the participant, and the remaining studies provided only general–categorical information about levels of intelligence (Connelly, 2004). Failure to provide information that can be used to help us understand how some treatments might be effective for one group and not another (e.g., individuals with high-functioning autism vs. those at the other end of the spectrum), is only one problem we face in trying to interpret treatment outcomes.

Lack of random assignment to treatments also makes it difficult to determine the relative benefits of one intervention over another, or the additive power of different combinations of interventions. Although using a control group can establish the efficacy of a given treatment, it does not address the relative merits of one treatment over other available interventions. This can only be accomplished when researchers undertake studies that go beyond the use of experimental group–no-treatment group comparisons. Random assignment or other procedures such as matching experimental and control groups ensure that systematic bias is not introduced into the outcomes. There is also a surprising lack of studies that provide detailed descriptions of treatment components, and a lack of evidence for the use of manualized treatment protocols, a gold standard for behavioral science research today. Not understanding the treatment is one problem, but oftentimes researchers do not even provide detailed information about the specific treatment procedures used. This raises questions as to the integrity of the treatment, that is, how reliably it was implemented (and how much it deviated from the intentions of the research protocol). Finally, researchers have not addressed the very important issue of maintenance and generalization of treatments for autism. Many important behaviors associated with ASD have not been found to generalize across settings and responses unless active generalization and maintenance strategies are incorporated into treatment protocols. For this reason, it is critical that future research evaluate the impact that specific "add-on" strategies (e.g., parent, sibling, and peer training components) have on a child's functioning in multiple contexts.

It may be that some of these methodological problems are responsible for the range of findings from research studies, that is, with some studies showing that with one type of treatment, children may make significant improvement, and others showing little or no gain (e.g., Schreibman, 2000). For this reason, readers are advised to evaluate the literature base carefully for selected interventions. A number of resources can be consulted for this, including the website for the Cambridge Center for Behavioral Studies (www.behavior.org). The Center has a section on autism, where current information can be found about empirically based treatments such as ABA. The Autism Biomedical Information Network (www.autism-biomed.org) is also a good website that provides information on scientifically supported methods and commentaries on ways to distinguish "good" science from pseudoscience. Last, readers may wish to review the autism section in the U.S. Surgeon General's report on mental health among children (www.surgeongeneral.gov). Given the complexity and unique features of ASD, it may be assumed that a "one-size-fits-all" treatment will not be found; instead, treatments tailored to specific problem behaviors, setting characteristics, intervention characteristics, functional levels, and other aspects of an individualized treatment program will prove to be the most effective. Such hypotheses need to be disproved or proved using sound empirical methods and replicated studies.

ACKNOWLEDGMENTS

We wish to acknowledge the following students who are part of the University of Utah Autism Meta-Analysis Project and contributed to the completion of this chapter: Elizabeth Christiansen, Julia Connelly, Lisa Goldy, Najmeh Hourmanesh, Lindsey Miller, and Eden Steffey.

REFERENCES

Adelinis, J. D., Piazza, C. C., & Goh, H. L. (2001). Treatment of multiply controlled destructive behavior with food reinforcement. *Journal of Applied Behavior Analysis, 34*, 97–100.
American Psychiatric Association. (2000). *Diagnostic and statistical manual of mental disorders* (4th ed., text rev.). Washington, DC: Author.
Anderson, S. R., & Romanczyk, R. G. (1999). Early intervention for young children with autism: Continuum-based behavioral models. *Journal of the Association for Persons with Severe Handicaps, 24*, 162–173.
Baker, M. J., Koegel, R. I., & Koegel, L. K. (1998). Increasing the social behavior of young children with autism using their obsessive behaviors. *Journal of the Association for Persons with Severe Handicaps, 23*, 300–308.
Becker-Cottrill, B., McFarland, J., & Anderson, V. (2003). A model of positive behavioral support for individuals with autism and their families. *Focus on Autism and Other Developmental Disabilities, 18*, 110–120.
Bird, F., Dores, P. A., Moniz, D., & Robinson, J. (1989). Reducing severe aggressive and self-injurious behaviors with functional communication training. *American Journal on Mental Retardation, 94*, 37–48.
Bondy, A., & Frost, L. (2001). The Picture Exchange Communication System. *Behavior Modification, 25*, 725–744.
Borthwick-Duffy, S. A. (1994). Epidemiology and prevalence of psychopathology in

people with mental retardation. *Journal of Consulting and Clinical Psychology, 62,* 17–27.

Braithwaite, K. L., & Richdale, A. L. (2000). Functional communication training to replace challenging behaviors across two behavioral outcomes. *Behavioral Interventions, 15,* 21–36.

Cafiero, J. M. (2001). The effect of an augmentative communication intervention on the communication, behavior, and academic program of an adolescent with autism. *Focus on Autism and Other Developmental Disabilities, 16,* 179–189.

Campbell, M., & Cueva, J. E. (1995). Psychopharmacology in child and adolescent psychiatry: A review of the past seven years. *Journal of the American Academy of Child and Adolescent Psychiatry, 34,* 1262–1271.

Carr, E. G., & Durand, V. M. (1985). Reducing behavior problems through functional communication training. *Journal of Applied Behavior Analysis, 18,* 111–126.

Charlop-Christy, M. H., Carpenter, M., Le, L., LeBlanc, L. A., & Kellet, K. (2002). Using the Picture Exchange Communication System (PECS) with children with autism: Assessment of PECS acquisition, speech, social–communicative behavior, and problem behavior. *Journal of Applied Behavior Analysis, 35,* 213–231.

Connelly, J. (2004). *Effectiveness of non-medication based treatments for the reduction of disruptive behavior in autism: A meta-analysis.* Unpublished masters thesis, University of Utah, Salt Lake City.

Dekeyzer, L. (2004). *Autism and the pervasive developmental disorders: Features of psychiatrically treated children and adolescents.* Unpublished masters thesis, University of Utah, Salt Lake City.

DeKlyen, M., & Odom, S. L. (1989). Activity structure and social interactions with peers in developmentally integrated play groups. *Journal of Early Intervention, 13,* 342–352.

DeLeon, I. G., Fisher, W. W., Herman, K. M., & Crosland, K. C. (2000). Assessment of a response bias for aggression over functionally equivalent appropriate behavior. *Journal of Applied Behavior Analysis, 33,* 73–77.

Delprato, D. J. (2001). Comparisons of discrete-trial and normalized behavioral intervention for young children with autism. *Journal of Autism and Developmental Disorders, 31,* 315–325.

Durand, V. M. (1999). Functional communication training using assistive devices: Recruiting natural communities of reinforcement. *Journal of Applied Behavior Analysis, 32,* 247–268.

Eikeseth, S., Smith, T., Jahr, E., & Eldevik, S. (2002). Intensive behavioral treatment at school for 4- to 7-year-old children with autism: A 1-year comparison controlled study. *Behavior Modification, 26,* 49–68.

Fernell, E., Watanabe, Y., Adolfsson, I., Tani, Y., Bergström, M., Hartwig, P., et al. (1997). Possible effects of tetrahydrobiopterin treatment in six children with autism: Clinical and positron emission tomography data: A pilot study. *Developmental Medicine and Child Neurology, 39,* 313–318.

Ferrara, C., & Hill, S. D. (1980). The responsiveness of autistic children to the predictability of social and nonsocial toys. *Journal of Autism and Developmental Disorders, 10,* 51–57.

Freeman, B. J. (1997). Guidelines for evaluating intervention programs for children with autism. *Journal of Autism and Developmental Disorders, 27*, 641–651.

Garrison-Harrell, L., & Kamps, D. (1997). The effects of peer networks on social–communicative behaviors for students with autism. *Focus on Autism and Other Developmental Disabilities, 12*, 241–255.

Goldstein, H. (2002). Communication intervention for children with autism: A review of treatment efficacy. *Journal of Autism and Developmental Disorders, 32*, 373–396.

Goldstein, H., & Ferrell, D. R. (1987). Augmenting communicative interaction between handicapped and nonhandicapped preschool children. *Journal of Speech and Hearing Disorders, 52*, 200–211.

Goldstein, H., Kaczmarek, L., Pennington, R., & Shafer, K. (1992). Peer-mediated intervention: Attending to, commenting on, and acknowledging the behavior of preschoolers with autism. *Journal of Applied Behavior Analysis, 25*, 289–305.

Gonzalez-Lopez, A., & Kamps, D. M. (1997). Social skills training to increase social interactions between children with autism and their typical peers. *Focus on Autism and Other Developmental Disabilities, 12*, 2–14.

Green, G. (1996a). Early behavioral intervention for autism: What does research tell us? In C. Maurice (Ed.), *Behavioral interventions for young children with autism: A manual for parents and professionals* (pp. 29–44). Austin, TX: Pro-Ed.

Green, G. (1996b). Evaluating claims about treatments for autism. In C. Maurice (Ed.), *Behavioral interventions for young children with autism: A manual for parents and professionals* (pp. 15–28). Austin, TX: Pro-Ed.

Green, G. (2004, March). *Autism treatments: The quality of the evidence*. Invited address to the Parents' Education as Autism Therapists—ABA Ireland Conference, Belfast, Northern Ireland.

Gresham, F. M., McIntyre, L. L., Olson-Tinker, H., Dolstra, L., McLaughlin, V., & Van, M. (2004). Relevance of functional behavioral assessment research for school-based interventions and positive behavioral support. *Research in Developmental Disabilities, 25*, 19–37.

Grossman, J. B., Carter, A., & Volkmar, F. R. (1997). Social behavior in autism. In C. S. Carter, I. I. Lederhendler, & B. Kirkpatrick (Eds.), The integrative neurobiology of affiliation [Special issue]. *Annals of the New York Academy of Sciences, 807*, 440–454.

Heathfield, L. T., Olympia, D., Clark, E., Jenson, W. R., Kircher, J., Connelly, J., Miller, L., & Steffey, E. (2004, July). *Effective interventions for children with autism: A summary of meta-analyses*. Paper presented at the American Psychological Association, Honolulu, HI.

Horner, R. H., Carr, E. G., Strain, P. S., Todd, A. W., & Reed, H. K. (2002). Problem behavior interventions for young children with autism: A research synthesis. *Journal of Autism and Developmental Disorders, 32*, 423–446.

Houlihan, D., Jacobson, L., & Brandon, P. K. (1994). Replication of a high-probability request sequence with varied interprompt times in a preschool setting. *Journal of Applied Behavior Analysis, 27*, 737–738.

Howlin, P., Goode, S., Hutton, J., & Rutter, M. (2004). Adult outcome for children with autism. *Journal of Child Psychology and Psychiatry, 45*, 212–227.

Iwata, B. A., Zarcone, J. B., Vollmer, T. R., & Smith, R. G. (1994). Assessment and treatment of self-injurious behavior. In E. Schopler & G. B. Mesibov (Eds.), *Behavioral issues in autism* (pp. 131–159). New York: Plenum Press.

Koegel, L. K., Camarata, S. M., Valdez-Menchaca, M., & Koegel, R. L. (1998). Setting generalization of question-asking by children with autism. *American Journal on Mental Retardation, 102,* 346–357.

Koegel, L. K., Koegel, R. L., & Surratt, A. (1992). Language intervention and disruptive behavior in preschool children with autism. *Journal of Autism and Developmental Disorders, 22,* 141–153.

Koegel, R. L., & Covert, A. (1972). The relationship of self-stimulation to learning in autistic children. *Journal of Applied Behavioral Analysis, 5,* 381–387.

Koegel, R. L., & Frea, W. D. (1993). Treatment of social behavior in autism through the modification of pivotal social skills. *Journal of Applied Behavior Analysis, 26,* 369–377.

Lainhart, J. E. (1999). Psychiatric problems in individuals with autism, their parents, and siblings. *International Review of Psychiatry, 11,* 278–298.

Lancioni, G. E., & Hoogeveen, G. R. (1990). Nonaversive and mildly aversive procedures for reducing problem behaviours in people with developmental disorders: A review. *Mental Handicap Research, 3,* 137–169.

Lee, S., & Odom, S. L. (1996). The relationship between stereotypic behavior and peer social interaction for children with severe disabilities. *Journal of the Association for Persons with Severe Handicaps, 21,* 88–95.

Lewis, M. H., & Bodfish, J. W. (1998). Repetitive behavior disorders in autism. *Mental Retardation and Developmental Disabilities Research Reviews, 4,* 80–89.

Lovaas, I., Newsome, C., & Hickman, C. (1987). Self-stimulatory behavior and perceptual reinforcement. *Journal of Applied Behavior Analysis, 20,* 45–68.

Malone, R. P. (1996). Stereotypies and neuroleptic-related dyskinesias in children with autism. In M. A. Richardson & G. Haugland (Eds.), *Use of neuroleptics in children* (pp. 121–136). Washington, DC: American Psychiatric Press.

Mastergeorge, A. M., Rogers, S. J., Corbett, B. A., & Solomon, M. (2003). Nonmedical interventions for autism spectrum disorders. In S. Ozonoff, S. J. Rogers, & R. L. Hendren (Eds.), *Autism spectrum disorders: A research review for practitioners* (pp. 133–160). Washington, DC: American Psychiatric Press.

McClannahan, L. E., & Krantz, P. J. (1999). *Activity schedules for children with autism: Teaching independent behavior.* Bethesda, MD: Woodbine House.

McConnell, S. R. (2002). Interventions to facilitate social interaction for young children with autism: Review of available research and recommendations for educational intervention and future research. *Journal of Autism and Developmental Disorders, 32,* 351–372.

McGee, G. G., Almeida, M. C., Sulzer-Azaroff, B., & Feldman, R. S. (1992). Promoting reciprocal interactions via peer incidental teaching. *Journal of Applied Behavior Analysis, 25,* 117–126.

Miller, L. (2005). *Interventions targeting social interaction skills in children and young adults with autism: A meta-analysis.* Unpublished doctoral dissertation, University of Utah, Salt Lake City.

Mirenda, P. (2003). Toward functional augmentative and alternative communication for students with autism: Manual signs, graphic symbols, and voice output communication aids. *Language, Speech, and Hearing Services in Schools, 34,* 203–216.

Myles, B. S., Simpson, R. L., Ormsbee, C. K., & Erickson, C. (1993). Integrating preschool children with autism with their normally developing peers: Research findings and best practices recommendations. *Focus on Autistic Behavior, 8,* 1–17.

National Research Council. (2001). *Educating children with autism.* Washington, DC: National Academy Press.

Odom, S. L., McConnell, S. R., McEvoy, M. A., Peterson, C., Ostrosky, M., Chandler, L. K., et al. (1999). Relative effects of interventions supporting the social competence of young children with disabilities. *Topics in Early Childhood Special Education, 19,* 75–91.

Ozonoff, S., & Rogers, S. J. (2003). From Kanner to the millennium. In S. Ozonoff, S. J. Rogers, & R. L. Hendren (Eds.), *Autism spectrum disorders: A research review for practitioners* (pp. 3–33). Washington DC: American Psychiatric Press.

Paisey, T. J., Fox, S., Curran, C., Hooper, K., & Whitney, R. (1991). Case study: Reinforcement control of severe aggression exhibited by a child with autism in a family home. *Behavioral Residential Treatment, 6,* 289–302.

Peck-Peterson, S. M., Caniglia, C., & Royster, A. J. (2001). Application of choice-making intervention for a student with multiply maintained problem behavior. *Focus on Autism and Other Developmental Disabilities, 16,* 240–246.

Pollard, N. L. (1998). Development of social interaction skills in preschool children with autism: A review of the literature. *Child and Family Behavior Therapy, 20*(2), 1–16.

Quill, K. A. (1997). Instructional considerations for young children with autism: The rationale for visually cued instruction. *Journal of Autism and Developmental Disorders, 27,* 697–714.

Reese, R. M., Richman, D. M., Zarcone, J., & Zarcone, T. (2003). Individualizing functional assessments for children with autism. *Focus on Autism and Other Developmental Disabilities, 18,* 87–92.

Rogers, S. J. (1998). Empirically supported comprehensive treatments for young children with autism. *Journal of Clinical Child Psychology, 27,* 168–179.

Rogers, S. J., Bennetto, L., McEvoy, R., & Pennington, B. F. (1996). Imitation and pantomime in high-functioning adolescents with autism spectrum disorders. *Child Development, 67,* 2060–2073.

Romano, J. P., & Roll, D. (2000). Expanding the utility of behavioral momentum for youth with developmental disabilities. *Behavioral Interventions, 15,* 99–111.

Rosenthal-Malek, A., & Mitchell, S. (1997). Brief report: The effects of exercise on the self-stimulatory behaviors and positive responding of adolescents with autism. *Journal of Autism and Developmental Disorders, 27,* 193–202.

Schlosser, R., & Lee, D. (2000). Promoting generalization and maintenance in augmentative and alternative communication: A meta-analysis of 20 years of effectiveness research. *Augmentative and Alternative Communication, 16,* 208–226.

Schopler, E. (1994). Behavioral priorities for autism and related developmental disorders. In E. Schopler & G. B. Mesibov (Eds.), *Behavioral issues in autism* (pp. 55–77). New York: Plenum Press.

Schopler, E., & Mesibov, G. B. (Eds.). (1994). *Behavioral issues in autism*. New York: Plenum Press.

Schreibman, L. (2000). Intensive behavioral/psychoeducational treatments for autism: Research needs and future directions. *Journal of Autism and Developmental Disorders, 30*, 373–378.

Sigman, M. (1994). What are the core deficits in autism? In S. H. Broman & J. Grafman (Eds.), *Atypical cognitive deficits in developmental disorders: Implications for brain function* (pp. 139–157). Hillsdale, NJ: Erlbaum.

Smith, T., Groen, A. D., & Wynn, J. W. (2000). Randomized trial of intensive early intervention for children with pervasive developmental disorder. *American Journal on Mental Retardation, 105*, 269–285.

Strain, P. S., & Schwartz, I. (2001). ABA and the development of meaningful social relations for young children with autism. *Focus on Autism and Other Developmental Disabilities, 16*, 120–128.

Sweeney, D. P., Forness, S. R., & Levitt, J. G. (1998). An overview of medications commonly used to treat behavioral disorders associated with autism, Tourette syndrome, and pervasive developmental disorders. *Focus on Autism and Other Developmental Disabilities, 13*, 144–150.

Symons, F. J., Koppekin, A., & Wehby, J. H. (1999). Treatment of self-injurious behavior and quality of life for persons with mental retardation. *Mental Retardation, 37*, 297–307.

Thorp, D. M., Stahmer, A. C., & Schreibman, L. (1995). Effects of sociodramatic play training on children with autism. *Journal of Autism and Developmental Disorders, 25*, 265–282.

Van Houten, R. V., & Rolider, A. (1988). Recreating the scene: An effective way to provide delayed punishment for inappropriate motor behavior. *Journal of Applied Behavior Analysis, 21*, 187–192.

Venter, A., Lord, C., & Schopler, E. (1992). A follow-up study of high-functioning autistic children. *Journal of Child Psychology and Psychiatry, 33*, 489–507.

Williams, P. G., Allard, A., Sears, L., Dalrymple, N., & Bloom, A. S. (2001). Brief report: Case report on naltrexone use in children with autism: Controlled observations regarding benefits and practical issues of medication management. *Journal of Autism and Developmental Disorders, 31*, 103–108.

Yeargin-Allsopp, M., Rice, C., Karapurkar, T., Doernberg, N., Boyle, C., & Murphy, C. (2003). Prevalence of autism in a U.S. metropolitan area. *Journal of the American Medical Association, 289*, 49–55.

15

Systems Interventions for Comprehensive Care

JANET E. FARMER
ELENA HARLAN DREWEL

Parents of children with neurodevelopmental disabilities are often faced with a daunting task—navigating the complex system of care to obtain comprehensive and coordinated services (Drotar, 2001; Krauss, Wells, Gulley, & Anderson, 2001). Whether their child has a congenital or an acquired condition, parents typically must learn how to access quality medical and mental health care, educational supports, financial assistance, and other resources from state and federal agencies. Inability to access adequate services places the child at risk for unwarranted disruptions in development, and the parents at risk for undue strain and distress.

The health service delivery system is a part of the social–ecological context in which children with chronic illness and disabilities function (Bronfenbrenner, 1979; Farmer, Clark, & Marien, 2003a; Kazak, Rourke, & Crump, 2003b). In the social–ecological conceptual framework, microsystems are proximal social and environmental factors that have an immediate influence on children's health and well-being, such as the family, school, hospital, and neighborhood contexts. At the next level of influence, mesosystems represent the overlap or interaction of two or more microsystems that form the more complex service delivery system. Linkages between microsystems may involve communication among individuals involved in the child's care in various settings, or actions in one microsystem that influence behaviors or attitudes in other care systems. For example, when a child sustains a significant traumatic brain injury, health care providers, educators, and families often must work together to develop a coordinated plan of care that promotes a successful transition from hospital to school (Deidrick & Farmer, in press; Semrud-Clikeman, 2001).

Many other conceptual models in pediatric and rehabilitation psychology acknowledge that multiple systems interact to influence child and family outcomes (e.g., Dunst, 1997; Wallander, Thompson, & Alriksson-Schmidt, 2003; World Health Organization, 2001). Theoretically, interventions that enhance coordinated and comprehensive care across these systems have the potential to promote healthy development and prevent secondary complications such as excessive hospitalizations, school failure, and poor child adjustment to disability. Yet pediatric psychologists have focused their intervention, research, and training efforts almost exclusively on direct service delivery to children and/or to their families rather than on improving aspects of the health care delivery system (Brown, 2004; Schneiderman & Speers, 1998; Spirito et al., 2003).

Our purpose in this chapter is to focus on mesosystems and how the interrelationships between microsystems may impact individual child and family outcomes. First, we review in more detail the systems of care that children and families must navigate. Then we present the results of an emerging body of research that examines child and family outcomes following interventions that improve the integration and coordination of health and related services.

COMPLEXITIES IN THE SYSTEM OF CARE

Children with special health care needs and disabilities receive services from a wide array of providers and programs that are often fragmented and inconsistently responsive to child and family needs (Drotar, 2001; Farmer et al., 2003a; Seid, Sobo, Gelhard, & Varni, 2004). The system of care has developed as a patchwork of disconnected services with differing and ever-changing eligibility criteria that challenge even the most experienced parents to access needed services in a timely way. To better understand the issues families face in getting their needs met, it is important to become familiar with the components of the health care delivery system. The next sections describe the three broad sectors that make up the structure of the health care system: personal health services, educational and other health-related support services, and community health services (Shi & Singh, 2001).

Personal Health Services

As shown in Figure 15.1, the care system for children with chronic health problems includes traditional medical and mental health services provided

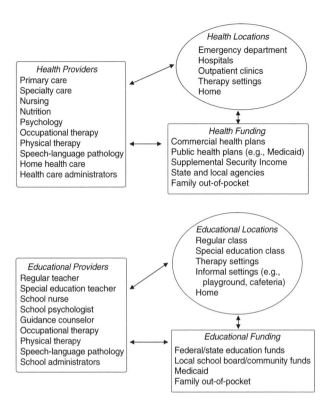

FIGURE 15.1. Complexities in the health and educational systems of care.

to individual children in a range of settings by a variety of primary and specialty care professionals. Traditional health service use in this group is much higher than that among children without chronic conditions (Lin & Lave, 2000; Newacheck, Inkelas, & Kim, 2004). For example, Newacheck and colleagues examined health care utilization among approximately 5 million children and youth with disabilities identified in a national survey of U.S. households conducted in 1999–2000. Compared to their peers without disabilities, these youngsters had more than four times the number of hospitalizations, more than twice as many physician visits, and five times as many visits to nonphysician health professionals, such as psychologists, social workers, nurse practitioners, and physical therapists. They also visited the emergency department twice as often and required approximately three times the number of prescription medications relative to children without disabilities.

Given the extent of care required, it comes as no surprise that the cost of personal health services for this group is quite high. The 1999–2000 national survey data showed that children with disabilities required nearly four times the annual total health care expenditures as those without disabilities (Newacheck et al., 2004). Their health care utilization accounted for 22.7% of health care costs for all children ages 0 to 17, even though they comprised only 7.3% of the population. Funding for these services comes primarily from private and public health insurance plans, but parents of children with chronic conditions often are underinsured and must contribute substantial out-of-pocket funds to obtain needed services, especially in the areas of mental health care and prescription medications (Krauss et al., 2001; McMenamy & Perrin, 2004; Newacheck et al., 2004). The greatest cost burden is on low-income families, who are approximately 19 times more likely than are higher income families to spend more than 5% of family income on out-of-pocket expenses (Newacheck et al., 2004).

Educational Services

In the health-related support services sector, the educational system has become a major source of care provision for children with neurodevelopmental disorders, addressing needs in the areas of health, cognition, behavior, and social–emotional development (Brown, 2004). Under the Individuals with Disabilities Education Act (IDEA), every child with a disability is entitled to a free and appropriate education that may include special education and related services (Shapiro & Manz, 2004; Wright & Wright, 2004). This federal mandate and others (e.g., Section 504 of the Rehabilitation Act of 1973) provide procedures for accessing special services and encourage individualized interventions that promote social inclusion in the least restrictive environment.

Like the medical system, the educational system is multifaceted and complex (see Figure 15.1). As Power and Blom-Hoffman (2004) point out, the school environment provides many opportunities for children with disabilities. Educational settings offer the expertise of multidisciplinary teams, a natural context that promotes healthy development and competence, and a venue for observing behavior and monitoring response to interventions over time. However, challenges in the school environment include a lack of specific professional training required to meet the needs of many children with chronic illnesses and disabilities, limited financial resources, and a variable level of commitment to and resources for social inclusion.

Community Health Services

Typically funded by state and federal agencies, the community health sector is designed to provide a safety net for children and families, sometimes funding services that are not covered elsewhere, such as service coordination or respite care. For example, the Maternal and Child Health Bureau (MCHB; funded by Title V of the Social Security Act) is a key agency charged with ensuring the health of children with chronic conditions and disabilities. Other agencies also provide families with financial supports and services, such as each state's Division of Mental Retardation/Developmental Disabilities or the federal Supplemental Security Income program. Public agency services can be especially hard to navigate due to varying eligibility requirements and changes in available services associated with fluctuations in the level of state and federal funding.

Another primary mission of these agencies is to implement population-wide, public health interventions aimed at prevention and early intervention. For instance, in the past 10 years, MCHB has shaped state and federal programs to improve identification of children with chronic conditions and to increase understanding of child and family needs. They have targeted a broad, noncategorical group of children with special health care needs (CSHCN) who have chronic physical, developmental, emotional, and/or behavioral concerns, and who require more health and related services than their peers (McPherson et al., 1998). Based on information gathered from large health surveys and other sources, MCHB has set an national agenda for CSHCN designed to encourage family-centered care that is accessible, comprehensive, coordinated, community-based, and culturally effective (U.S. Department of Health and Human Services, 1999). Such policies are a part of the ecological context for children with chronic illness and disabilities and have led to explorations of how to improve the service delivery system for CSHCN.

IMPROVING THE SYSTEM OF CARE

Increasing awareness of the complexities in the service delivery system has led to substantial growth in efforts to build comprehensive and coordinated systems of care for children with chronic health conditions and their families (American Academy of Pediatrics, 2002; Drotar, 2001; Farmer et al., 2003a; Silva, Sofis, & Palfrey, 2000; Stille & Antonelli, 2004). Based on a consensus meeting of an interdisciplinary group of researchers and practitioners, Drotar (2001) described comprehensive care as "the coordinated provision of a broad range of health-related services as needed to maintain health and well-being of children with a chronic illness or health condition in the context of a coordinated partnership with the family who actively participates in decision making about the child's care" (p. 159). Pediatricians have mounted a major initiative to encourage comprehensive and coordinated care as a part of the "Medical Home" model, which states that all children should have a primary care provider who provides continuity in care and ensures that families have access to needed medical and nonmedical services (American Academy of Pediatrics, 2002; Cooley, 2004). Such care requires collaborative communication among health care and community providers, as well as the provision of family supports to promote effective coping with the emotional and physical demands of caring for the child.

Potential barriers to comprehensive care are numerous, beyond the fact that the system of care itself is complex and difficult to navigate (Seid et al., 2004). For example, the structure of health care financing is based on an acute care model in which symptoms are managed, but there is limited financial support for services that support long-term functioning, prevention of secondary disability, or overall quality of life (Drotar, 2001; Stein, 2001). Health care providers rarely are reimbursed for care coordination activities and also lack training in chronic care management (Davidson, Silva, Sofis, Ganz, & Palfrey, 2002). Furthermore, a national survey about CHSCN indicated that there is uneven access to care coordination services (Weller, Minkovitz, & Anderson, 2003). For example, 65% of children received medical care coordination (e.g., oversight of medical treatments, therapies, and prescription medications), but only 30% received nonmedical care coordination (e.g., assistance with access to social services). Those children who were insured were more likely than uninsured children to receive medical care coordination, while those who experienced more limitations in activities of daily living were more likely to receive nonmedical care coordination compared to those with less impairment in everyday functioning. Children from racial/ethnic minorities were less likely to receive care coordination services compared to white children. Rural children may be more vulnerable to fragmented care because of health care provider shortages and the increased likelihood that they are uninsured (Coburn, McBride, & Ziller, 2002; Nordahl, Copans, & Stamm, 2003).

As the problems in the health care delivery system have been recognized, a few demonstration projects have developed in an effort to promote change. Table 15.1 presents an overview of community-based studies identified in the recent literature that sought to increase comprehensive care for CSHCN and their families. The early studies by Stein and colleagues (Stein, 2001) took place when hospital-based care was still the norm for children with complex chronic health conditions. These studies forged the way for the transition to community-based care, which is now the standard for most children, and they were innovative in their thorough assessment of the health and well-being of children and families. Like this early work, subsequent interventions tended to have common elements, such as engagement of the family as a partner, interdisciplinary team interactions, information about resources and services, emotional support, advocacy and problem

TABLE 15.1. Intervention Studies That Enhance Comprehensive and Coordinated Care for Children with Chronic Health Conditions

Study	Purpose	Sample and design	Key elements	Results
Stein (2001)	To present results of the Pediatric Ambulatory Care Treatment Study conducted during the 1970s and 1980s, with a review of several studies investigating the impact of a home care program	219 families of children with complex chronic health conditions living at home Pre-post randomized study of enhanced care versus standard care groups	• Interdisciplinary team approach • Community-based • Care coordination • Patient advocacy • Family education	• Increased parent satisfaction with care • Decreased unmet health needs • Improved maternal mental health • Improved child mental health
Pless et al. (1994)	To determine whether a specialized nursing intervention aimed at optimizing family functioning would improve psychosocial outcomes in children	267 families of children with mixed chronic physical conditions Randomized control of enhanced care vs. routine nursing services	• Nurses interact with families • Identification of resources and services • Assistance with problem solving about unmet needs • Emotional support • Family education	• Improved parent report of child adjustment • Improved scholastic competence, behavioral conduct, and self-worth among older children
Liptak, Burns, Davidson, & McAnarney (1998)	To examine the effects of a comprehensive care program on medical resource utilization and cost	Descriptive study of 10,715 admissions of children with chronic conditions	• Interdisciplinary team approach • Care coordination • Access to therapists, psychologists, and social workers	• Decreased length of stay, annual admissions, and inpatient hospital charges • Fewer children readmitted • Increased use of ambulatory services

(*continued*)

TABLE 15.1. (continued)

Study	Purpose	Sample and design	Key elements	Results
Ireys, Chernoff, DeVet, & Kim (2001); Chernoff, Ireys, DeVet, & Kim (2002)	To determine whether community-based parent-to-parent and child-directed supports improve maternal and child adjustment	136 mothers, and children with diabetes mellitus, sickle cell anemia, cystic fibrosis, or moderate to severe asthma	• Experienced mothers matched with target mothers • Information about resources and services • Emotional support and affirmation • Child life specialist intervention to promote coping and self-esteem in children	• Decrease in maternal anxiety • Improvements in child adjustment
Naar-King, Siegel, Smyth, & Simpson (2003)	To evaluate a program that integrates mental and physical health services in hospital-based clinics	116 parents, and children with complex medical conditions Compared outcomes from traditional versus integrated clinics	• Interdisciplinary team approach • One comprehensive team evaluation per year • Individual plan of care • Access to psychologists, social workers, and dieticians	• Children in integrated clinics showed fewer behavior problems and better school adjustment

Palfrey et al. (2004)	To assess outcomes from the Pediatric Alliance for Coordinated Care, a medical home intervention to improve care coordination	150 children with chronic conditions from six primary care practices Pre–post design	• Nurse practitioner assigned to a primary care practice • Assistance with care coordination • Individual health plan	• Easier access to care and services • Improved communication among health professionals • Decreased parent work absences • Decreased hospitalizations
McMenamy & Perrin (2004)	To assess outcomes from the Guiding Appropriate Pediatric Services (GAPS) program, a medical home intervention that provided expanded care and care coordination	98 families of children with chronic health conditions Posttreatment assessment of success at getting needs met	• Individual Family Service Plan to identify top three medical and nonmedical needs • Problem solving about ways to address these needs • Parent advisory groups identified ways to improve care	• Needs for information and specific help were often met • Needs for parent-to-parent contact and counseling were met less often
Farmer, Clark, Marien, Sherman, & Selva (2005)	To assess outcomes from the Missouri Partnership for Enhanced Delivery of Services (MO-PEDS), a medical home intervention in a more rural area than other studies	51 families of children with chronic health conditions Pre–post assessment of child and family outcomes	• Nurse, physician, and family addressed child and family needs • Individualized care plan • Care coordination, including information and resource identification • Problem-solving assistance • Emotional support and advocacy	• Improved satisfaction with care coordination • Improved access to mental health services • Decreased family needs and caregiver strain • Decreased parent work absences • Improved school attendance

solving, and improved communication among care providers (e.g., via a written Individual Health Care Plan). Outcome variables differed across studies but, in general, families reported improved satisfaction with services, easier access to needed services, and better child and family functioning. Some studies found decreased utilization of services (e.g., hospitalizations) and resulting decline in costs.

MISSOURI PARTNERSHIP FOR ENHANCED DELIVERY OF SERVICES

To illustrate this approach in more detail, the Missouri Partnership for Enhanced Delivery of Services (MO-PEDS) is a medical home demonstration project designed to improve comprehensive and coordinated care for a noncategorical group of CSHCN in the central Midwest (Farmer et al., 2003a; Farmer, Marien, Clark, Sherman, & Selva, 2004; Farmer, Clark, Marien, Sherman, & Selva, 2005). In the first phase of this initiative, children and youth with chronic conditions ($N = 83$) were identified in three primary care practices in a nine-county area that included a small metropolitan area of 79,000 population and eight surrounding rural counties. They ranged in age from less than 1 year to 17 years ($M = 7.1$ years, $SD = 5.0$), and 72% had two or more chronic conditions. Although all children had some type of health insurance and a source of primary care, most were from low-income families (52% earned less than $20,000 per year). In addition to frequent contact with primary and specialty care providers for medical services, children also received services from multiple nonmedical sources, as shown in Table 15.2. These data illustrate the variability in services provided to children with differing chronic conditions, which is likely associated with factors such as time of onset, level of severity, program eligibility criteria, and the family's ability to navigate the system of care. At the point of enrollment in the project, parents reported an average of nine unmet family needs, most commonly in the areas of need for information, social support, and community services (Farmer et al., 2004).

The MO-PEDS intervention was based on the Medical Home model of care adapted from leading pediatricians in the field of primary care for CSHCN (Silva et al., 2000). The care team consisted of a nurse practitioner, who partnered with physicians and family members in their communities to ensure comprehensive and coordinated care for the child. The nurse conducted an assessment in the child's home to clarify unmet medical and nonmedical needs, identified health and community resources for meeting the needs, wrote an Individual Care Plan with short-term goals, and provided family supports (e.g., emotional support, assistance with solving complex problems). A parent consultant (a paid family member of a

TABLE 15.2. Agencies Providing Services to Children with Chronic Conditions, by Primary Diagnosis

Diagnostic category (ICD-9-CM codes)	N	SSI n (%)	MR/DD n (%)	MH n (%)	Title V n (%)	Early intervention[a] n (%)	Special education[b] n (%)
Perinatal, congenital, and nervous system conditions (320–389, 740–779)	42	20 (48)	22 (52)	11 (26)	21 (42)	16 (80)	23 (92)
Mental health conditions (290–319)	9	4 (44)	4 (44)	5 (56)	1 (11)	0 (0)	6 (75)
Organ-specific conditions (001–289, 390–739, 800–999)	29	7 (24)	3 (10)	6 (21)	2 (7)	1 (25)	14 (58)
Ill-defined signs or symptoms (780–799)	3	1 (33)	1 (33)	0 (0)	0 (0)	0 (0)	1 (100)
Total	83	32 (39)	30 (36)	22 (27)	24 (29)	17 (63)	44 (76)

Note. Unpublished data from Janet E. Farmer. SSI, Supplemental Security Income; MR/DD, Division of Mental Retardation/Developmental Disabilities (Department of Mental Health); MH, mental health services; Title V, Bureau of Special Health Care Needs (Department of Health and Senior Services).
[a]Young children only (0 to 36 months); percentages based on the number reported in this age range.
[b]School-age children only (3 to 18 years); percentages based on the number reported in this age range.

CSHCN) assisted with family-to-family supports. The nurse and parent consultant also made presentations to physicians regarding topics related to chronic care management, family-centered care, and so forth.

Care coordination interventions typically fell into four broad categories: (1) health/medical, (2) mental health and family supports, (3) educational consultation, and (4) interagency collaboration. Each child and family had an individual plan of care tailored to their needs, but the following are a few examples of specific activities that the nurse, family, and physician facilitated:

- Educational consultation to obtain health-related accommodations (e.g., an accessible classroom, assistive technology).
- Referral to health professionals who could address unmet needs (e.g., dentist, neuropsychologist, behavioral specialist).
- Identification of creative ways to fund needed services through untapped public and private sources.
- Housing modifications to ensure the safety of a child with developmental delays and severe behavior problems.
- Arrangements for medical treatment from specialists in other states (e.g., Medicaid insurance authorization for out-of-state treatment).
- Interagency care conferences to design collaborative and coordinated health plans for children with very complex needs.
- Identification of resources for basic family needs such as food and clothing.
- Contact with children's wish-granting organizations.
- Clarification of risks for health complications (e.g., family watering down food supplement because of inadequate supply for an infant with a gastrostomy tube) and arrangements for corrective action (e.g., changes in physician's order for these supplements).

After approximately 1 year of intervention by the MO-PEDS staff, 95% of the 51 families who completed a follow-up survey felt that the MO-PEDS intervention was helpful to them (Farmer et al., 2005). Analysis of data from the project showed improvements in family satisfaction with care coordination, decreased family needs, and lower perceptions of family strain. Parents also reported better access to mental health services and better school attendance for their children. Fewer parents missed over 10 days of work, and families of children with greater functional impairments were more likely to experience a decrease in needs. In this study, improvements on key outcome variables were not related to geographic location (i.e., rural vs. urban) or to socioeconomic status, suggesting that this type of intervention may be useful for a wide range of families of children with chronic conditions.

CLINICAL IMPLICATIONS

The outcomes from multifaceted programs that encourage comprehensive care should capture the attention of psychologists and other mental health professionals, since enhancements in the care delivery system show the potential to improve psychosocial outcomes for children with chronic health conditions and their families. Although traditional mental health interventions may be warranted under some circumstances, not every child or parent will need this type of service in order improve their overall adjustment. To illustrate, Kazak and colleagues (2003a) examined risk factors associated with family need for psychosocial interventions in children newly diagnosed with cancer. Over half (59%) of the families reported few or no risk factors, indicating good potential for adjustment to illness and the need only for standard psychosocial supports provided by the oncology team (termed "universal" care; Mrazek & Haggerty, 1994). About one-third (34%) identified four to seven risk factors, suggesting the need for increased interventions such as support groups, educational programs, or regular access to social workers or child life specialists to problem-solve about specific needs ("selected" care). The other 7% reported 8–16 risk factors, placing them in the "targeted" care group that would likely require intensive therapeutic supports from a psychologist. Programs such as those described in Table 15.1 may be most appropriate for families requiring "selected" care, though such programs may also help the "targeted" care group to access direct mental health services.

Taken as a whole, these findings suggest that psychologists must consider expanding the scope of their intervention paradigms to include strategies that modify contextual barriers to care and produce change in the organization and processes of service delivery (Drotar et al., 2001; King, King, & Rosenbaum, 2004; Schneiderman & Speers, 1998; Seid et al., 2004). This paradigm shift places an emphasis on health promotion and prevention of unwarranted disability through supportive environments, builds on family strengths rather than simply remediating deficits, and has the potential to improve the care of entire patient populations rather than single individuals or families. The expanded service delivery model requires clinicians to consider the following aspects of care: (1) family-centered care; (2) universal screening in primary care settings; (3) interdisciplinary team interactions; (4) systematic program development; and (5) funding changes.

Family-Centered Care

This approach to clinical care emphasizes the importance of building partnerships with families and assessing not only child and family functioning but also the social and environmental context in which they live. Taking the family's perspective results in an increased awareness of contextual factors that create family strain, such as educators who are not familiar with effective ways to develop an individualized plan for children with acquired brain injuries, health insurance plans that refuse or delay the purchase of standard medical equipment for children with physical impairments, or health care specialists who recommend conflicting treatment strategies and fail to resolve these differences. Such contextual barriers are potentially modifiable. For example, a child neuropsychologist practicing family-centered care might find that an 8-year-old girl born at very low birth weight has unidentified neurocognitive problems that require special education supports, and that her single mother is overwhelmed by other health problems and financial strain in the family. Specific recommendations might include ways educators can address the child's learning and behavioral needs, and strategies for the parent to access community resources and supports (e.g., respite care through public agency sources or other informal supports from coworkers or at church). By facilitating linkages across microsystems in this way, the neuropsychologist promotes comprehensive, family-centered care. Naar-King and Donders (Chapter 9, this volume) provide more information about this model of service delivery.

Universal Screening

Although not every child and family will require intensive services, all children with chronic conditions and their families should be screened for medical, mental health, educational, vocational, and social needs to provide adequate supports (Drotar et al., 2001; Farmer et al., 2004; Kazak et al., 2003a). Primary care providers, such as pediatricians and school nurses, may be the optimal professionals to conduct such screenings, since they are most likely to see the full range of children with chronic conditions, but any clinic that interacts regularly with this group of children may engage in the screening process to ensure comprehensive care. Psychologists can play an important role in the development and use of screening instruments to identify those who need referral for more in-depth, interdisciplinary care (Drotar et al., 2001; Farmer, Marien, & Frasier, 2003b; Seid et al., 2004).

Interdisciplinary Teams

Interdisciplinary teams encourage thorough assessment of child and family needs, effective communication regarding treatment plans across disciplines, and partnerships across systems of care (e.g., between hospital and school personnel; mental health and primary care providers). Psychologists are well qualified to facilitate the development of collaborative teams and to encourage shared leadership roles based on the specific needs of the child and family (Frank, Hagglund, & Farmer, 2004). For individual children, psychologists can promote team interactions by consulting with other health professionals, educators, and agency personnel during the assessment process. Furthermore, staffings prior to discharge from rehabilitation or interpretive feedback sessions following neuropsychological assessment are key opportunities to include the child's community service providers, and to identify common goals and treatment strategies across systems of care.

Program Development

At the program level, psychologists can shape the development and evaluation of service delivery practices that encourage comprehensive, family-centered care (Illback, Cobb, & Joseph, 1997). As an example, Farmer and Muhlenbruck (2001) described the programmatic use of telehealth technologies to change the structure and process of care for children with special health care needs. These advanced telecommunication systems are especially useful for children who live in rural and underserved areas, since they increase access to specialty care. They also allow coordinated treatment planning with community providers and family members who otherwise would be unlikely to participate due to geographic distance from the tertiary care center.

Funding Changes

Equally important is the identification of new mechanisms to fund care coordination, interdisciplinary team interactions, telehealth contacts, and other systems interventions that promote health and prevent unwarranted disability. To accomplish these kinds of changes, psychologists will need to become more involved in at the "macrosystem" level, where legislative action determines public policy related to reimbursement for innovative health services (Bronfenbrenner, 1979; Kazak et al., 2003b). Alternative sources of funding may need to be sought, such as from managed care organizations and other public agencies that have a stake in promoting the health and well-being of children with chronic conditions.

FUTURE RESEARCH DIRECTIONS

Although research findings from programs that provide comprehensive and coordinated care suggest improvements in child and family outcomes, these studies have many methodological limitations (Drotar et al., 2001; Smith,

Layne, & Garell, 1994; Liptak, Burns, Davidson, & McAnarney, 1998). The studies typically use convenience samples with unknown selection biases, and like many other programs in pediatric psychology, most have not met standard research design criteria for intervention studies (Stinson, McGrath, & Yamada, 2003). Common treatment components exist, but there is no standard approach to intervention or evaluation, which makes it challenging to compare results across studies. It is also unclear which of the components account for the improvements observed. Furthermore, very few studies investigate the maintenance of treatment effects, though the available evidence suggests that there may be a long-term impact on children's mental health (e.g., Stein & Jessop, 1991). Future research must address these methodological shortcomings.

In addition, in the current context of limited resources for health service delivery, it is essential to identify differing levels of psychosocial supports that can be tailored to the various needs of families of children with chronic conditions. Some studies, but not all, suggest that families of children with more complex needs may benefit most from intensive care coordination interventions (Farmer et al., 2005; Palfrey et al., 2004; Stein, 2001). Other studies show that family needs are related not only to level of child functioning but also to variables such as social support and perceptions of burden (e.g., Farmer et al., 2004; Kazak et al., 2003a). In the study of children with cancer, Kazak and colleagues found that family psychosocial risk factors may determine whether supports such as care coordination are adequate, or if more intensive individualized mental health treatment is likely to be needed. Additional research on how to tailor each family's level of support is likely to result in quality improvements in the systems of care that maximize child health and functioning at a manageable cost.

REFERENCES

American Academy of Pediatrics. (2002). Policy statement: The medical home. *Pediatrics, 110*, 184–186.

Bronfenbrenner, U. (1979). *The ecology of human development.* Cambridge, MA: Harvard University Press.

Brown, R. T. (2004). Introduction: Changes in the provision of health care to children and adolescents. In *Handbook of pediatric psychology in school settings* (pp. 1–19). Mahwah, NJ: Erlbaum.

Chernoff, R., Ireys, H. T., DeVet, K. A., & Kim, Y. J. (2002). A randomized, controlled trial of a community-based support program for families of children with chronic illness: Pediatric outcomes. *Archives of Pediatric and Adolescent Medicine, 156*, 533–539.

Coburn, A. F., McBride, T. D., & Ziller, E. C. (2002). Patterns of health insurance coverage among rural and urban children. *Medical Care Research and Review, 59,* 272–292.

Cooley, W. C. (2004). Redefining primary pediatric care for children with special health care needs: The primary medical home. *Current Opinion in Pediatrics, 16,* 689–692.

Davidson, E. J., Silva, T. J., Sofis, L. A., Ganz, M. L., & Palfrey, J. S. (2002). The doctor's dilemma: Challenges for primary care physicians caring for the child with special health care needs. *Ambulatory Pediatrics, 2,* 218–223.

Deidrick, K. M., & Farmer, J. E. (in press). School reentry following traumatic brain injury. *Preventing School Failure.*

Drotar, D. (2001). Promoting comprehensive care for children with chronic health conditions and their families: Introduction to the special issue. *Children's Services: Social Policy, Research, and Practice, 4,* 157–163.

Drotar, D., Walders, N., Burgess, E., Nobile, C., Dasari, M., Kahana, S., et al. (2001). Recommendations to enhance comprehensive care for children with chronic health conditions and their families. *Children's Services: Social Policy, Research, and Practice, 4,* 251–265.

Dunst, C. J. (1997). Conceptual and empirical foundations of family-centered practice. In R. J. Illback, C. T. Cobb, & H. M. Joseph, Jr. (Eds.), *Integrated services for children and families: Opportunities for psychological practice* (pp. 75–91). Washington, DC: American Psychological Association.

Farmer, J. E., Clark, M. J., & Marien, W. E. (2003a). Building systems of care for children with chronic health conditions. *Rehabilitation Psychology, 48,* 242–249.

Farmer, J. E., Clark, M. J., Marien, W. E., Sherman, A., & Selva, T. J. (2005). Comprehensive primary care for children with special health care needs in rural areas. *Pediatrics, 116,* 1–8.

Farmer, J. E., Marien, W. E., Clark, M. J., Sherman, A., & Selva, T. J. (2004). Primary care supports for children with chronic health conditions: Identifying and predicting unmet family needs. *Journal of Pediatric Psychology, 29,* 355–367.

Farmer, J. E., Marien, W., & Frasier, L. (2003b). Quality improvements in primary care for children with special health care needs: Use of a brief screening measure. *Children's Health Care, 32,* 273–285.

Farmer, J. E., & Muhlenbruck, L. (2001). Telehealth for children with special health care needs: Promoting comprehensive systems of care. *Clinical Pediatrics, 40,* 93–98.

Frank, R. G., Hagglund, K., & Farmer, J. E. (2004). Chronic illness management in primary care: The cardinal symptoms model. In R. G. Frank, S. H. McDaniel, J. H. Bray, & M. Heldring (Eds.), *Primary care psychology* (pp. 159–275). Washington, DC: American Psychological Association.

Illback, R. J., Cobb, C. T., & Joseph, H. M. (1997). *Integrated services for children and families: Opportunities for psychological practice.* Washington, DC: American Psychological Association.

Ireys, H. T., Chernoff, R., DeVet, K. A., & Kim, Y. (2001). Maternal outcomes of a randomized controlled trial of a community-based support program for families of children with chronic illness. *Archives of Pediatric and Adolescent Medicine, 155,* 771–777.

Kazak, A. E., Cant, C., Jenson, M. M., McSherry, M., Rourke, M. T., Hwang, W., et al. (2003a). Identifying psychosocial risk indicative of subsequent resource use in families of newly diagnosed pediatric oncology patients. *Journal of Clinical Oncology, 21,* 3220–3225.

Kazak, A. E., Rourke, M. T., & Crump, T. A. (2003b). Families and other systems in pediatric psychology. In M. C. Roberts (Ed.), *Handbook of pediatric psychology* (3rd ed., pp. 159–175). New York: Guilford Press.

King, S., King, G., & Rosenbaum, P. (2004). Evaluating health service delivery to children with chronic conditions and their families: Development of a refined measure of processes of care (MPOC-20). *Children's Health Care, 33,* 35–57.

Krauss, M. W., Wells, N., Gulley, S., & Anderson, B. (2001). Navigating systems of care: Results from a national survey of families of children with special health care needs. *Children's Services: Social Policy, Research, and Practice, 4,* 165–187.

Lin, C. J., & Lave, J. R. (2000). Utilization under children's health insurance programs: Children with vs. without chronic conditions. *Journal of Health Social Policy, 11,* 1–14.

Liptak, G. S., Burns, C. M., Davidson, P. W., & McAnarney, E. R. (1998). Effects of providing comprehensive ambulatory services to children with chronic conditions. *Archives of Pediatric and Adolescent Medicine, 152,* 1003–1008.

McMenamy, J. M., & Perrin, E. C. (2004). Integrating psychology into pediatrics: The past, the present, and the potential. *Family Systems and Health, 20,* 153–160.

McPherson, M., Arango, P., Fox, H., Lauver, C., McManus, M., Newacheck, P. W., et al. (1998). A new definition of children with special health care needs. *Pediatrics, 102,* 137–140.

Mrazek, P. G., & Haggerty, R. J. (Eds.). (1994). *Reducing risks for mental disorders: Frontiers for preventive intervention research.* Washington, DC: National Academy Press.

Naar-King, S., Siegel, P. T., Smyth, M., & Simpson, P. (2003). An evaluation of an integrated health care program for children with special needs. *Children's Health Care, 32,* 233–243.

Newacheck, P. W., Inkelas, M., & Kim, S. E. (2004). Health services use and health care expenditures for children with disabilities. *Pediatrics, 114,* 79–85.

Nordahl, K. C., Copans, S. A., & Stamm, B. H. (2003). Children and adolescents in rural and frontier areas. In B. H. Stamm (Ed.), *Rural behavioral health care* (pp. 159–170). Washington, DC: American Psychological Association.

Palfrey, J. S., Sofis, L. A., Davidson, E. J., Liu, J., Freeman, L., & Ganz, M. L. (2004). The Pediatric Alliance for Coordinated Care: Evaluation of a medical home model. *Pediatrics, 113,* 1507–1516.

Pless, I. B., Feeley, N., Gottlieb, L., Rowat, K., Dougherty, G., & Willard, B. (1994). A randomized trial of a nursing intervention to promote the adjustment of children with chronic physical disorders. *Pediatrics, 94,* 70–75.

Power, T. J., & Blom-Hoffman, J. (2004). The school as a venue for managing and preventing health problems: Opportunities and challenges. In R. T. Brown (Ed.), *Handbook of pediatric psychology in school settings* (pp. 37–48). Mahwah, NJ: Erlbaum.

Schneiderman, N., & Speers, M. A. (1998). Behavioral science, social science, and public health in the 21st century. In N. Schneiderman, M. A. Speers, J. M. Silva, J. Tomes, & J. H. Gentry (Eds.), *Integrating behavioral and social sciences with public health* (pp. 3–28). Washington, DC: American Psychological Association.

Seid, M., Sobo, E. J., Gelhard, L. R., & Varni, J. W. (2004). Parent reports of barriers to care for children with special health care needs: Development and validation of the Barriers to Care Questionnaire. *Ambulatory Pediatrics, 4*, 323–331.

Semrud-Clikeman, M. (2001). *Traumatic brain injury in children and adolescents: Assessment and intervention.* New York: Guilford Press.

Shapiro, E. S., & Manz, P. H. (2004). Collaborating with schools in the provision of pediatric psychological services. In R. T. Brown (Ed.), *Handbook of pediatric psychology in school settings* (pp. 49–64). Mahwah, NJ: Erlbaum.

Shi, L., & Singh, D. A. (2001). *Delivering health care in America: A systems approach* (2nd ed.). Gaithersburg, MD: Aspen.

Silva, J. M., Sofis, L. A., & Palfrey, J. S. (2000). *Practicing comprehensive care: A physician's operations manual for implementing a medical home for children with special health care needs.* Boston: Institute for Community Inclusion.

Smith, K., Layne, M., & Garell, D. (1994). The impact of care coordination on children with special health care needs. *Children's Health Care, 23*, 251–266.

Spirito, A., Brown, R. T., D'Angelo, E., Delmater, A., Rodrigue, J., & Lawrence, S. (2003). Society for pediatric psychology task force report: Recommendations for the training of pediatric psychologists. *Journal of Pediatric Psychology, 28*, 85–98.

Stein, R. E. K. (2001). Home-based comprehensive care services for children with chronic conditions. *Children's Services: Social Policy, Research, and Practice, 4*, 189–201.

Stein, R. E. K., & Jessop, D. J. (1991). Long-term mental health effects of a pediatric home care program. *Pediatrics, 88*, 490–496.

Stille, C. J., & Antonelli, R. C. (2004). Coordination of care for children with special health care needs. *Current Opinion in Pediatrics, 16*, 700–705.

Stinson, J. N., McGrath, P. J., & Yamada, J. T. (2003). Clinical trials in the *Journal of Pediatric Psychology*: Applying the CONSORT statement. *Journal of Pediatric Psychology, 28*, 159–167.

U.S. Department of Health and Human Services, Health Resources and Services Administration (1999). *Measuring success for Healthy People 2010: National agenda for children with special health care needs.* Washington, DC: Author.

Wallander, J. L., Thompson, R. J., Jr., & Alriksson-Schmidt, A. (2003). Psychosocial adjustment of children with chronic physical conditions. In M. C. Roberts (Ed.), *Handbook of pediatric psychology* (3rd ed., pp. 141–158). New York: Guilford Press.

Weller, W. E., Minkovitz, C. S., & Anderson, G. F. (2003). Utilization of medical and health-related services among school-age children and adolescents with special health care needs (1994 National Health Interview Survey on Disability [NHIS-D] Baseline Data). *Pediatrics, 112,* 593–603.

World Health Organization. (2001). *International classification of functioning, disability, and health: ICF.* Geneva: Author.

Wright, P. W. D., & Wright, P. D. (2004). *Wrightslaw: Special education law.* Hartfield, VA: Harbor House Law Press.

16

Cultural Perspectives in Pediatric Rehabilitation

RUBEN J. ECHEMENDÍA
MICHAEL WESTERVELD

The United States is becoming increasingly ethnoculturally diverse. Population statistics reveal that the white population is growing at a much slower rate than other groups. According to U.S. census data (U.S. Bureau of the Census, 2000), the white population in the U.S. grew at a rate of 8.6% between 1990 and 2000. In contrast, the black population grew by 21.5%, Hispanics/Latinos grew by 57.9%, American Indian/Alaska Natives grew by 110.3%, the Asian population increased its numbers by 72.2%, and Native Hawaiians increased by 139.5%. These numbers clearly emphasize the growing diversity within our culture. Importantly, the numbers of ethnic and racially diverse children are growing at a much faster rate than their white counterparts, and minority children comprise a significantly higher proportion of their respective populations than do white children. The 2000 census data indicate that 23.5% of the white population is under the age of 18, whereas 31.4% of blacks, 33.9% of American Indians/Alaska Natives, 24.1% of Asians, 31.9% of Native Hawaiians. and 35% of Hispanics/Latinos are 17 years of age or younger (U.S. Bureau of the Census, 2000).

As the numbers of racial and ethnic minorities grow, the number of these children with developmental or acquired neurological impairments will also grow. This presents a significant challenge to neuropsychology in general but to pediatric neuropsychology in particular, simply because the vast majority of U.S. neuropsychologists are white and English-speaking, and rely largely on Eurocentric models of mind–body relationships (Echemendía, 2004). Eurocentric models emphasize the importance of the individual as opposed to collective models in which the welfare of the group (family, tribe, community) takes precedence over the needs of the individual. In order to best serve these children and their families, we need to gain an appreciation for the cultural diversity within all of us, while becoming cognizant of the impact of these differences on injury rates, diagnoses, survival, assessment, and rehabilitation. Often, there exists as much or more variability within a cultural group than between cultural groups. Manly and her colleagues 2005, as well as others (Lucas, 1998; Kennepohl, Shore, Nabors, & Hanks, in press) have demonstrated that differences in neuropsychological test scores among elders of the same ethnic group are related to a variety of cultural factors. For example, Manly et al. (1998b) found that scores on the Wechsler Adult Intelligence Scale–Revised (WAIS-R) among neurologically intact African Americans varied as a function of level of acculturation with those who were less acculturated obtaining lower scores than those with higher levels of acculturation. Similarly, Arnold, Montgomery, Casteneda, and Langoria (1994) found that performance on the Halstead–Reitan Neuropsychological Test Battery varied in relation to levels of acculturation among Hispanic college students.

Understanding cultural variability within and between groups is not simply a matter of sensitivity and making patients comfortable, but an issue of efficacy in health care provision. Although there has been minimal research directly addressing the role of cultural sensitivity in treatment and rehabilitation of pediatric brain injury, there is some general evidence that cultural sensitivity training programs not only improve awareness and sensitivity of health care providers to patient needs but also improve health outcomes (Majumdar Browne, Roberts, & Carpio, 2004). To this end, we review the role of cultural influences on the assessment and rehabilitation process. Rather than discuss and describe issues that are specific to only one group of people, (e.g., blacks or Latino/as), we focus on issues that are common among most cultural groups. These issues include acculturation, socioeconomic status, language, and education.

THE INDIVIDUAL IN CONTEXT

Most texts of cultural neuropsychology have chapters that describe the major ethnic and racial groups in the United States, and the similarities and differences among these groups and in comparison to a reference white group. This approach is useful in helping a reader become acquainted with some of the nuances that exist between cultures. However, just as group data cannot always be applied to a specific individual, knowledge of general group characteristics is insufficient for understanding the role of culture in any given patient. The use of group terms often obscures the variability that exists within groups. For example, Wong and Fujii (2004) estimate that there are 32 distinct cultural groups within the category of Asian and Pacific Islander, each with its own customs and practices that augment similarities in racial features and cultural values. Similarly, Harris, Echemendía, Ardila, and Rosselli (2001) point out that there are 556 American Indian tribes and Alaska Native entities with 135 American Indian and 20 Alaska Native languages. Hispanics and Latinos in the United States hail from a broad range of countries that share a common language but differ greatly in their sociocultural and sociopolitical perspectives. When differences in immigration patterns and in race, identification with native culture, and other factors are added, the complexity of understanding the individual's cultural history begins to unfold.

An often disregarded aspect of cultural differences is the variability within what is considered to be white America. Although we tend to focus on the historically identified "minority" groups, consider that there exist marked differences within the broad U.S. culture. These differences are evident across geographic regions (e.g., North vs. South, rural vs. urban), political perspectives, religious beliefs and practices, education, and socioeconomic status, to name but a few. These differences transcend ethnic and racial classification. Thus, differences in cultural variables are the rule rather than the exception, and we must attempt to understand the extent to which our patients are similar to, or different from, the cultural group to which they are being compared.

Many of the variables associated with culture are quite complex. This complexity may result in definitional ambiguity at best, and at worst, inaccurate attributions that may result in misdiagnosis and inadequate or inappropriate treatment. Helms (1995, 1997) has argued convincingly that race is a poorly defined variable, since it conveys a biological distinctiveness that has yet to be found. Zuckerman (1990) asserts that race is a construct in search of scientific support. Scientific data have shown that there is more genetic variability within races than between them (Wilkinson & King, 1987). Given its lack of biologically identifiable distinctiveness, race appears to be best understood as a sociopolitical construct.

Our challenges in grasping the variability in cultural expressions are magnified by the variability that exists in individual expression of neuropathology. As Heaton and Pendleton (1981) have observed, "No two brain damaged patients are alike in terms of their pattern of ability deficits and strengths, the requirements of their daily lives, or other factors (past experiences, social support system, financial resources, etc.) that may influence success in everyday functioning" (p. 815). Taken together, these individual differences in culture and neuropathology emphasize the need for comprehensive and detailed assessment of the patient in order to develop a truly individualized plan for rehabilitation.

ASSESSMENT

For children with neurodevelopmental conditions, assessment of neuropsychological status often plays a critical role in planning and conducting rehabilitation. It should be obvious, then, that issues pertaining to cultural and ethnic differences in assessment also become relevant to treatment. Consider that interventions often employ a deficit reduction model (e.g., improvement in the deficient skill through practice and training), a compensatory model (e.g., improvement in functional status through development of compensation using areas of strength), or a combination of these. If the assessment of deficits and skills is biased, or reflects issues (e.g., language differences) other than the neuropsychological status of the individual, it will be difficult to plan the most effective interventions.

Neuropsychological assessment within a multicultural context presents a formidable challenge. Many variables must be considered, including the patient's familiarity and comfort with the testing situation, test construction, normative data, test translation and adaptation, and the functional equivalence of cognitive tasks across cultural groups. A thorough discussion of these factors is beyond the scope of this chapter (see Bracken & Barona, 1991; Ferraro, 2002; Geisinger, 1994); however, there are specific issues related to test selection, normative data, and test translation that we wish to underscore.

First, there is the issue of test selection and the use of appropriate normative data. It is routine for U.S. neuropsychologists to use measures developed and normed in one culture with individuals from a different culture (Echemendía & Julian, 2002). For example, Echemendía and Harris (2004) surveyed U.S. neuropsychologists and found that the tests used with bilingual and monolingual Spanish speakers did not differ from those used with English speakers. Moreover, these practitioners usually applied norms that were developed on English speakers, irrespective of the linguistic status of the patient being tested. Geisinger (1994) argues that the use of U.S. norms with linguistically and culturally different populations should be avoided. If it must occur, then a very good (preferably empirically supported) reason must be offered. This issue is particularly salient with children, since cultural variables may differentially affect cognitive development.

The use of culturally specific norms is not without controversy. Manly, Byrd, Touradji, and Stern (2004) argue that the use of separate norm groups "may leave ethnic differences in test performance unexplained, unexamined, and thus not understood" (p. 38), although they do concede that the use of ethnic-specific norms will likely reduce misdiagnosis of cognitive impairment. Similarly, it may be argued that it is important to use English norms when assessing the cognitive or academic skills of a child in relation to his or her classmates. Although there are no easy answers to this issue, it appears that the most parsimonious approach is to use the referral question or reason for testing to guide the test selection process. If the purpose of the evaluation is to understand the child's cognitive strengths and weaknesses following a neurological event, then the use of culture-specific tests and norms is warranted. If, on the other hand, the purpose of the assessment is to determine this child's ability in a given content area relative to his or her peers in school, then standard English normative data (to the extent they reflect the local culture) would be most appropriate. In the latter situation, there needs to be careful interpretation of the test data, since children's test scores may represent not only their knowledge of the content area but also their familiarity with the testing situation, their approach to the tests, and their ability to understand and follow directions.

Test translation and adaptation remain crucial issues in cultural neuropsychology. Echemendía and Harris (2004) found that it was common practice for U.S. neuropsychologists who evaluate monolingual Spanish speakers to translate tests extemporaneously while testing the patient, or to translate a test and then use this translated version with Spanish speaking patients. Our experience is that this practice is not limited to the evaluation of Spanish speakers but is widespread when testing linguistically diverse populations. Although this practice usually results from frustration with the lack of formally translated tests, it remains quite problematic. Specifically, extemporaneous or idiosyncratic translations by neuropsychologists or translators employed by them do not provide the required careful study of test items and their cultural nuances; there is no opportunity to pilot or adapt the items, there is no back translation to ensure equivalence, and there are no psychometric data to assess the validity and reliability of the items. Similarly, direct translation of a measure often is problematic, because many words and phrases cannot be translated directly (Bracken & Barona, 1991). Many have argued that cultural adaptation and modification of a test are superior to the process of direct translation and back translation (cf. Padilla, 1979; Geinsinger, 1994). Van de Vijver and Hambleton (1996) have published guidelines from the International Test Commission for the translation and adaptation of tests from one culture to another. In addition to stating that the translation process should avoid bias and be guided by a thorough understanding of the culture and language, they stress that the materials, methods, and techniques of administration should be familiar to the target population, and that ecological validity must be statistically determined.

An associated topic involves the use of translators. This is a highly controversial area in psychology, with passionate discourse on each side of the discussion (e.g., Artiola, Fortuny, & Mullaney, 1998). There is little argument that in an ideal world, every bilingual/bicultural patient would be assessed by a bilingual/bicultural neuropsychologist who has access to well-developed and well-normed neuropsychological instruments. Reality imposes upon us the fact that because the number of bicultural/bilingual neuropsychologists is miniscule relative to the number of patients needing services, translators need to be employed. However, it is critical that the neuropsychologist spend time training the translator on neuropsychological test practices. The difference between assessment and rehabilitation also brings forth an interesting issue regarding the use of translators. Although the inclusion of family members during the course of rehabilitation has been shown to be a key predictor of outcomes (see Chapter 9; this volume), the use of family members in the role of translators during neuropsychological assessment should be strongly discouraged because of their natural desire to "help" the child when he or she is unsure of an answer or even to correct the child's incorrect answer.

ACCULTURATION

Acculturation is the process by which individuals from one culture are exposed to and begin to integrate the behaviors, modes of communications, thoughts, and feelings of a new culture. According to Harris et al. (2001), the values and expectations expressed within a given culture will have a significant impact on "the process and outcome of cognitive and neuropsychological assessment (p. 395)." We will argue that culture also plays a significant role in the process of rehabilitation and that well-conceived culturally oriented plans of intervention lead to better outcomes. Berry (1988) asserts that cognitive values are "the set of cognitive goals which are collectively shared and toward which children are socialized in a particular society. It is essential to understand these goals, since one cannot assess how far a person has gotten unless one understands where he is going" (p. 12). Consider the development of an Individualized Education Plan for a child from a culturally diverse background. There are some approaches whereby either knowingly or unknowingly, increased acculturation is one of the goals of rehabilitation in a brain injured child. The goal is to help them to "fit" better within school, which has become the primary method for integrating children into the dominant culture, and increasingly in our society includes teaching of values and so forth. Through formal schoolwork and peer contact at school, the child begins to adopt the host culture's attitudes, beliefs, and values. While this approach may help a child become a better student and increase peer relationships, it may also create alienation and even rebellion against parents who wish to maintain their traditional cultural values. This source of conflict may serve to undermine the recovery–treatment process.

As we emphasize throughout this chapter, the extent to which a child has incorporated a new culture, abandoned an old culture, or is identified with an existing culture or subculture is critical in understanding test scores and planning successful rehabilitation strategies. Any discussion of acculturation requires a few definitions. Marín (1992) differentiates between assimilation and biculturality. "Assimilation" is a unidirectional process by which the individual moves away from the original culture and toward the new culture. "Biculturality", on the hand, involves learning the values, behaviors, and qualities of the new culture, while simultaneously maintaining all or part of the cultural components of the original culture. Biculturality allows the child to function effectively within both cultures, while not feeling the need to distance him- or herself from the host culture. However, it is important to underscore the fact that pressure to assimilate is often intensely experienced by children and adolescents who seek to be less "different" than their majority culture peers. This pressure differs developmentally as a function of age, social pressures, the degree to which the child is "different from" peers, and his or her self-view.

Acculturation involves a highly individualized, dynamic interaction of variables whose outcome is neither static nor complete. Rehabilitation is also a dynamic complex process that is significantly affected by the individual's view of him- or herself not only in relation to his or her own development and relationships with others, but also with respect to changes in personality and self-identity that stem from the brain injury. An individual's view of him- or herself is also complicated by racial and ethnic identity. Identification with one's race differs from identification with one's ethnicity, yet both have an impact on the acculturation process. As we have stated earlier, although race is believed to be biologically determined, it has virtually no independent behavioral, biological, or social implications (Casas, 1984). An individual's or group's beliefs and feelings about a racial group can have profound implications for intrapersonal and interpersonal functioning (Helms, 1990). Ethnic identity is not biologically based. It relates to an individual's identification with "a group of individuals who share a unique social and cultural heritage (customs, language, religion, and so on) passed on from generation to generation" (Casas, 1984, p. 787). Both racial identity and ethnic identity are not static and usually progress along a developmental continuum. Furthermore, identification with a racial or ethnic group varies as a matter of degree for each person. Since race and ethnicity are not equivalent, a young patient may struggle with issues related to both. For example, a young, dark-skinned Latino patient may struggle with acceptance from his black friends because he is judged to be Latino and not black. On the other hand, he is judged to be black and not Hispanic by his Latino friends. Now, add to this conundrum the fact that this young man has suffered a traumatic brain injury, which makes him even more different than his peers. This is further complicated by the fact that cultural factors influence our understanding of brain dysfunction. Ackerman and Banks (2002) observed that a person's understanding of neurological impairment may be strongly influenced by cultural values and by spiritual and religious beliefs. These beliefs may determine whether the brain dysfunction is "a challenge to be overcome, a deserved punishment or fate" (p. 388). Racial and ethnic groups may also vary widely in their ability to accept cognitive, physical, and motor limitations in a brain-injured person. For example, traditional Latino males view the role of the male as being strong and independent, neither needing nor requesting assistance, even when it is needed. This oftentimes fiercely independent streak collides with the needs of the neurologically impaired adolescent, who now must rely on others for activities of daily living. Here the cultural and developmental issues interact in a way that further intensifies the individual's challenges, since the adolescent is also likely to be struggling with issues of independence that are orthogonal to the cultural expression of independence. A failure to identify these struggles will lead to needless complications in the rehabilitation process and missed opportunities for important work with the adolescent and his family, who may also be struggling differentially with their son's traumatic brain injury, because of their own culturally laden views of independence, self-worth, and sex role identification. Thus, the impact of acculturation, and racial and ethnic identification, on an individual's intra- and interpersonal functioning should not be underestimated.

The Measurement of Acculturation

The assessment and measurement of acculturation is complex, although several scales are available for use in rehabilitation settings (e.g. Sabogal, Marín, Otero-Sabogal, & Perez-Stable, 1987; Helms, 1990; Wong, Strickland, Fletcher-Janzen, Aidila, & Reynolds, 2000). Unfortunately, there are few empirically derived, developmentally appropriate scales of acculturation for use with children, although some do exist (Barona & Miller, 1994; Cuellar, Harris, & Jasso, 1980; Epstein et al., 1996; Tropp et al., 1999). However, careful interviewing and data collection from multiple sources will allow the pediatric neuropsychologist to generate a comprehensive view of the child's level of acculturation, as well as the level of acculturation of family members. Important variables to assess are as follows:

Cultural Perspectives in Pediatric Rehabilitation

- To what extent do the child and parent share the same cultural values?
- What language does the child speak at home, with friends, at school?
- How comfortable is the child with the English language? To what extent is he or she bilingual?
- With whom does the child play/hang out?
- Is the neighborhood ethnically and racially diverse or culturally homogeneous? Is the school ethnically and racially diverse? Are there resources for English as a second language? Are there bilingual/bicultural counselors?
- What music does the child listen to? How does he or she dress?
- At what age did the child immigrate to the United States?

In assessing the parents, the following variables are important:

- Why did the family emigrate? How did it immigrate?
- What is the parents' level of education?
- What was their socioeconomic status in their native country?
- What is the parents' occupational history?
- What are the parents' attitudes toward education?
- What is their familiarity with U.S. school systems?
- What are their expectations for their child's education?
- What is the role of the child in the family?
- What resources (financial, social, health insurance, etc.) are available to the parents?
- To what extent are the parents familiar with and what are their attitudes toward the health care system, service providers, and neuropsychological testing?
- Do they understand the child's injury, the course of recovery, and the goals of rehabilitation? Do they share those goals?
- What are the parents' views of physical, motor, and cognitive limitations, and how do these views interact with their ability to support and accept their child?

SOCIOECONOMIC STATUS

The socioeconomic status (SES) of parents is an important variable to evaluate. The data are clear that ethnic and racially diverse groups are overrepresented at lower SES levels compared to their white counterparts (Echemendía & Julian, 2002). The data are also quite clear that SES has direct impact on neuropsychological test functioning and, hence, the pattern of strengths and deficits that are the targets of the rehabilitation process. SES can have an impact on cognitive performance in myriad ways, a review of which is beyond the scope of this chapter. However, it is important to recognize that SES can affect a child at the very basic levels of nutrition and safety, which can have long-term consequences in cognitive development. SES also has an impact on the value, quality, and attitudes that children and their parents have toward education. These attitudes can have dramatic influences on an individual's perception of neurological dysfunction. For example, it is not unusual for adolescents with sports-related traumatic brain injuries to place their goals for a future in professional sports ahead of their neurological integrity. In one situation, a young, very promising high school football player, with a history of multiple sports-related concussions and persistent postconcussion symptoms, said, "Doc, I really don't care about my brain. You can care about my brain if you want to, but football is the only way I can get out of this place [rural, poor]."

It is also important to underscore that there is much variability within ethnic and racial groups in SES. Although membership in a racial or ethnic minority increases the probability of being represented in a lower tier socioeconomically, there are many affluent, well-educated members of these groups as well.

EDUCATION

On the surface, it would appear that formal education is a relatively easy variable to operationalize. The most common measure of education is the number of years of formal schooling. Unfortunately, this variable is complicated by the significant variability that exists within and between educational systems. This is particularly true if a child has received part of his or her education in a school system outside of the United States. Puente, Sol Mora, and Muno-Cespedes (1997) have urged caution in interpreting the educational level of those educated outside of the United States, because of the lack of equivalence in educational systems. Not only do differences exist between foreign-educated students and U.S.-educated students, but there are also significant differences within countries. For example, the educational systems that exist in most urban centers are distinctly different than those in rural areas. There are also significant differences in the degree to which cultures place an emphasis on private versus public education. For example, affluent parents in Latin America expose their children to an educational system in which they learn English at a very early age. Students are also exposed to and have the resources to obtain United States fashion, music, and pop culture. Students in rural areas rarely have these opportunities. Even within the United States, there are marked differences among urban, suburban, rural, public and private schools. Indeed, Manly et al. (1998a, 1998b, 1999, 2004) have conducted elegant research that demonstrates how the quality of education can explain cognitive test score differences between black and white elders matched on years of education. Their data also demonstrate that age, years of education, acculturation, and reading ability each contribute independent sources of variance to neuropsychological test scores across many cognitive domains.

Education has been related to cultural factors and neuropsychological test performance in a variety of cross-cultural studies (Pontón et al., 1996; Ardila, Rosselli, & Otrosky, 1992; Ardila, Rosselli, & Rosas, 1989; Lecours, Mehler, & Parente, 1987). An often promulgated key misconception is that patients with limited formal education, literacy, and linguistic skills will perform poorly on measures of verbal functioning, but their performance on nonverbal tasks will be unaffected. Ardila et al. (1989), and Rosselli, Ardila, and Rosas (1990) have demonstrated that illiterate individuals perform worse on a wide range of neuropsychological measures, including measure of visuospatial functioning, when compared to their literate counterparts. Similarly, Manly and her colleagues (1999) found that illiterate elders performed poorly on measures of visual matching and recognition relative to their literate peers.

Perez-Arce and Puente (1996) discuss differential maturation of functional scholastic behaviors. They posit that stages of readiness to learn and readiness to acquire literary skills are facilitated by the stimulation that occurs in literate environments. Consequently, children who have been raised in illiterate or "transient" environments may be significantly delayed when they enter U.S. schools. Similarly, the development of writing skills has been thought to facilitate a variety of cognitive tasks and is not limited to facilitating visuomotor, visuospatial, fine motor, and graphomotor skills (Harris et al., 2001).

Piaget's (1928) theory assumes homogeneity in cognitive development across cultures. Empirical evidence suggests that this assertion is incorrect. Shade (1991) has shown that black children show differences in categorization (e.g. word lists, pictures, etc.) when compared to whites. These culturally based differences regarding the emphasis on details versus Gestalt, perceptual (attributes of an object) versus conceptual (categorical), and functional versus descriptive factors may have profound implications for scores on neuropsychological tests (Manly & Jacobs, 2004). For example, Bruner, Oliver, and Greenfield (1966) compared uneducated, rural Senegalese children with urban, educated (French-style) children on quantity conservation. The uneducated children relied on perceptual explanations of the phenomenon, whereas the educated children relied on conceptual explanations. Interestingly, the uneducated children were able to learn the conceptual manner of explanation after a short period of formal training. Similarly, de Lemos (1965) studied Aboriginal children and found that they exhibited differential levels of cognitive development when compared to other children. These findings suggest that cultural factors can have an impact on the cognitive development of children. In support of this observation, Kaufman (1990) has commented that cognitive abilities which presumably progress along similar lines of development across cultures, are highly dependent on factors such as verbal exchange.

Taken together, these studies underscore the importance of evaluating a child's education experience using a multifaceted approach that includes the quality, nature, and extent of those experiences, as well as the child's and parents' attitude toward education.

LANGUAGE

Speaking a language that is different from that spoken in the majority culture is probably the most readily apparent index of cultural differences. It does not require scientific training to recognize the challenges faced by individuals who are unable to communicate their wishes, needs, and desires effectively to the majority of people around them. In the rehabilitation context, language plays a very significant role since many patients experience disturbances in expressive and receptive language as a result of either brain trauma or neurodevelopmental delays.

Although an important first step, asking whether the child speaks English is not sufficient. It is important to assess how long the child has been speaking English; his or her proficiency in speaking, reading, and writing English; and when he or she speaks English, with whom and how often. The fact that the child does speak English does not mean that he or she can speak English and his or her native language equally well. Research has demonstrated that the so-called "balanced bilingual" may not exist, since bilinguals tend to have greater facility with one language or the other (Manuel-Dupont, Ardila, Rosselli, & Puente, 1992; Hickey, 1972; Harris, Cullum, & Puente, 1995). It is important to formally assess a child's relative proficiency in both English and their native language. Several measures have been developed for this purpose. For example, based on a normative sample of 5,602 subjects, the Bilingual Verbal Ability Test (BVAT; Riverside Publishing Co.) allows an examiner to generate English language proficiency scores and bilingual verbal ability scores in 18 languages plus English in children age 5 through adulthood. The BVAT is easily administered in approximately 15–20 minutes and consists of two stages; first, the patient is asked the meaning of words of English (which yields the English proficiency score) and then given the opportunity to define any words missed in English in his or her native language, yielding the bilingual verbal ability score.

The assessment of a child's language proficiency in both languages is important in both the diagnostic and rehabilitation phase. In order to determine whether a child is experiencing difficulty with the English language simply due to lack of exposure, or whether the difficulty reflects an underlying neurodevelopmental dysfunction, a thorough assessment in both languages must be conducted. Data should be gathered from multiple sources of information, including past school records, parent reports, and teacher reports. If available, an examination of a child's writing prior to entering the rehabilitation process is often quite helpful. Generally, neurodevelopmental deficits are apparent in both languages and persist across settings, whereas language difficulties due to lack of acculturation are apparent only in the second language. The results of measures such as the BVAT can also be used as outcome measures to assess the child's progression toward proficiency in both languages.

Understanding a child's premorbid language function, whether due to bilingual upbringing or differences in dialect, is also critical, in that it influences the manifestation and recovery of acquired language disturbance (aphasia). Conventional wisdom suggests that the more robust language is that with which the child is most familiar, or the "native" language. However, more recent information suggests that this may not always be the case, and that language disturbance (and subsequent recovery from impairment) may be based on biological factors (e.g., nature and location of the lesion; Moretti et al., 2001; Aglioti, Beltramello, Girardi, & Fabbro, 1996) or linguistic factors (e.g., the structure of the language or the specific nature of the deficit) (Fabbro, 2001) rather than which language was acquired first or that with which the child is most familiar. Thus, awareness of language differences also has practical implications for treatment and recovery.

FAMILY BURDEN/COPING

The family has been referred to regularly throughout this chapter. Some of the most effective models of rehabilitation involve not only treatment of the patient but also working with the patient's family and other environmental influences. This is particularly important for a child (in contrast to an adult) in need of rehabilitation, because the parent/primary family unit is often the main resource for care coordination. There is evidence that cultural and ethnic differences in the family perception and response to injury may affect the level of family involvement, which ultimately affects long-term outcome. These changes in long-term outcome are independent of socioeconomic factors that contribute to differences in the availability of resources. One aspect of cultural differences in this regard is the recognition of and tolerance for differences in manifestation of cognitive and/or behavioral problems that may accompany traumatic brain injury. According to Kendall and Hatton (2002), there are significant differences in treatment patterns between white majority families and ethnic minority families, even after controlling for SES and insurance differences. They suggest that problems such as attention-deficit/hyperactivity disorder, academic underachievement, and even delinquency are more likely to be viewed in a medical context by white families.

Health perceptions also differ among families from various cultural and ethnic groups, and these in turn have been shown to affect coping strategies and long-term outcome. Coping strategies are an important variable in determining outcome, with strategies that suggest disengagement/denial from issues related to the injury associated with significantly worse outcome than acceptance and more active coping strategies (Wade et al., 2001). These traits may differ among cultural/ethnic minorities. For example, Yeates (2002) et al. found that black and white parents reported different coping strategies following pediatric traumatic brain injury, independent of SES. In their study, Yeates et al. found that black families tended to use avoidant coping strategies, such as mental disengagement and denial. There was also a greater reliance on religion. In contrast, white families relied more on acceptance, a more emotion-focused strategy. Brown, McCauley, Levin, Contant, and Boake (2004) found that ethnicity may play a significant role in the perception of current health functioning in patients with mild to moderate traumatic brain injury. They found a significant interaction between ethnicity and injury with minority traumatic brain injury groups reporting significantly worse health, namely, in the form of physical functioning, than patients who sustained general trauma. Specifically, African Americans reported significantly worse physical symptoms and greater difficulties performing activities of daily living when compared to their Hispanic or European American counterparts.

Cultural/ethnic differences in health perceptions and family relations may also bear upon willingness to access mental health and other supportive services, independent of their availability. There may be an increased tendency to rely on informal networks (e.g., extended family, religious network) in dealing with the consequences of injury. Other factors include cultural and institutional barriers to service acceptance, including attribution of symptoms and difficulty acknowledging coping difficulties (Armengol, 1999). Armengol also notes that service delivery is critical; rapport may depend on sensitivity to the core values and attitudes of the family, and follow-up may be dependent on the degree to which this rapport can be established. Thus, it is critical to gain a thorough understanding of family members' views of the injury, their response to the injury, as well as their coping strategies (which may be culturally influenced; e.g., religion) in order to maximize potential outcome.

CONCLUSIONS

The recognition of cultural differences in pediatric patients undergoing rehabilitation for acquired or neurodevelopmental disorders adds complexity to a multifaceted and dynamic process. This chapter has briefly touched on some of the salient issues regarding the role of cultural variables in the rehabilitation process. We have talked about the roles of acculturation, education, language, SES, health perceptions, and the family. Throughout all of these discussions, one common theme seems to emerge: A well-conceived plan for rehabilitation can only occur in the context of a comprehensive understanding of our individual patients in relation to themselves, their families, their friends, and their cultural beliefs and values. This process takes time and effort, and requires that we move beyond our usual approaches to assessment and rehabilitation. It requires us to be creative and to be open to the possibility that our "tried and true" methods may not be fully applicable to a culturally diverse population. Although effortful, the recognition that multicultural forces play an important role in our rehabilitative efforts will maximize our patients' outcomes and most likely enhance our own world views.

REFERENCES

Ackerman, R., & Banks, M. (2002). Looking for threads: Commonalities and differences. In F. Ferraro (Ed.), *Minority and cross cultural aspects of neuropsychological assessment* (pp. 387–415). Lisse, The Netherlands: Swets & Zeitlinger.

Ardila, A., Rosselli, M., & Ostrosky, F. (1992). Sociocultural factors in neuropsychological assessment. In A. E. Puente & R. J. McCaffrey (Eds.), *Psychobiological factors in clinical neuropsychological assessment* (pp. 181–192). New York: Plenum Press.

Ardila, A., Rosselli, M., & Puente, A. E. (1994). *Neuropsychological evaluation of the Spanish speaker.* New York: Plenum Press.

Ardila, A., Rosselli, M., & Rosas, P. (1989). Neuropsychological assessment in illiterates: Visuospatial and memory abilities. *Brain and Cognition, 11*, 147–166.

Aglioti, S., Beltramello, A., Girardi, F., & Fabbro, F. (1996). Neurolinguistic and follow-up study of an unusual pattern of recovery from bilingual subcortical aphasia. *Brain, 119*, 1551–1564.

Armengol, C. G. (1999). A multimodal support group with Hispanic traumatic brain injury survivors. *Journal of Head trauma Rehabilitation, 14*, 233–246.

Arnold, B. R., Montgomery, G. T., Castaneda, I., & Longoria, R. (1994). Acculturation and performance of Hispanics on selected Halstead–Reitan neuropsychological tests. *Assessment, 1,* 239–248.

Artiola-i-Fortuny, L., & Mullaney, H. (1998). Assessing patients whose language you do not know: Can the absurd be ethical? *Clinical Neuropsychologist, 12,* 113–126.

Barona, A., & Miller, J. A. (1994). Short acculturation scale for Hispanic youth (SASH-Y): A preliminary report. *Hispanic Journal of the Behavioral Sciences, 16,* 155–162.

Berry, J. W. (1988). Cognitive values and cognitive competence among bricoleurs. In J. W. Berry & S. H. Irvine (Eds.), *Endogenous cognitive functioning in cultural contexts.* NATO NSI Series D: Behavioural and Social Sciences, No. 41. Dordrecht, Netherlands: Martimus Jijhof.

Berry, J. W., Trimble, J., & Olmedo, E. L. (1988). Assessment of acculturation. In W. J. Lonner & J. W. Berry (Eds.), *Field methods in cross-cultural research* (pp. 291–324). Beverly Hills, CA: Sage.

Brown, S., McCauley, S., Levin, H., Contant, C., & Boake, C. (2004). Perception of health and quality of life in minorities after mild-to-moderate traumatic brain injury. *Applied Neuropsychology, 11,* 54–64.

Bracken, B., & Barona, A. (1991). State of the art procedures for translating, validating, and using psychoeducational tests in cross-cultural assessment. *School Psychology International, 12,* 119–132.

Bruner, J. S., Oliver, R. R., & Greenfield, P. M. (1966). *Studies in cognitive growth.* New York: Wiley.

Cuellar, I., Harris, L., & Jasso, R. (1980). An acculturation scale for Mexican American normal and clinical populations. *Hispanic Journal of Behavioral Sciences, 2,* 199–217.

de Lemos, M. M. (1965). The development of conservation in Aboriginal children. *International Journal of Psychology, 4,* 2155–2169.

Echemendía, R. J. (2004). Cultural diversity and neuropsychology: An uneasy relationship in a time of change. *Applied Neuropsychology, 11,* 1–3.

Echemendía, R. J., & Harris, J. G. (2004). Neuropsychological test use with Hispanic/Latino populations in the United States: Part II of a national survey. *Applied Neuropsychology, 11,* 4–12.

Echemendía, R. J., & Julian, L. (2002). Neuropsychological assessment of Latino children. In F. Ferraro (Ed.), *Minority and cross cultural aspects of neuropsychological assessment* (pp. 181–203). Lisse, The Netherlands: Swets & Zeitlinger.

Epstein, J. A., Botvin, G. J., Dusenbury, L., & Diaz, T. (1996). Validation of an acculturation measure for Hispanic adolescents. *Psychological Reports, 79,* 1075–1079.

Fabbro, F. (2001). The bilingual brain: Bilingual aphasia. *Brain and Language, 7,* 201–210.

Ferraro, F. (2002). *Minority and cross cultural aspects of neuropsychological assessment.* Lisse, The Netherlands: Swets & Zeitlinger.

Geisinger, K. (1994). Cross-cultural normative assessment: Translation and adaptation issues influencing the normative interpretation of assessment instruments. *Psychological Assessment, 6,* 304–312.

Harris, J. G., Cullum, C. M., & Puente, A. E. (1995). Effects of bilingualism on verbal learning and memory in Hispanic adults. *Journal of the International Neuropsychological Society, 1*, 10–16.

Harris, J. G., Echemendía, R. J., Ardila, A., & Rosselli, M. (2001). Cross cultural cognitive and neuropsychological assessment. In J. J. Andrews & D. Saklofske (Eds.), *Handbook of psychoeducational assessment* (pp. 392–414). San Diego: Academic Press.

Heaton, R. K., & Pendelton, M. O. (1981). Use of neuropsychological tests to predict adult patient's everyday functioning. *Journal of Clinical and Consulting Psychology, 49*, 807–821.

Helms, J. E. (1990). *Black and white racial identity: Theory, research and practice*. Westport, CT: Greenwood Press.

Helms, J. E. (1995). Why there is no study of cultural equivalence in standardized cognitive ability testing? In N. R. Goldberger & J. B. Vernoff (Eds.), *The culture and psychology reader* (pp. 674–719). New York: New York University Press.

Helms, J. E. (1997). The triple quandary of race, culture, and social class in standardized cognitive ability testing. In D. P. Flanagan, J. L. Genshaft, & P. L. Harrison (Eds.), *Contemporary intellectual assessment: Theories, tests, and issues* (pp. 517–532). New York: Guilford Press.

Hickey, T. (1972). Bilingualism and the measurement of intelligence and verbal learning ability. *Exceptional Children, 39*, 24–28.

Kaufman, A. S. (1990). *Assessing adolescent and adult intelligence*. Needham, MA: Allyn & Bacon.

Kendall, J., & Hatton, D. (2002). Racism as a source of health disparity in families with children with attention deficit hyperactivity disorder. *Advances in Nursing Science, 25*, 22–39.

Kennepohl, S., Shore, D., Nabors, N., & Hanks, R. (2005). African American acculturation and neuropsychological test performance following traumatic brain injury. *Journal of the International Neuropsychological Society, 10*(4), 556–577.

Lecours, R. L., Mehler, J., & Parente, M. A. (1987). Illiteracy and brain damage-1: Aphasia testing in culturally contrasted populations (control subjects). *Neuropsychologia, 25*, 231–245.

Lucas, J. A. (1998). Acculturation and neuropsychological test performance in elderly African Americans. *Journal of the International Neuropsychological Society, 4*, 77.

Majumdar, B., Browne, G., Roberts, J., & Carpio, B. (2004). Effects of cultural sensitivity training on health care provider attitudes and patient outcomes. *Journal of Nursing Scholarship, 36*, 161–166.

Manly, J. J., Byrd, D. A., Touradji, P., & Stern, J. (2004). Acculturation, reading level, and neuropsychological test performance among African American elders. *Applied Neuropsychology, 11*, 37–46.

Manly, J. J., & Jacobs, D. M. (2004). Future directions in neuropsychological assessment with African Americans. In F. Ferraro (Ed.), *Minority and cross cultural aspects of neuropsychological assessment* (pp. 79–96). Lisse, The Netherlands: Swets & Zeitlinger.

Manly, J. J., Jacobs, D. M., Sano, M., Bell, K., Merchant, C. A., Small, S. A., et al. (1999). African American acculturation and neuropsychological test performance among nondemented community elders. *Journal of the International Neuropsychological Society, 5*, 191–202.

Manly, J. J., Jacobs, D. M., Sano, M., Bell, K., Merchant, C. A., Small, S. A., et al. (1998b). Cognitive test performance among nondemented community elders and whites. *Neurology, 50*, 1238–1245.

Manly, J. J., Jacobs, D. M., Sano, M., Bell, K., & Merchant, C. A. (1998b). Cognitive test performance among non-demented elderly African Americans and Whites. *Neurology, 50*, 1238–1245.

Manuel-Dupont, S., Ardila, A., Rosselli, M., & Puente, A. (1992). Bilingualism. In A. E. Puente & R. J. McCaffrey (Eds.), *Handbook of neuropsychological assessment: A biopsychosocial perspective* (pp. 193–210). New York: Plenum Press.

Marín, G. (1992). Issues in the measurement of acculturation among Hispanics. In K. F. Geisinger (Ed.), *Psychological testing of Hispanics* (pp. 235–251). Washington, DC: American Psychological Association.

Marín, G., Sabogal, F., Marín, B. V., Otero-Sabogal, R., & Perez-Stable, E. J. (1987). Development of a short acculturation scale for Hispanics. *Hispanic Journal of Behavioral Sciences, 9*, 183–205.

Moretti, R., Bava, A., Torre, P., Antonello, R. M., Zorzon, M., Zivadinov, R., & Cazzato, G. (2001). Bilingual aphasia and subcortical–cortical lesions. *Perceptual & Motor Skills, 92*, 803–814.

Munoz-Sandoval, A. F., Cummins, J., Alvardo, C. G., & Reuf, M. (1998). *The bilingual verbal ability tests.* Itasca, IL: Riverside Publishing.

Padilla, A. M. (1979). Crucial factors in the testing of Hispanic-Americans: A review and some suggestions for the future. In R. W. Tyler & S. H. White (Eds.), *Testing, teaching and learning: Report of a conference on testing.* Washington, DC: National Institute of Education.

Perez-Arce, P., & Puente, A. E. (1996). Neuropsychological assessment of ethnic minorities: The case of Hispanics living in North America. In R. J. Sbordonen, & C. J. Long (Eds.), *Ecological validity of neuropsychological testing* (pp. 283–300). Delray Beach, FL: GR Press/St. Lucie Press.

Piaget, J. (1928). *Judgment and reasoning in the child* (M. Worden, Trans.). New York: Harcourt, Brace & World.

Pontón, M. O., Satz, P., Herrera, L., Urrutia, C. P., Ortiz, F., Young, R., D'Elia, L., Furst, C. J., & Namerow, N. (1996). The Neuropsychological Screening Battery for Hispanics: Initial report. *Journal of the International Neuropsychological Society, 2*, 96–104.

Puente, A. E., Sol Mora, M., & Munoz-Cespedes, J. M. (1997). Neuropsychological assessment of Spanish-speaking children and youth. In C. R. Reynolds & E. Fletcher-Janzen (Eds.), *Handbook of clinical child neuropsychology* (2nd ed., pp. 371–383). New York: Plenum.

Rosselli, M., Ardila, A., & Rosas, P. (1990). Neuropsychological assessment in illiterates II: Language and praxic abilities. *Brain and Cognition, 12*, 281–296.

Shade, B. J. (1991). African American patterns of cognition. In R. L. Jones (Ed.), *Black psychology* (3rd ed., pp. 231–247). Berkeley, CA: Cobb & Henry.

Tropp, L. R., Erkut, S., Coll, C. G., Alarcon, O., Garcia, H., & Vazquez, H. (1999). Psychological acculturation development of a new measure for Puerto Ricans on the U.S. mainland. *Educational and Psychological Measurement, 59*, 351–367.

U.S. Bureau of the Census. (2000). *Population estimate*. Retrieved January 10, 2004, from *www.census.gov*.
Van de Vijver, F., & Hambleton, R. K. (1996). Translating tests: Some practical guidelines. *European Psychologist, 1*, 89–99.
Wilkinson, D. Y., & King, G. (1987). Conceptual and methodological issues in the use of race as a variable: Policy implications. *Milbank Quarterly, 65*(Suppl. 1), 56–71.
Wong, T., & Fujii, D. (2004). Neuropsychological assessment of Asian Americans: Demographic factors, cultural diversity and practical guidelines. *Applied Neuropsychology, 11*, 23–36.
Wong, T., Strickland, T. L., Fletcher-Janzen, E., Ardila, A., & Reynolds, C. (2000). Theoretical and practical issues in the neuropsychological assessment and treatment of culturally dissimilar patients. In E. Fletcher-Janzen, T. L. Strickland, & C. R. Reynolds (Eds.), *Handbook of cross-cultural neuropsychology* (pp. 3–18). New York: Kluver Academic/Plenum Press.
Yeates, K. O., Taylor, H. G., Woodrome, S. E., Wade, S. L., Stancin, T., & Drotar, D. (2002). Race as a moderator of parent and family outcomes following pediatric traumatic brain injury. *Journal of Pediatric Psychology, 27*, 393–403.
Zuckerman, M. (1990). Some dubious premises in research and theory on racial differences: Scientific, social, and ethical issues. *American Psychologist, 45*, 1297–1303.

17

Epilogue

IDA SUE BARON

The term "neurodevelopmental disabilities" encompasses an exceptionally broad array of conditions. Disturbance, or presumption of disturbance, at some location within the central nervous system is a common underlying feature of each neurodevelopmental disorder. Since many diagnoses are subsumed under this umbrella term, these diverse conditions may have both commonalities that link them and uniquely individual features that distinguish them. It is a natural evolution to investigate systematically with increasing sophistication the overlapping, as well as distinctive, features that characterize each condition falling under this overarching disability rubric. The aims of further defining, understanding, and expanding our knowledge about these many conditions are worthy goals in the service of developing effective, empirically based, ecologically appropriate treatment strategies and systems interventions that ensure optimal outcome for each child, to the best of our science and practice. This volume accomplishes an important mission in providing the reader with substantial didactic and practical information about relevant psychosocial issues related to a multitude of disabilities, a discussion about both their typical and idiosyncratic presentations, and an explication of the range of intervention options that can be employed for children who fall along the broad spectrum of neurodevelopmental disability. The authors' clear focus on the importance of context or milieu, emphasizing child, family, biomedical, and socioenvironmental factors, deservedly elevates the influence of this volume for the reader.

HISTORICAL CONTEXT

A look backward is worthwhile to appreciate better how rapid and dramatic changes in science and practice have expanded our knowledge about the child who has a neurodevelopmental disability. Contrary to current emphases, psychosocial issues and system interventions were not prominently discussed in the early disability-related literature, when breadth of coverage but insufficient depth of knowledge were natural consequences of relatively narrow diagnostic capability. Limited empirical data regarding the full medical and psychological impact of a disability on both the child and family were further restricting. In retrospect, differential diagnosis for a child with known or suspected central nervous system (CNS) disorder was hindered greatly by early diagnostic techniques that provided only basic or preliminary information about CNS structure and often were unable to provide insight about function. A clinical science that merged brain and behavior was in its infancy. Furthermore, neurodiagnostic procedures and clinical appraisals of function were often viewed independently and unscientifically, in isolation from a consideration of the relevant psychosocial factors that were influential determinants of behavior and deserving of consideration. With focus often placed on diagnostic specificity, a host of critical contributory moderating variables were likely to be overlooked or minimized.

Consequently, there was an unduly heavy dependence on clinical acumen to bridge the gap between brain structure and functional behavioral repertoire. Clinical management and treatment approaches were more likely to achieve fleeting prominence despite being unsupported by scientific evidence. Too often, a gap remained between the many presumptive etiological factors that were distinctive to the condition of interest and the recognition of their importance and interactions in effecting behavioral change. As this volume makes clear, there is a welcome and needed shift toward rigorous experimental investigation of critical child, family, and socioenvironmental factors that may play a major role in determining developmental course, treatment choice, timing and effectiveness of interventions, and outcome parameters and expectations. As a result, there is clear movement toward ever-better management, treatment, and rehabilitation strategies representing a more appropriate standard of care than ever was previously endorsed. The result is that the child with a neurodevelopmental disability is now assured of a more thorough understanding by treating professionals and a more rigorous appraisal of the range of factors that ultimately influences diagnosis, management, intervention, and outcome.

CONTRIBUTIONS TO ADAPTIVE CHILD FUNCTION

The increased knowledge base that now benefits the child with a neurodevelopmental disability is consequent to a confluence of developments in related fields of scientific inquiry. Included among these are the many revolutionary investigational and clinical advances in medical methodology and practice, significant advances in health care and psychological science, increasingly sophisticated psychological instrumentation and broader clinical practice responsibilities, a clearer appreciation for the extended range of critical socioenvironmental variables, and an emphasis on both the child's and family's unique and individualized circumstances. Together, these many developments contribute to substantially changed roles of professionals who work with the child with a neurodevelopmental disability. They also result in greater ability to magnify the attention paid to even the youngest patients in novel ways, as well as to children of any age with emergent neurodevelopmental disorders.

The numerous technological and methodological innovations are not replacements for behavioral and psychosocial investigations of the expression of an underlying pathology. In fact, they strengthen the roles of those who undertake such investigations and are engaged in evaluation, treatment, and education. Their substantial contribution is exemplified by innovations in neuroimaging techniques, such as positron emission tomography (PET), magnetic resonance imaging (MRI), and its derivations such as functional magnetic resonance imaging (fMRI). Such methods hold promise for increasingly precise delineation of the nature and extent of a lesion, for correlating neural network interference with behavior or treatment outcomes, and for enabling monitoring of a normal or abnormal developmental course relative to accompanying behavioral expression. For example, fMRI studies not only led to greater appreciation of the trajectory of normal brain development in healthy children and adolescents (Hertz-Pannier et al., 1997; Giedd et al., 2004; Gogtay et al., 2004) but also provided useful data identifying subtle varieties of developmental abnormalities (Barkovich, 2005). Such techniques provide information about brain regional activation patterns across the various childhood conditions associated with neurodevelopmental disability and about brain function correlated with performance on specific cognitive test instruments. Various factors contribute to the success of these applications, including an appreciation for developmental theory and practice in the study of child brain–behavior relationships, distinct from knowledge accumulated through adult investigations (Baron, 2004; Fletcher & Taylor, 1984). When considering the individual child, it is essential to weigh alternative models of inference (Fennell & Bauer, 1997), to partition out the component behaviors that most likely influence performance (Johnstone & Farmer, 1997; Johnstone & Wilhelm,

1997), and to refine methods and develop innovative techniques to assess behavior and facilitate recovery (Farmer & Muhlenbruck, 2000).

As this volume makes explicitly clear, it is now possible to evaluate more assuredly the impact of interventions at critical developmental junctures. This, in turn, will aid in educational and vocational planning, and assist in educating family members about etiology, diagnosis, and treatment. The succession of scientific and clinical advances also helps to delineate the most productive ways to aid the child in learning to accommodate and to compensate. They offer the professional the means to plan and conduct investigative trials, and to evaluate the child's developmental progress and any deviations from the expected trajectory associated with diverse treatment protocols. The latter has particular relevance in regard to the elucidation of practical consequences of interventions that directly affect neurobehavioral outcome for the actively maturing child. These functional tasks are not supplanted by neuroimaging advances but, rather, are made more sophisticated by their advent. Brain–behavior studies remain distinctive and critical to progressively refine our understanding about subtle manifestations of neurodevelopmental disorders in infancy, childhood, and adolescence.

Whether for a congenital or an acquired disability, the diagnosing and treating professionals have an important collaborative role to play in providing insights about the nature of the impairment, its impact on the psychological well-being of the child, and strategies that will best ameliorate any consequent delay or impairment. As the authors in this volume emphasize, there is a prepotent need to combine information from multiple sources to understand best the complexity of the child's individual needs, and to plan and intervene accordingly. Although etiology is highly relevant and may appear defining initially, it does not solely determine an intervention approach or dictate which strategy will prove most efficacious for the child. Rather, the context of the child's special individualized circumstances must be considered. It is only through combining the data from various data sources that a more comprehensive understanding about inherent residual capacities and preserved functions will be obtained. Multiple data sources also inform about the available resources in the child's immediate environment. Together, these diverse sources contribute the data required to ensure the child's continued developmental progression and advancement through an expected maturational trajectory.

How to enhance the daily life experiences of the child with a neurodevelopmental disability, and encourage continued gains, maintains a deservedly high priority. There is a clear role for the professional who has responsibility for such children, whether it is an immediate challenge for a well defined CNS disorder or a sequence of challenges that eventually manifests as late appearing dysfunction (i.e., one that becomes apparent only when the vulnerability is finally challenged by emerging social, cognitive, behavioral, or academic circumstances). As one reads this volume, it is apparent that an even greater focus than ever before is placed on hypothesizing, experimentally testing, validating, and establishing the most useful ways to provide optimal circumstances that encourage the child's adaptive growth and development. These applications are often best when grounded in a theoretical basis, including a developmental model, and then applied within a context of empirical sophistication and validation. One important goal is to provide the child with the means to respond successfully to the intrinsic demands at each subsequent developmental stage or adaptive level. A second goal is to ensure that the child's competencies are encouraged sufficiently to enable eventual mastery of the competing demands emerging in adolescence and adulthood, to the best of that child's ability.

SURVIVAL RATES AND DEVELOPMENTAL COURSE

These goals of successful mastery to the best of the child's ability and effective integration into society attain special prominence in light of the increased survival rates associated with many populations of children who once had exceptionally poor prognoses. Many factors contribute to the increasing success of multidisciplinary efforts expended on behalf of children with neurodevelopmental disabilities. We have seen innovative medical advances and elegant clinical trials contribute to an extended lifespan, greater preservation of neuropsychological integrity, and greater acceptance of the conditions associated with neurodevelopmental disability, along with more forceful attempts to intervene and enhance quality of life for both the child and family. However, improved survival may not always be accompanied by more favorable cognitive and behavioral prognosis due to disease specifics, treatment choices, socioenvironmental factors, or a combination of related determinant factors.

The concern with facilitating the continued progress and outcome of children with various neurodevelopmental conditions who survive longer consequent to medical advances over the last few decades is well documented in this volume. For example, discussion includes those children with sensorimotor deficits due to spinal cord injury (Chapter 3); pre-, peri-, or neonatal insult and prematurity (Chapter 4); cerebral palsy, spina bifida, and hydrocephalus (Chapter 5); chronic illness (Chapter 6); hearing loss (Chapter 7) or visual impairment (Chapter 8); acquired brain injury (Chapters 2, 10, and 12); leukemia or brain cancer (Chapter 11); and autism (Chapter 14). Accordingly, there is a need for even greater emphasis on the therapeutic, cognitive, and societal consequences of long-term survival for those with neurodevelopmental disorders. Planning for adulthood is now the reasonable intent of interventions that before might have been palliative and intended for a brief time interval.

As given credence in this volume, a thorough professional places emphasis on "evaluation," which supersedes "testing." Evaluation is aided by a complete history taking, record review, interview with the child and family members; personal contact with others knowledgeable about the child, such as physicians, diagnosticians, therapists, caregivers, or teachers; and a summary written report that serves as a tangible resource for all concerned with the child's functioning. Whenever possible, an informative interpretive session is helpful to compare systematically the child's observed neurobehavioral and interpersonal functioning in various settings to the expressed problem areas, to further elucidate current problems not yet well articulated, and to anticipate the likelihood of future problems, in order to recommend proactively a preventive course of action. Choosing ecologically valid measures to predict real-world behaviors remains a valid enterprise (Ready, Stierman, & Paulsen, 2001). A balanced, multisource data collection has a higher likelihood of providing indices of the child's inherent strengths and integrity of family factors, elements that are essential components in developing the most meaningful treatment or rehabilitation plan.

As part of the efforts to balance the child's weaknesses by rigorously employing the child's strengths, there is not only a need to protect the family from ill-advised treatments and unsupported, unreliable lay advice, but also a responsibility to encourage a search for sources that provide reputable information. The informational exchange now possible electronically can be a major force to empower family members to advocate successfully for their child, but flawed when the source is not scientifically grounded. Supportive of gains made for both the professional and lay individual is greater access to an ever-increasing, complex literature on the intricacy of neurodevelopmental maturation that informs about how a child progresses, stabilizes, or regresses in response to a multitude of biomedical, psychological, and environmental factors. An informational network of both professional organizations and lay groups that share an interest in disabilities and transmit their information electronically has developed. Furthermore, the importance of educating family members sufficiently and at their level of understanding should be foremost in any intervention strategy. Family members need assistance in maneuvering through the competing systems that are put in place for their child but can be the child's strongest advocate when informed and encouraged to be active on their child's behalf. They can serve as a first line of defense regarding safety and treatment effects, and be the first to recognize a halt in progress (e.g., when a treatment is not working or when a modification is needed).

PSYCHOSOCIAL CONTRIBUTIONS TO ADAPTIVE CHILD FUNCTIONING

It is increasingly recognized that the child is embedded in a world of multiple "social–emotional feedback loops" that position the child at any point in time to respond either adaptively or ineffectively. There is an ever-growing appreciation for the immense value of strong and cohesive social support systems (Kinsella, Ong, Murtaugh, Prior, & Sawyer, 1999; Taylor et al., 2001; Sines, 1987; Yeates et al., 1997), and the need to evaluate these longitudinally and support their maintenance when effective. The emergence of a more focused appraisal of component factors that might influence outcome has resulted in a greater appreciation for some critical nonmedical determinants, several of which were too long relegated to minor roles or neglected in research. This volume contains numerous references to the importance of these determinants, many of which relate to family, cultural, and socioenvironmental factors. One such variable is parent involvement. Parental roles are wide-ranging but include, at a minimum, supportive caretaker, role model, informal therapist, unofficial tutor, and advocate negotiating the complicated health care and academic settings in order to ensure the provision of needed services.

Sibling relationships and the role of the child with a disability vis-à-vis all other family members is a second familial variable. The child's assumed or assigned position or role within the family is an important component, and the reactive responses of other family members to the child may be crucial determinants of outcome. Their support can be a positive force, but their resentment or lack of comprehension may take the family in a negative direction. A critical appraisal about how well a child can cope with the medical and psychosocial factors that distinguish their sibling's neurodevelopmental disability, along with their insight, is valuable when the family is in emotional disarray, when external supports are weakened, or when family cohesiveness is subsumed to the disorder. Family members adapt and shift to accommodate the presence of a child with an illness or developmental challenge. Evaluation of existing supports for the child in each environment and from each family member is helpful. Asking the child through informal or objective means can be illuminating and provide a perspective not easily obtained in another way. Even a very young child has insight and sensitivity about his or her condition that can be appreciated if asked for in a developmentally appropriate way (e.g., through play, art, words, or demonstrable actions).

Cultural context or ethnicity represents a third variable. Acceptance of the doctor–patient role is not universal for the families of the children encountered in private practice or a hospital setting. Different customs and beliefs shape the responses of family members to the medical or psychological establishment. There are those whose cultural beliefs engender resistance despite a loving, well-meaning attitude toward their child. Reasons for potential noncompliance must be understood if they are to be addressed effectively. Often, obstacles to care may be based on rituals or superstitions that are communicated through generations but alien to the treater. Clear communication and transparent methods are most likely to result in meaningful exchanges in the context of family members' educational level and cultural background. This becomes another essential step in the development and implementation of any treatment or rehabilitation plan.

A fourth important influence relates to peer relationships, which may be either positive or negative. While it is important to assist children in building supportive friendships and engaging in age-appropriate peer interactions, it is also important to minimize the likelihood that children will experience the detrimental impact of negative peer contacts due to the perceptions of others about their disability, such as the destructive bullying or teasing with which they may be less able to cope. Children with neurodevelopmental disabilities may be especially subject to the negative repercussions of problematic social–emotional relationships, even when these are considered "normal" and a typical part of the repertoire of children of a particular developmental age. Direct instruction and role modeling are among the essential supplemental techniques that will enable the child to understand, cope, and respond appropriately.

The child's temperament and personality structure is a fifth variable that strongly influences coping abilities and adaptability. Temperament and personality are variables that determine and can alter outcome for an individual child relative to another child with superficially similar features. The influence of these factors in interpersonal relationships, motivation, persistence, and willingness or resistance to work toward the rehabilitative goals can be profound.

One of the greater challenges is to balance concern about independent function within the context of a supportive social–environmental structure, psychosocial functioning, and interpersonal relationships, in order to expect the most successful and healthy experiences possible for the child, the family, and the society. This volume includes important informational chapters on acquired and congenital conditions that potentially result in long-term disability. The authors pay particular attention to condensing this vast literature into meaningful chapters that highlight essential aspects, including some aspects not given due consideration in the past. Given that the behavioral, cognitive, emotional, psychosocial, and educational effects of these disorders and their impact on the maturational trajectory may have commonalities between them, the distinct phenotypes evident for many of these conditions have not always received a sufficient degree of deserved attention. By focusing on those points typically neglected or relegated to less substantial consideration in the past, the chapters in this volume provide a valuable context for understanding the range of factors inherent within this broad disability classification. Of special value, the section on innovative treatment strategies (Part III) provides needed insight into how our colleagues charged with the daily battle to remediate and rehabilitate effectively face their many challenges.

FUTURE DIRECTIONS

Diverse professionals concentrating their interests and experiences in equally diverse ways ultimately benefit the child with a neurodevelopmental disability. Yet many tasks have only recently surfaced, and much remains to be accomplished. The wide collection of conditions under the neurodevelopmental disorder rubric, many of which are addressed in this volume, appears overwhelmingly complex when considered at only a superficial level. However, each requires parsing and a thorough mastery of specific identifying features in order to better understand consequent immediate and long-term effects on the developing infant or child, and family members. Such critical knowledge is the substance of this volume, and its authors have kept these fundamental objectives in mind.

Understanding how brain regions or circuits adapt, realign, or redistribute function, or essentially "cross-cover" for dysfunctional regions or networks, is critical knowledge for those involved in rehabilitation (Frank & Elliott, 2000). Treatment and rehabilitation are intimately linked to the basic concepts of neuroplasticity and cognitive reserve (Aram & Eisele, 1992; Goldman & Lewis, 1978; Huttenlocher, 1994; Levin, 2003), which provide a core foundation for all rehabilitative efforts with children. As steps are taken toward improving the range of treatment choices for children with well-defined neurodevelopmental disabilities and consequent secondary cognitive and behavioral problems, data are also emerging about various applications that facilitate evaluation of functional changes in response to neurodevelopmental insult (Anderson & Pentland, 1998; Levisohn, Cronin-Golomb, & Schmahmann, 2000; Michaud, Rivara, Jaffe, Fay, & Dailey, 1993). How these will influence one child but not another is an area of special interest. Since individual brains vary in their specific area of representation of function, one cannot assume that a single brain regional template applies to all individuals (Johnson, 2005). Thus, the commonalities and distinctive differences that characterize the complexity of neurodevelopmental disabilities at a macroscopic level also have an impact at a microscopic level, and the appreciation for this is ever-increasing.

Often, data that illuminate child issues still arise from the results of adult studies or analyses of the application of therapies that have an established empirical basis for the rehabilitation of adults. Yet these may sometimes prove applicable to some degree in theory or practice to children. Recognition of emerging productive theories and applications from the adult literature remains important as efforts are expended toward a future that is based on those theories and applications formulated and generated, with developmental issues as central and decisive.

It is also important to implement conditions for optimal outcome and provide a full range of needed resources for the child without discernable physical impairments, whose cognitive or behavioral impairments are not easily appreciated in a casual personal encounter. While a child may have obvious physical manifestations, such as those that may be apparent secondary to a diagnosis of spina bifida or cerebrovascular disorder, there are other children (e.g., those with autistic spectrum disorders) whose more covert problems make them appear unimpaired to naive individuals, despite the fact that their disabilities are far from subtle when fully appreciated. The symptomatology of these children requires just as much attention as that given the child with an overt disability, and steps need to be taken to ease the transition of such children into social–environmental circumstances, making sure that others are well educated about their abilities and disabilities.

It is apparent that traditional diagnostic nomenclature for established psychiatric or psychological diagnoses creates a situation in which many children fall within borderline or undefined areas. In turn, their access to interventional services is limited, prevented, or labored. Without formal recognition, access to medical care reimbursement for their disorder may be denied, and the ability to obtain other supplemental resources may be subsequently limited as well. Yet, in practice, one encounters many such children for whom a diagnosis is clear and for whom intervention is warranted, with the aim of creating the circumstances for greater proficiency in activities of daily living, interpersonal adeptness, and higher cognitive skills building. A taxonomy based on a pragmatic recognition of children's efficiency in their personal, individual settings would be far more acceptable for the children and the community than limited or restrictive definitions that unfortunately result in a mandated exclusion of children needing assistance. The authors of this volume also support the recognition of the need to amend and develop classification systems that better serve the purpose of facilitating a child's full development.

It is clear that grouping varied neurodevelopmental conditions together under a broad rubric has led to an underappreciation of the nature of these diverse conditions and thus, of their potential outcome parameters. By focusing on both basic, essential features in these populations and the opportunities for treatment, the authors in this volume have made a significant contribution to our growing understanding of many key issues that should receive prominent attention. These distinctive features associated with specific disorders, or applicable to multiple disorders, need to be embedded in a dynamic maturational plan that realistically varies from child to child and from disorder to disorder. As a result, the detail provided in these chapters adds rich data to the information base that must be integrated if one is to better appreciate needed direction in treatment, monitoring, and adjustment of the regimen to best advantage.

A continued broadening of scientific knowledge is a core need if we are to bridge the divide between understanding a child's normal development or deficits consequent to a congenital or acquired condition: whether the family possesses the full range of coping skills, whether the child has the foundation of personal strengths enabling successful adaptation, whether the immediate societal environment in which that child functions will provide the systems and support necessary to see these strengths optimized, whether our means for determining the strengths of these essential component factors exist in a sufficiently useful way, and whether applied treatments have proven ecological validity. The gains that have rapidly accumulated in recent years are described well within this volume. In reading this book, the preponderance of cited references that address these points are notably current, attesting to the recency with which many of these important influences have accelerated.

Among the future studies that hold exceptional potential for broadening our knowledge are those that focus on the youngest child with a neurodevelopmental disability. There is a clear need to understand better the influences of the many contributory influences on physical and mental development. The moderating influences of genetic predisposition and cognitive reserve remain constructive lines of investigation, including which factors can be utilized most effectively to effect substantial change, and which remain more resistant to adaptation. Which procedures will enable the most reliable estimation and characterization of a premorbid profile of strengths and weaknesses remain to be determined. There is a continued need to emphasize the moderating effects of age, socioeconomic status, gender, wellness, and maturational level, and to learn how these can influence outcome singly or in combination. In addition, there is value in continuing to extend investigations downward to the youngest ages, then to prospectively follow these children over a lengthy time course, considering how each stage is differentially affected by the relevant etiological and treatment factors (Baron & Gioia, 1998). The literature providing prospective data from infancy on to childhood regarding risk factors, guidelines for management and intervention to ensure optimal neurodevelopmental outcome, and late neurodevelopmental outcome is relatively sparse but expanding. Study of infants and very young children, who only recently are receiving much deserved attention with respect to their neurodevelopmental outcome (Hack & Taylor, 2000; Taylor, Minich, Bangert, Filipek, & Hack, 2004), and in response to medical interventions (Ment et al., 2000), along with enhanced recognition of the substantial impact of social and environmental factors (Vohr et al., 2003), holds enormous potential for investigators across all related disciplines. Collaborative investigation that seeks to illuminate why some infants succeed optimally and others do not is an exciting and useful line of potential study. The integrated combination of knowledge from child neuropsychology and developmental cognitive neuroscience, for example, can result in exceptionally rich paradigms. Timing of intervention and its relation to eventual outcome often remains unknown or is not considered. Yet it is increasingly shown that greater vulnerability is associated with times of rapid rates of neural development, and that these occur at younger ages (Limperopoulos et al., 2005). Continued close examination of these and other, related influences represent especially powerful directions in clinical practice and empirical research. As this volume makes strikingly clear, the aims of prediction, prevention, effective intervention, and prognosis should be uppermost for the professional encountering a child with neurodevelopmental disability.

REFERENCES

Anderson, V., & Pentland, L. (1998). Residual attention deficits following childhood head injury: Implications for ongoing development. *Neuropsychological Rehabilitation, 8,* 283–300.

Aram, D., & Eisele, J. A. (1992). Plasticity and recovery of higher cognitive functions following early brain injury. In I. Rapin & S. J. Segalowitz (Eds.), *Handbook of neuropsychology: Vol. 6. Child neuropsychology* (pp. 73–92). Oxford, UK: Elsevier Science.

Barkovich, A. J. (2005). Magnetic resonance in epilepsy: Neuroimaging techniques. In R. I. Kuzniecky & G. D. Jackson (Eds.), *Magnetic resonance in epilepsy* (2nd ed., pp. 221–248). Burlington, MA: Elsevier.

Baron, I. S. (2004). *Neuropsychological evaluation of the child.* New York: Oxford University Press.

Baron, I. S., & Gioia, G. A. (1998). Neuropsychology of infants and young children. In G. Goldstein, P. D. Nussbaum, & S. R. Beers (Eds.), *Handbook of human brain function: Assessment and rehabilitation: Vol. III. Neuropsychology* (pp. 9–34). New York: Plenum Press.

Farmer, J. E., & Muhlenbruck, L. (2000). Pediatric neuropsychology. In R. G. Frank & T. G. Elliott (Eds.), *Handbook of rehabilitation psychology* (pp. 377–397). Washington, DC: American Psychological Association.

Fennell, E. B., & Bauer, R. M. (1997). Models of inference and evaluating brain–behavioral relationships in children. In C. R. Reynolds & E. Fletcher-Janzen (Eds.), *Handbook of clinical child neuropsychology* (2nd ed., pp. 204–215). New York: Plenum Press.

Fletcher, J. M., & Taylor, H. G. (1984). Neuropsychological approaches to children:

Towards a developmental neuropsychology. *Journal of Clinical Neuropsychology, 6,* 39–56.
Frank, R. G., & Elliott, T. R. (Eds.). (2000). *Handbook of rehabilitation psychology.* Washington, DC: American Psychological Association.
Giedd, J. N., Rosenthal, M. A., Rose, A. B., Blumenthal, J. D., Molloy, E., Dopp, R. R., Clasen, L. S., Fridberg, D. J., & Gogtay, N. (2004). Brain development in healthy children and adolescents: Magnetic resonance imaging studies. In J. K. M. Keshavan & R. Murray (Eds.), *Neurodevelopment and schizophrenia* (pp. 35–44). Cambridge, UK: Cambridge University Press.
Gogtay, N., Giedd, J. N., Lusk, L., Hayashi, K. M., Greenstein, D. A., Vaituzis, C., Herman, D. H., Nugent, T. F., III, Clasen, L., Toga, A. W., Rapoport, J. L., & Thompson, P. M. (2004). Dynamic mapping of human cortical development during childhood through early adulthood. *Proceedings of the National Academy of Sciences of the USA, 101,* 8174–8179.
Goldman, P. S., & Lewis, M. (1978). Developmental biology of brain damage and experience. In C. W. Cotman (Ed.), *Neuronal plasticity* (pp. 291–310). New York: Raven Press.
Hack, M., & Taylor, H. G. (2000). Perinatal brain injury in preterm infants and later neurobehavioral function. *Journal of the American Medical Association, 284,* 1973–1974.
Hertz-Pannier, L., Gaillard, W. D., Mott, S. H., Cuenod, C. A., Bookheimer, S. Y., Weinstein, S., Conry, J., Papero, P. H., Schiff, S. J., Le Bihan, D., & Theodore, W. H. (1997). Noninvasive assessment of language dominance in children and adolescents with functional MRI: A preliminary study. *Neurology, 48,* 1003–1012.
Huttenlocher, P. R. (1994). Synaptogenesis, synapse elimination, and neural plasticity in human cerebral cortex. In C. A. Nelson (Ed.), *Threats to optimal development: Integrating biological, psychological, and social risk factors* (pp. 35–54). Hillsdale, NJ: Erlbaum.
Johnson, M. H. (2005). *Developmental cognitive neuroscience* (2nd ed.). Oxford, UK: Blackwell.
Johnstone, B., & Farmer, J. E. (1997). Preparing neuropsychologists for the future: The need for additional training guidelines. *Archives of Clinical Neuropsychology, 12,* 523–530.
Johnstone, B., & Wilhelm, K. L. (1997). The construct validity of the Hooper Visual Organization Test. *Assessment, 4,* 243–248.
Kinsella, G., Ong, B., Murtaugh, D., Prior, M., & Sawyer, M. (1999). The role of the family for behavioral outcome in children and adolescents following traumatic brain injury. *Journal of Consulting and Clinical Psychology, 67,* 116–123.
Levin, H. S. (2003). Neuroplasticity following non-penetrating traumatic brain injury. *Brain Injury, 17,* 665–674.
Levisohn, L., Cronin-Golomb, A., & Schmahmann, J. D. (2000). Neuropsychological consequences of cerebellar tumour resection in children: Cerebellar cognitive affective syndrome in a paediatric population. *Brain, 123,* 1041–1050.
Limperopoulos, C., Soul, J. S., Gauvreau, K., Huppi, P. S., Warfield, S. K., Bassan, H., Robertson, R. L., Volpe, J. J., & du Plessis, A. J. (2005). Late gestation cerebellar growth is rapid and impeded by premature birth. *Pediatrics, 115,* 688–695.

Ment, L. R., Vohr, B. R., Allan, W., Westerveld, M., Sparrow, S. S., Schneider, K., Katz, K., Duncan, C. C., & Makuch, R. W. (2000). Outcome of children in the indomethacin intraventricular hemorrhage prevention trial. *Pediatrics, 105,* 485–491.

Michaud, L. J., Rivara, F. P., Jaffe, K. M., Fay, G., & Dailey, J. L. (1993). Traumatic brain injury as a risk factor for behavioral disorders in children. *Archives of Physical Medicine and Rehabilitation, 74,* 368–375.

Ready, R. E., Stierman, L., & Paulsen, J. S. (2001). Ecological validity of neuropsychological and personality measures of executive functions. *The Clinical Neuropsychologist, 15,* 314–323.

Sines, J. O. (1987). Influence of the home and family environment on childhood dysfunction. In B. B. Lahey & A. E. Kazdin (Eds.), *Advances in clinical child psychology* (pp. 1–54). New York: Plenum Press.

Taylor, H. G., Minich, N., Bangert, B., Filipek, P. A., & Hack, M. (2004). Long-term neuropsychological outcomes of very low birth weight: Associations with early risks for periventricular brain insults. *Journal of the International Neuropsychological Society, 10,* 987–1004.

Taylor, H. G., Yeates, K. O., Wade, S. L., Drotar, D., Stancin, T., & Burant, C. (2001). Bidirectional child–family influences on outcomes of traumatic brain injury in children. *Journal of the International Neuropsychological Society, 7,* 755–767.

Vohr, B. R., Allan, W., Westerveld, M., Schneider, K., Katz, K., Makuch, R. W., & Ment, L. R. (2003). School-age outcomes of very low birth weight infants in the indomethacin intraventricular hemorrhage prevention trial. *Pediatrics, 111,* e340–e346.

Yeates, K. O., Taylor, H. G., Drotar, D., Wade, S., Stancin, T., & Klein, S. (1997). Preinjury family environment as a determinant of recovery from traumatic brain injury in school-age children. *Journal of the International Neuropsychological Society, 3,* 617–630.

Index

Academic achievement (*see also* Educational settings)
  achievement tests, 214
  cancer survivors, 193–194
  chronic illnesses, 102–103
  cognitive-behavioral interventions, 193–194
  preterm birth, 69–70
  qualitative assessment, brain injury, 215–217
  visual impairments, 140–141
Access to health care
  chronic illness, 110
  ethnic minorities/rural areas, 110–111
  future directions, 182
  as intervention barrier, 174–175
  online approach, 181
Acculturation, 294–297
  definition, 295
  measurement, 296–297
  and neuropsychological test performance, 290
  racial and ethnic identity issues, 295–296
  and rehabilitation goals, 299
Acquired brain injury, 208–233 (*see also* Traumatic brain injury)
  abstract verbal skills, brain injury, 25
  apoptosis, preterm infants, brain injury, 64
  developmental considerations, 211–212
  educational interventions, 219–222
  educational planning, 218–219
  future research directions, 225–227
  incidence, 209
  long-term impact, 212
  psychoeducational assessment, 213–215
  qualitative assessment, 215–217
  school setting, 208–233
  rehabilitation in, 220–223
  screening recommendations, 225–226
  transition planning, 223–225
African Americans (*see also* Ethnic minorities)
  avoidant coping, families, 302
  culture-based cognitive development, 299–300
  visual impairments, 135–136
Age effects, chronic illness, 108
Aggression
  autism interventions, 259–261
  multimodal interventions, 189
American Sign Language, 122–123
Antecedent behavior management, 178–179, 222
Applied behavioral analysis (ABA), 256
  and "discrete trial training," 256
  empirical support, autism, 250–256
Articulation rate, cerebral palsy, 84–85

323

Asperger syndrome, stereotypical behavior, 259
Assertiveness
  assessment needs, 91
  physically disabled, 237–238
  social skills training, 240
Assessment (see Neuropsychological assessment; Qualitative assessment)
"Assimilation," versus biculturality, 295
Assistive communication devices, autism, 258
Asthma, academic outcomes, 102
Attachment relationship, and deafness, 122
Attention-deficit/hyperactivity disorder
  assessment needs, 90
  and preterm birth, 72–73
Attention impairment
  cancer survivors, 191–193
  cognitive remediation program, 193
  metacognitive intervention, 189
  myelomeningocele, 87–88
  pharmacologic treatment, 198–200
"Attention process training," 191–192
Autism spectrum disorders, 249–268
  aggression interventions, 259–261
  applied behavioral support, 250, 256
  aversive interventions, autism, 260
  behavioral disorder interventions, 259–261
  communication skill interventions, 255–259
  functional equivalence training, 256
  future research directions, 261–263
  interventions, 249–268
  nonaversive disorders, 260–261
  peer-mediated interventions, 251–253
  prevalence, 249
  social skills training, 251–255
  structured environmental interventions, 256–257
Autism Biomedical Information Network, 263
Avoidance coping
  chronic illness, 108
  family cultural differences, 302

B

Back translation, 293
"Balanced bilingual," 300
Behavior Rating Inventory of Executive Function
  premature birth, 72
  traumatic brain injury, 28
Behavioral functioning
  chronic illness, 101–102
  educational challenges, brain injury, 212–213
  and family adjustment, 173–174
  overview, 9–10
  preterm birth, 72–73
  spinal cord injury, 45–48
  traumatic brain injury, 27–28, 173–174, 212–213
Behavioral management strategies, brain injury, 178–179
Behavioral momentum intervention, 254
Behavioral rehabilitation
  and ecological interventions, 190
  family environment interaction, 201–202
  future directions, 201–203
  and stimulant medications, 198–200
  brain injury, 178–179
"Biculturality," 295
Bilingual Verbal Ability Test, 300–301
Blindness
  clinical implications, 139–143
  definitions, 133–135
  developmental factors, 138–139
  educational needs, 140
  employment, 142–143
  epidemiology, 134–136
  future research directions, 143–144
  independent living skills, 137–138
  Individualized Education Plans, 142
  and motor impairment, 141
  neuropsychological status, 141–142
  psychological assessment, 141–142
  rehabilitation services, 142
  social outcomes, 136–139
Brain injury (see Traumatic brain injury)

Brain tumors (see Cancer survivors)
Building Friendships program, 241–242

C

California Verbal Learning Test—
  Children's Version, 26–27
Cambridge Center for Behavioral Studies,
  262–263
Cancer survivors
  academic impairments, 103
  assertiveness training, 240
  "attention process training," 171–172
  cognitive-behavioral therapy, 192
  cognitive remediation program, 192–
    193
  compensatory memory system, 194
  coordinated health care systems, 281
  gender issues, 107
  metacognitive intervention, 192
  rehabilitation strategies, 190–195
  school re-entry programs, 195–196
  stimulant medication, 199–200
CanChild website, 150
Capacity ratings, impairment determination, 8–9
Caregiving stress, overview, 13–14
Care coordination interventions, 280
Case management, in transition planning, 225
Catheterization, spinal cord injury, 55
Cerebellar volume, preterm infants, 67
Cerebral palsy, 81–83, 88–91
  assessment and intervention needs, 90–91
  dependency–autonomy issue, 89
  epidemiology, 81–82
  and epilepsy, 83–84
  etiology, 82–83
  future research directions, 90–91
  neuropsychology, 84–85
    subtype risks, 85
  pathophysiology, 83
  psychosocial outcomes, 88
Chiari type II malformation, 86–87
Child abuse, and brain injury, 30
Child Perceptions of Specialty Care, 153

Children with special health care needs
  prevalence estimates, 5–6
  service delivery for, 273
Children's Category Test, 26–27
Cholinergic agonists, 200
Chronic illness, 98–118
  academic and cognitive outcomes,
    102–103
  age factors, 108
  clinical implications, 112–113
  coping style, 108–109
  developmental changes, 104–105
  disease severity role, 106
  and duration of disease, 107
  epidemiology, 99
  ethnic minorities, 110–111
  familial outcomes, 103–104
  family-centered care outcome, 157
  functional status role, 106–107
  future research directions, 113–114
  gender factors, 107
  longitudinal studies, 105
  parental adjustment, 111
  pathophysiology, 99
  peer relationships, 111–112
  psychological outcomes, 99–102
  in rural areas, 110
  socioeconomic factors, 109
Circle of friends approach, 222
Classification
  multidimensional systems, 8–9
  neurodevelopmental disabilities, 3–9
  research need, 318
Client Satisfaction Questionnaire, 153,
  155
Cochlear implants, 122
Cognitive appraisal
  chronic illness adjustment, 108–109
  traumatic brain injury stress, 172
Cognitive-behavioral therapy
  cancer survivors, 191–192
  school setting, 220–221
  therapeutic relationship component,
    198
  in traumatic brain injury, 222
Cognitive development, cultural factors,
  299–300

Cognitive impairment
　acquired brain injury, 211–212
　assessment, 213–217
　chronic illnesses, 102–103, 108
　deafness and hard-of-hearing, 120–121
　diabetes mellitus, 102, 108
　and duration of disease, 107
　ecological interventions, 190
　educational challenges, brain injury, 212–213
　monitoring of, 215
　psychoeducational assessment, 213–215
　qualitative assessment, 215–217
　rehabilitation, 186–207
　traumatic brain injury, 25–27, 211–212
　and visual impairments, 136–137, 140
Cognitive rehabilitation, 186–207
　cancer survivors, 191–193
　and ecological intervention, 190
　and family environment, 201–202
　future research directions, 201–203
　and stimulant medications, 198–200
　therapeutic relationship component, 198
Cognitive remediation program, 192–193
　cancer survivors, 192–193
　individualized approach in, 198
　parental involvement role, 193
Coma duration, cognitive effects, 26–27
Communication skills training
　applied behavior analysis in, 256
　autism, 255–259, 261
　structured environmental interventions in, 256–257
　traumatic brain injury, 178–180
Community participation/integration, 234–246
　conceptual model, 235
　coordinated care studies, 274–278
　emerging approaches, 242–244
　and health care systems, 272–273
Compensatory memory system, 194
Consumer satisfaction
　measures, 153
　family-centered care, 156–164

"Coordinator," transitional services, 225
Coping style
　chronic illness, 108
　cultural factors, families, 301–303
　targeted intervention, 170–172
　and temperament, 316
　traumatic brain injury, 172–173
　　and family problem-solving, 178–181
Corpus callosum
　myelomeningocele, 87–88
　preterm infants, 66–67
Critical periods, and preterm birth, 64
Cued English method, deafness, 123
Cultural context, 289–307 (see also Ethnic minorities)
　assessment, 292–294
　　norm group issues, 292–293
　cognitive developmental influences, 299–300
　educational history influences, 298–300
　family burden/coping, 301–303
　and health care delivery, 302–303
　health perceptions, 302, 315–316
　individual factors in, 290–292
　and language, 300–301
　socioeconomic factors, 297–298
Culture-specific tests, 293
Cystic fibrosis, adjustment problems, 105

D

Daily planners, 223
"Deaf" culture
　definition, 120
　and self-esteem, 124
Deaf parents, 122
Deafness, 119–131
　age-at-diagnosis, 121
　clinical implications, 124–127
　cognitive outcomes, 120–121
　developmental outcomes, 120–124
　educational issues, 122–124
　future research directions, 127–128
　psychiatric disorders, 124–125
　psychological assessment, 125–126

psychosocial impact, 120–124
psychotherapy, 126–127
Dependency–autonomy issue
  assessment needs, 90–91
  nonverbal populations, 89
Depression
  and cerebral palsy, 88
  and duration of disease, 107
  psychotherapy, 197
Developmental factors
  acquired brain injury, 211–212
  chronic illness, 104–105
  deafness and hard-of-hearing, 120–124
  overview, 14–15
  preterm birth, 64, 74
  spinal cord injury, 46–47
  traumatic brain injury, 30, 211–212
  visual impairments, 128–129
Diabetes mellitus
  age-of-onset effect, 108
  cognitive impairments, 102
  longitudinal studies, 105
  peer support, 111
Diagnostic nomenclature, 318
Direct Instruction approach, 219
Direct social skills interventions, autism, 254–255
Discrete trial training, autism, 256
Drug treatment (see Pharmacologic treatment)
Duration of disease, and psychosocial outcome, 106–107
Dyskinetic cerebral palsy, 83, 85

E

Education history, cultural issues, 298–300
Educational factors (see also School functions/settings)
  acquired brain injury, 208–227
  family involvement, 218–219
  overview, 11–13
  preterm birth, 69–70
  spinal cord injury, 53–54
  systems aspects, 272
  traumatic brain injury, 28–29, 208–227

Electronic speech output devices, autism, 258
Emotional functioning
  chronic illness, 101
  overview, 9–10
  spinal cord injury, 45–48
  traumatic brain injury, 27–28
  visual impairment, 128–129
Employment
  acquired brain injury, 196–197
  overview, 11–13
  spinal cord injury, 52–54
  visual impairment, 142–143
Environmental factors
  and intervention, 190
  overview, 61–63
  and premature birth, 61–75
  in social participation model, 235
Epidemiology, overview, 3–9
Epilepsy
  and cerebral palsy, 83–84
  cognitive impairment, 102
Ethnic minorities, 289–307
  access to health care, 110
  acculturation, 294–297
  assessment, 294–297
  brain injury perceptions, 296
  cognitive developmental influences, 299–300
  educational experience evaluation, 298–300
  family burden/coping, 301–303
  health care delivery, 302–303
  health perceptions, families, 302
  identity issues, 295–296
  individual context, 290–292
  language, 300–301
  neuropsychological assessment, 292–294
  norm groups, 292–293
  population statistics, 289
  socioeconomic status, 297–298
  and traumatic brain injury, 31
  visual impairments, 135–136
Eurocentric cultural model, 290
"Evaluation," emphasis on, 314

Executive function
  preterm birth, 71–72
  spastic cerebral palsy, 85
  traumatic brain injury, 28
Extremely low birth weight
  academic achievement, 69–70
  assessment, 73–74
  attention-deficit/hyperactivity disorder, 72–73
  and brain insult, 64–67
  executive function, 71–72
  intelligence quotients, 68–69
  language disabilities, 70–71
  major and minor disabilities, 62–63
  pathogenesis, 63–67
  survival rates, 62
  visual–motor skills, 71

F

Family-centered care (*see also* Pediatric family-centered rehabilitation)
  barriers to implementation, 158, 165–166
  comprehensive systems approach, 281–282
  evaluation, 151–156
  future research directions, 166
  key principles, 149–150, 281–282
  outcomes, 156–164
Family-Centered Care Questionnaire—Revised, 152, 154
Family-Centered Program Rating Scale, 152, 154
Family functioning
  behavior problems link, 173–174
  and child's recovery, brain injury, 173–174
  chronic illness, 103–104
  cultural factors, 301–303
  overview, 13–14, 315–317
  preterm birth, 74
  in social participation model, 235
  social support role, 315–316
  spina bifida, 89
  spinal cord injury, 50–51

  traumatic brain injury, 29, 31, 171–174, 201–202
  interventions, 170–185
  risk and protective factors, 172–173
  tailored approach, 177–181
  visual impairments, 140–141
Family satisfaction with care
  family-centered care, 156–164
  family problem-solving program, 180–181
  measures, 153, 155
Fathers, in family problem-solving program, 180
Folate supplementation, 86
Foreign-educated students, 298–299
Friendships, and assertiveness, 238
Frontal lobe dysfunction, 212
Functional analysis, intervention selection, 261
Functional disabilities, 5–7
Functional equivalence training, autism, 256
Functional magnetic resonance imaging, 311
Functional status, and outcome, 106–107

G

Gender factors, chronic illness adjustment, 107
Generalization
  autism interventions, 262
  social sills training, 239–240, 253
  structured environmental interventions, 257
Glasgow Coma Scale, 24
Glutamate, and preterm birth, 64, 66
Gray matter volume, preterm birth, 66–67
Guiding Appropriate Pediatric Services program, 277

H

"Habilitation," 220
Hard-of-hearing, 119–131
  age-at-diagnosis, 121
  clinical implications, 124–127

cognitive outcomes, 120–124
developmental outcomes, 121–124
educational issues, 122–124
future research directions, 127–128
identity problems, 124
psychiatric disorders, 124–125
psychological assessment, 125–126
psychosocial impact, 120–124
psychotherapy, 126–127
Health care accessibility (*see* Access to health care)
Health care delivery system, 269–288
  barriers to comprehensive care, 274
  collaboration in, 273–280
    clinical implications, 281–283
    community-based studies, 274–278
  components, 270
  cost, 271–272
  cultural/ethnic factors, 302–303
  family-centered care in, 281–282
  funding, 283
  future research directions, 283–284
  interdisciplinary teams in, 282–283
  program development, 283
  social–ecological framework, 269–270
  utilization, 270–271
Hearing loss, 119–131
Hemiplegic cerebral palsy, 85
Hemophilia, cognitive impairment, 103
High school, graduation rates, 12
Hippocampus, preterm infants, 66–67
Hispanics (*see also* Ethnic minorities)
  individual context, 291
  neuropsychological impairment perceptions, 296
  visual impairments, 135–136
HIV/AIDS, school functioning, 102
Hydrocephalus
  and functional status, 106
  and myelomeningocele, 86–88
  neuropsychology, 87–88
Hypoxic–ischemic encephalopathy, 61, 64–65

I

Identity problems, in hard-of-hearing, 124
Illiteracy, cognitive development effects, 299
Independent living skills, visually impaired, 137–138
Individualized Education Plans
  brain injury rehabilitation, 195
  school re-entry, 224
  visual impairments, 142
Individualized interventions (*see* Tailored approaches)
Individuals with Disabilities Education Act, 4, 6, 272
Infants, research directions, 319–320
Informational support, traumatic brain injury, 175–176
Institute for Family-Centered Care, 150
Instructional programming
  acquired brain injury, 218–222
  strategies, 219–222
Insulin-dependent diabetes mellitus
  age-of-onset effect, 108
  cognitive impairments, 102
  peer support, 111
Intelligence quotient (*see* IQ)
Intelligence tests
  and deafness, 125–126
  in psychoeducational assessment, 214–215
Interdisciplinary teams, health care, 282–283
International Classification of Functioning, Disability, and Health, 8–9
Interpreters, and deafness, 126–127
Intrauterine infection, and cerebral palsy, 82
Intraventricular hemorrhage, preterm infants, 61, 65
IQ
  cerebral palsy, 84–85
  myelomeningocele, 87
  preterm birth, 68–69
    socioeconomic factors, 69
  psychoeducational assessment, brain injury, 214–215

L

Language
  applied behavior analysis intervention, 256
  in autism, 253, 255–259
  cultural factors in proficiency of, 300–301
  and preterm birth, 70–71
Learned passivity
  physically disabled, 237–238
  social consequences, 237–238
Learning disorders, and preterm birth, 69–70
Leukemia (see Cancer survivors)
Life Needs Model, 242
Lipomyelomeningocele, 86
Literate environments, cognitive effects, 299–300
Longitudinal studies, chronic illness, 105
Low birth weight, 61–75
  academic achievement, 69–70
  ADHD/behavioral issues, 72–73
  assessment, 73–74
  brain insult, 64–67
  and cerebral palsy, 82–83
  executive function, 71–72
  intelligence quotients, 68–69
  language disabilities, 70–71
  major and minor disabilities, 62–63
  pathogenesis, 63–67
  survival rates, 62
  visual–motor skills, 71

M

Magnetic resonance imaging, 311
Maintenance of gains
  autism interventions, 262
  social skills training, 239–240, 253
Manualized treatment, 262
Marital distress, and chronic illness, 104
Massed practice technique, 191
Maternal and Child Health Bureau, 273
Mathematics deficit, preterm birth, 69
Measures of Processes of Care, 152, 154
"Medical Home" model, 273–274, 278
Memory deficits, cancer survivors, 194

Mental retardation, cerebral palsy, 84
Mesosystems, in health care, 269–270
Metacognitive strategies
  attentional processes improvement, 189
  cancer survivors, 191–192
  in pediatric populations, 189
  traumatic brain injury, 222
Methylphenidate hydrochloride, 199
  cancer survivors, 199–200
  rehabilitation adjunct, 199
Microsystems, and health care, 269–270
Mild acquired brain injury
  educational challenges, 212–213
  educational planning, 218–219
  functional recovery, 213
Missouri Partnership for Enhanced Delivery of Services, 278–280
  care coordination interventions, 280
  family satisfaction, 280
  intervention model, 278, 280
  purpose of, 278
Mitrofanoff procedure, 55
Moderating variables
  risk and protective factors, 171–173
  traumatic brain injury, 30–31, 171–174
  interventions, 176–177
Mothers, caregiving stress, overview, 13
Motor deficits
  preterm birth, 71
  visual impairment, 141
MPOC for Service Providers, 154
MPOC—Short Form, 154
Multimodal approaches, effectiveness, 189
Multiple births, and cerebral palsy, 83
Myelination, preterm infants, 64–65
Myelomeningocele, 86–88

N

Neural tube deficits, 85–91
  assessment and intervention needs, 90–91
  epidemiology, 86
  psychosocial outcomes, 88–89
  risk factors, 86

Neurodevelopmental, overview
    definition, 3
    classification, 3–9
    epidemiology, 3–9
Neuroimaging techniques, 311–312
Neuropsychological assessment
    and acculturation, 296–297
    acquired brain injury, 214
    cultural issues, 290, 292–298
    norm groups, 292–293
    preterm birth, 73–74
    test translation issue, 293
    visual impairments, 141–142
Necrosis, preterm infants, brain injury, 64
Nonaversive interventions, autism, 260–261
Nonverbal intelligence tests, and deafness, 126
Nonverbal learning disabilities, preterm birth, 69–70
Nonverbal population
    assessment and intervention needs, 90–91
    dependency–autonomy issue, 89
Norm groups, cultural factors, 292–293
Nutritional factors, 190

O

Oligodendrocytes, and preterm birth, 64–65
Online interventions, families, 180–181
Operant conditioning, in autism, 260–261
Oral–aural communication methods, 123
Outcome monitoring, family-centered care, 152–153

P

Parent–child relationship
    and chronic illness, 104
    deafness and hard-of-hearing, 121–122
    targeted intervention, brain injury, 177
Parent Perceptions of Specialty care, 153, 155

Parents
    acculturation assessment, 297
    chronic illness adjustment, 111
    collaboration with professionals, barriers, 165
    ethnic and racial group influences, 297–298
    involvement of, 218–219, 315
    overprotectiveness, spina bifida, 89
    overview, 13–14
    satisfaction with care, 156–164
        measures, 153, 155
    social facilitation methods, 243
    traumatic brain injury adjustment, 171–174
    targeted interventions, 176
Passive behavior
    physically disabled, 237–238
    social consequences, 237–239
Patient satisfaction with care
    family-centered care, 153, 156–164
    family problem-solving, brain injury, 180–181
    measures, 153
Patient Satisfaction Questionnaire, 153, 155
Pediatric Alliance for Coordinated Care, 276
Pediatric Ambulatory Care Treatment Study, 275
Pediatric cancer (see Cancer survivors)
Pediatric family-centered rehabilitation, 149–169
    barriers to implementation, 158, 165–166
    core elements, 149–151
    evaluation, 151–156
    future research directions, 166
    outcomes, 156–164
    principles, 150
Peer relationships, 234–246
    and assertiveness, 237–238
    autism interventions, 251–253
    chronic disease adjustment, 111–112
    influence of, 316
    and mentoring, 242
    social inclusion facilitation, 241–242

Peer relationships (*continued*)
  spinal cord injury, 52
  visual impairments, 138–139
Perceptual organization, brain injury, 26–27
Performance IQ
  myelomeningocele, 87
  preterm birth, 70
Perinatal causes, overview, 4–5
Periventricular/intraventricular
    hemorrhage, 65
Periventricular leukomalacia
  cerebral palsy, neuropsychology, 84–85
  preterm infants, 65
Personal data assistant, memory aid, 223
Personality, and adaptation, 316
Pharmacologic treatment
  cancer survivors, 199–200
  in rehabilitation, 198–201
Picture-based schedules, autism aid, 257
Picture Exchange Communication
    System, 257–258
Pivotal response training, autism, 257
Play
  autism intervention, 253–254
  social integration function, 241
  stigma consequences for, 236–237
Positron emission tomography, 311
Postnatal causes, overview, 4–5
Postsecondary education
  and brain injury, 196, 223–225
  overview, 12
  transition planning, 223–225
Posttraumatic stress, spinal cord injury,
    47–48
Premature birth, 61–75
  academic achievement, 69–70
  assessment, 73–74
  basal ganglia, preterm infants, 66
  brain insult, 64–67
  developmental course, 74
  family-centered care outcomes, 157
  family functioning, 74
  intelligence quotients, 68–69
  language disabilities, 70–71
  neuropsychological outcomes, 71–73
  pathogenesis, 63–67
Prenatal causes, overview, 4–5

Preventive intervention, chronic illness,
    112–113
Primary care interventions, 278–280
Primary prevention, chronic illness, 112
PRISM project, 135–136
Private education, cultural differences,
    298–299
Problem-solving therapies
  ABCs of, 179
  online version, 180–181
  and traumatic brain injury, families,
    176–181
  satisfaction data, 180–181
Process evaluation
  components, 151–152
  family-centered care, 151–152
  measures, 154–155
Professional satisfaction, 153, 155–164
Project PRISM, 135–136
Protective factors, brain injury stress, 172–173
Provigil, 200
Psychiatric disorders
  deaf and hard-of-hearing, 124–125
  overview, 9–10
Psychoeducational assessment, brain
    injury, 213–215
Psychosocial outcomes (*see* Social adjustment/outcomes)
Psychotherapy
  brain injury, 197–198
  cancer survivors, 198
  and deafness, 126–127
Public education, cultural differences,
    298–299

Q

Qualitative assessment
  in educational settings, brain injury,
    215–217, 226
  monitoring function, 216–217
  teacher empowerment for, 226

R

Racial issues (*see also* Ethnic minorities)
  as construct, 291
  identity problems, 295–296

Randomization, in treatment evaluation, 262
Readiness to learn, and literacy, 299
Reading difficulties, preterm birth, 69
"Recovery" indexes, brain injury, 212–213
Religion, and coping, ethnic groups, 302
Repetitive behaviors, autism, 259–261
Residential schools, and deafness, 123
Response cost technique, autism, 260
Retinopathy of prematurity, 132, 140, 142
Risk factors, brain injury coping, 171–173
Rural areas
  fragmented care, 274
  health care access, 110

S

Satisfaction with care
  family problem-solving program, 180–181
  measures, 153
  Missouri Partnership services, 280
  patients, 153, 156–164, 180–181
  professionals, 153, 155–164
School functions/setting
  acquired brain injury, 208–227
  identification of, 210–211
  assessment teams in, 217–218
  cancer survivors, 195–196
  and deafness, 122–124
  psychoeducational assessment, brain injury, 213–215
  qualitative assessment, 215–217
  re-entry, 223–224
  social integrative interventions, 240–242
  spinal cord injury, 48–50
    accessibility, 49–50
  systems aspect, 272
School psychologists, assessment role, 217
School re-entry
  acquired brain injury, 223–224
  transition planning, 224

Screening recommendations
  acquired brain injury, 225–226
  health care delivery systems, 282
Secondary prevention, chronic illness, 112
Seizure disorders, cognitive impairment, 102
Self-efficacy, and social problem solving, 237–238
Self-esteem, and deafness, 124
Self-injurious behavior
  autism interventions, 259–261
  spinal cord injury, 48
Self-stimulating behaviors, autism, 259–261
Services Satisfaction Questionnaire, 153, 155
Severe acquired brain injury
  educational challenges, 212–213
  educational planning, 218–219
Sexuality, spinal cord injury, 52–53
Sibling relationships
  and chronic illness, 104
  overview, 13–14, 315
  spinal cord injury, 51
  stress in, 13–14
  traumatic brain injury, 29
Sickle cell disease
  cognitive impairment, 103
  follow-up study, adjustment problems, 105
  and gender, 107
  parental adjustment, 111
Sign language training, autism, 258–259
Signed English method, 123
Sleep patterns, 190
Social adjustment/outcome, 234–246
  cerebral palsy, 88
  chronic illness, 99–101, 106–112
  conceptual model, 235
  deafness and hard-of-hearing, 120–124
  interventions, 238–243
  overview, 10–11, 315–317
  social information processing role, 237–239
  spina bifida, 88–89
  spinal cord injury, 45–48

Social adjustment/outcome (*continued*)
  traumatic brain injury, 27–28
  treatment needs, 236–238
  visual impairments, 136–139
Social information processing, 232–238
  physically disabled, 237–238
  social functioning consequences of, 237–239
Social integration, 234–236
  conceptual model, 235
  emerging approaches, 242–243
  future research directions, 243–244
  interventions, 236–243
Social problem solving
  and learned passivity, 237–238
  physically disabled, 237–238
  traumatic brain injury, 27–28
Social skills training, 239–240
  autism spectrum disorders, 251–255
  generalization/maintenance of gains problem, 239–240
  physically disabled, 239–240
  technique, 240
  traumatic brain injury, 190
Socioeconomic disadvantage
  chronic illness, 109
  ethnic minorities, 297–298
  and preterm birth, IQ, 69–70
  and traumatic brain injury, 30–31
Spastic cerebral palsy
  executive functions, 85
  pathophysiology, 83
Special education services
  and brain injury severity, 213
  in educational planning, 218
  overview, 11–12
  traumatic brain injury, 28–29, 213
  visual impairments, 140
Speech–language disabilities
  autism, 255–259
    intervention, 255–259
  preterm birth, 70–71
Speech output devices, 258
Spina bifida, 85–91
  assessment and intervention needs, 90–91
  future research directions, 90–91

neuropsychology, 87–88
psychosocial outcomes, 88–89
risk factors, 86–87
Spinal cord injury, 42–60
  anatomical and physiological features, 44
  concomitant head injury, 45
  developmental factors, 46–47, 51–52
  educational outcomes, 53–54
  emotional and behavioral issues, 45–48
  etiology, 43–44
  family issues, 50–51
  long-term outcomes, 53–54
  overview, 42–45
  poor outcome risk factors, 53–54
  research needs, 55–56
  school issues, 48–50
  sexuality, 52–53
  social issues, 45–48
  treatment implications, 54–55
Staff Perceptions of Specialty Care, 153, 155
Staff satisfaction
  family-centered care, 156–164
  measures, 153, 155
Stereotypical behaviors, autism, 259–261
Stigma
  physical disabilities, 236–237
  social consequences, 236–237
Stimulant medications
  cancer survivors, 199–200
  in rehabilitation, 198–200
Strattera, 200
Stress
  appraisal of, brain injury, 172–173
  targeted intervention, 176–177
  in families, overview, 13–14
Stress management program
  problem-solving approach, 178–181
  and traumatic brain injury, 176
Structured environmental interventions
  autism, 254, 256–257
  techniques, 257
Subplate neurons, preterm infants, 66–67
Supplemental Security Income program, eligibility, 4–5
Survival rates, 313–314

Symbol boards, 258
Symbolic communication strategies, autism, 257–258
Systems of care (see Health care delivery system)

T

Tailored approaches
  family intervention, brain injury, 177–181
  research needs, 182, 284
TEACCH intervention, 250
Teachers
  cancer survivors, school re-entry, 195
  qualitative assessment empowerment, 226
  social integration facilitation, 240–242
Team approach
  classroom-based social intervention, 241–242
  family-centered care model, 151
Telehealth technologies, 283
Temperament, and adaptation, 316
Tertiary prevention, chronic illness, 112–113
Tetrahydrobiopterin, 251
Tetraplegia (see Spinal cord injury)
Text-based schedule, autism, 257
Therapeutic relationship, in rehabilitation, 198
Time-out procedure, autism, 260
Total communication training, autism, 259
Training, school-based assessment teams, 217
Transition planning
  acquired brain injury, 223–225
  and case management, 225
  community participation approach, 242–243
  postsecondary school period, 224–225
  school re-entry, 224
Translation, neuropsychological tests, 293
Translators, in testing, 294

Traumatic brain injury, 23–41, 170–191
  behavior therapy and drug treatment, 190
  and child abuse, 30
  clinical implications, 31–32
  cognitive and behavioral rehabilitation, 186–191
  cognitive sequelae, 25–27, 211–212
  and coma duration, 26
  and cultural values, 296, 302
  developmental changes, 30, 211–212
  educational planning/interventions, 218–222
  epidemiology, 23–24, 170
  family adjustment, 29–31, 171–174, 201–202
  family interventions, 170–185
    research review, 175–181
  future research directions, 32–33, 225–227
  identification in school setting, 210–211
  informational support, 175–176
  long-term impact, 212
  moderating variables, 30–31
  online family-based intervention, 180–181
  pathophysiology, 23–24
  perceptions of, ethnic factors, 302
  psychoeducational assessment, 213–215
  psychosocial outcomes, 27–29, 238
  psychotherapy, 197–198
  qualitative assessment, 215–217
  school setting, 208–227
  severity classification, 24
  social problem solving, 238
  spinal cord injury, 45
  transition planning, 223–225
Twins, and cerebral palsy, 83

U

Universal screening, health care system, 282
Utilization of health care, ethnic minorities, 110–111

V

Ventricular volume, preterm infants, 67
Verbal communication training, autism, 255
Verbal IQ, myelomeningocele, 87
Very low birth weight, 61–75
  academic achievement, 69–70
  ADHD/behavioral issues, 72–73
  assessment, 73–74
  and brain insult, 64–67
  and cerebral palsy, 82–83
  executive function, 71–72
  intelligence quotients, 68–69
  language disabilities, 70–71
  major and minor disabilities, 62–63
  pathogenesis, 63–67
  survival rates, 62
  and visual impairments, 140–141
  visual–motor skills, 71
Victimization, physically disabled, 236
Videoconferences, family problem-solving, 180–181
"Visual acuity," 133
Visual impairments, 132–146
  clinical implications, 139–143
  cognitive development, 136–137
  definition, 133–135
  developmental factors, 138–139
  educational needs, 140
  employment, 142–143
  epidemiology, 134–136
  future research directions, 143–144
  independent living skills, 137–138
  Individualized Education Plans, 142
  neuropsychological status, 141–142
  psychological assessment, 141–142
  rehabilitation services, 142
  social outcomes, 136–139
Visual–motor skills, preterm birth, 71
Visual perception, spina bifida, 88
Vocational services/outcome
  brain injury rehabilitation, 196–197
  overview, 11–13
  transition planning, 224

W

Web-based intervention
  family problem-solving, 180–181
  future directions, 202
Wechsler Intelligence Scale for Children—3rd ed.
  and deafness, 125
  traumatic brain injury, 26
Wheelchair children, social consequences, 237
White matter volume, preterm infants, 66–67
Work schedules, autism intervention, 257

Y

Youth En Route, 242–243